Pediatric Otolaryngology

THE REQUISITES IN PEDIATRICS

SERIES EDITOR

Louis M. Bell, MD

Patrick S. Pasquariello, Jr. Chair in General Pediatrics
Professor of Pediatrics
University of Pennsylvania School of Medicine
Chief, Division of General Pediatrics
Attending Physician, General Pediatrics and Infectious Diseases
The Children's Hospital of Philadelphia
Philadelphia, Pennsylvania

OTHER VOLUMES IN
THE REQUISITES IN PEDIATRICS SERIES

Orthopaedics and Sports Medicine
Endocrinology
Nephrology and Urology
Pulmonology
Cardiology

COMING SOON IN
THE REQUISITES IN PEDIATRICS SERIES

Gastroenterology
Adolescent Medicine
Infectious Diseases
Hematology and Oncology

Pediatric Otolaryngology

THE REQUISITES IN PEDIATRICS

Ralph F. Wetmore, MD
Professor of Otorhinolaryngology:
Head and Neck Surgery
University of Pennsylvania School of Medicine
Senior Surgeon
The Children's Hospital of Philadelphia
Philadelphia, Pennsylvania

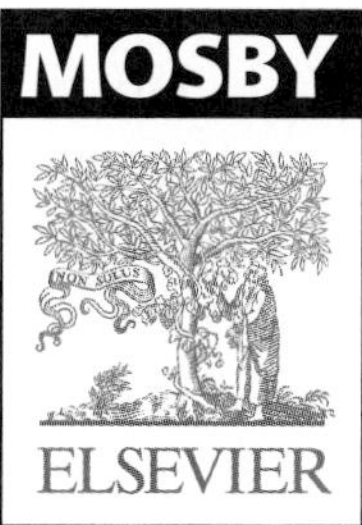

MOSBY
ELSEVIER

1600 John F. Kennedy Boulevard
Suite 1800
Philadelphia, PA 19103-2899

PEDIATRIC OTOLARYNGOLOGY: THE REQUISITES IN PEDIATRICS ISBN: 978-0-323-04855-2

Notice

Knowledge and best practice in this field are constantly changing. As new research and experience broaden our knowledge, changes in practice, treatment, and drug therapy may become necessary or appropriate. Readers are advised to check the most current information provided (i) on procedures featured or (ii) by the manufacturer of each product to be administered, to verify the recommended dose or formula, the method and duration of administration, and contraindications. It is the responsibility of the practitioner, relying on their own experience and knowledge of the patient, to make diagnoses, to determine dosages and the best treatment for each individual patient, and to take all appropriate safety precautions. To the fullest extent of the law, neither the Publisher nor the Editor assumes any liability for any injury and/or damage to persons or property arising out of or related to any use of the material contained in this book.

The Publisher

Library of Congress Cataloging-in-Publication Data
Pediatric otolaryngology / [edited by] Ralph F. Wetmore. — 1st ed.
p. ; cm.—(The requisites in pediatrics)
Includes bibliographical references.
ISBN 978-0-323-04855-2
1. Pediatric otolaryngology. I. Wetmore, Ralph F. II. Series.
[DNLM: 1. Otorhinolaryngologic Diseases. 2. Child.
3. Neck—physiopathology. WV 140
P37086 2007]
RF47. C4P386 2007
618.92′09751—dc22

2006033359

Publishing Director: Judith Fletcher
Developmental Editor: Kristina Oberle
Publishing Services Manager: Frank Polizzano
Senior Project Manager: Robin Hayward
Marketing Manager: Laura Meiskey

Printed in the United States of America.

Last digit is the print number: 9 8 7 6 5 4 3 2 1

Contributors

Eric D. Baum, MD
Connecticut Pediatric Otolaryngology
Madison, North Haven, and New Haven, Connecticut

Jennifer R. Burstein, MA
Manager, Speech-Language Pathology
Center for Childhood Communication
The Children's Hospital of Philadelphia
Philadelphia, Pennsylvania

Joseph G. Donaher, MA
Instructor, Temple University
Center for Childhood Communication
The Children's Hospital of Philadelphia
Philadelphia, Pennsylvania

Lisa M. Elden, MD
Assistant Professor of Otorhinolaryngology: Head and Neck Surgery
University of Pennsylvania School of Medicine
The Children's Hospital of Philadelphia
Philadelphia, Pennsylvania

Kevin H. Franck, PhD, MBA
Assistant Professor of Otorhinolaryngology: Head and Neck Surgery
University of Pennsylvania School of Medicine
Director, Cochlear Implant Program
Center for Childhood Communication
The Children's Hospital of Philadelphia
Philadelphia, Pennsylvania

John A. Germiller, MD, PhD
Assistant Professor of Otorhinolaryngology: Head and Neck Surgery
University of Pennsylvania School of Medicine
Attending Surgeon, Department of Pediatric Otolaryngology
The Children's Hospital of Philadelphia
Philadelphia, Pennsylvania

Judith S. Gravel, PhD
Director, Center for Childhood Communication
The Children's Hospital of Philadelphia
Philadelphia, Pennsylvania

Steven D. Handler, MD, MBE
Professor of Otorhinolaryngology: Head and Neck Surgery
University of Pennsylvania School of Medicine
Associate Director, Department of Otolaryngology
The Children's Hospital of Philadelphia
Philadelphia, Pennsylvania

Ian N. Jacobs, MD
Associate Professor of Otorhinolaryngology: Head and Neck Surgery
University of Pennsylvania School of Medicine
Director, Center for Pediatric Airway Disorders
The Children's Hospital of Philadelphia
Philadelphia, Pennsylvania

Ken Kazahaya, MD, MBA
Assistant Professor of Otorhinolaryngology: Head and Neck Surgery
University of Pennsylvania School of Medicine
Director, Pediatric Skull Base Surgery
Medical Director, Cochlear Implant Program
The Children's Hospital of Philadelphia
Philadelphia, Pennsylvania

Jeffrey L. Keller, MD
Assistant Clinical Professor of Otolaryngology
Mount Sinai School of Medicine
Attending Physician
Northern Westchester Hospital Center
Mount Kisco, New York

Carol Knightly, AuD
Director, Clinical Operations
Center for Childhood Communication
The Children's Hospital of Philadelphia
Philadelphia, Pennsylvania

Iman Naseri, MD
Resident
Emory University School of Medicine
Atlanta, Georgia

William P. Potsic, MD
Professor of Otorhinolaryngology: Head and Neck Surgery
University of Pennsylvania School of Medicine
Director, Pediatric Otolaryngology and Human Communication
The Children's Hospital of Philadelphia
Philadelphia, Pennsylvania

Daniel S. Samadi, MD
Clinical Professor of Otolaryngology
Director, Department of Pediatric Otolaryngology
Hackensack University Medical Center
Hackensack, New Jersey

Udayan K. Shah, MD
Assistant Professor of Otorhinolaryngology: Head and Neck Surgery
University of Pennsylvania School of Medicine
Director, Otolaryngology Innovative Techniques Program
Associate Director, Trauma (Otolaryngology)
The Children's Hospital of Philadelphia
Philadelphia, Pennsylvania

Davinder J. Singh, MD
Director of Research, Barrow Craniofacial Center
Barrow Neurological Institute
Attending Surgeon
Phoenix Children's Hospital
Phoenix, Arizona

Steven E. Sobol, MD
Director, Department of Pediatric Otolaryngology
Emory University School of Medicine
Chief, Department of Otolaryngology
Children's Healthcare of Atlanta
Atlanta, Georgia

Cynthia Solot, MA
Senior Speech Language Pathologist
The Children's Hospital of Philadelphia
Philadelphia, Pennsylvania

Lawrence W. C. Tom, MD
Associate Professor of Otorhinolaryngology: Head and Neck Surgery
University of Pennsylvania School of Medicine
Associate Surgeon, Pediatric Otolaryngology
The Children's Hospital of Philadelphia
Philadelphia, Pennsylvania

Ralph F. Wetmore, MD
Professor of Otorhinolaryngology: Head and Neck Surgery
University of Pennsylvania School of Medicine
Senior Surgeon
The Children's Hospital of Philadelphia
Philadelphia, Pennsylvania

Amy White, AuD
Audiologist
Center for Childhood Communication
The Children's Hospital of Philadelphia
Philadelphia, Pennsylvania

Steven G. Wolfe, MD
Instructor, Department of Otorhinolaryngology: Head and Neck Surgery
University of Pennsylvania School of Medicine
Philadelphia, Pennsylvania

Karen B. Zur, MD
Assistant Professor of Otorhinolaryngology: Head and Neck Surgery
University of Pennsylvania School of Medicine
Director, Pediatric Voice Program
Associate Director, Center for Pediatric Airway Disorders
The Children's Hospital of Philadelphia
Philadelphia, Pennsylvania

Foreword

As a general pediatrician and an infectious diseases specialist, I often rely on my pediatric otolaryngology colleagues for their help and expertise in managing a host of diseases that are both common and unique to infants and children. The rationale for and importance of this partnership is most apparent as one reads through this, the sixth volume of **The Requisites in Pediatrics**, entitled *Pediatric Otolaryngology*.

Dr. Wetmore offers a carefully edited volume that meets the goal of The Requisites series. The editors and authors were asked to consider and discuss the common pediatric conditions within their specialty and include practical information that would guide primary care providers, resident physicians, nurse practitioners, and students in the care of their patients and families. Indeed, the contents of this volume include the most important diseases and conditions that can affect the head and neck in infants and children and much more.

The volume includes 16 chapters, beginning with Congenital Malformations of the Head and Neck and Diseases of the External Ear in Chapters 1 and 2. Chapters 3 and 4 are also outstanding, dealing with the vital issues of disorders of communication (hearing loss; speech and language; swallowing and feeding). The importance of a multidisciplinary approach to the diagnosis and management of these conditions is stressed.

Otitis media, sinusitis, pharyngitis, the common cold, and prolonged cough illnesses are common conditions that all primary care providers diagnose and manage every working day. All of these diseases require careful and judicious use of antibiotics and sometimes referral to a pediatric otolaryngologist. Chapters 5 through 11 detail the pathophysiology of these conditions, the management issues, and the resulting (often suppurative) complications of these conditions that require referral.

The final chapters are all excellent, dealing with pediatric issues about sleep disorders, aerodigestive foreign bodies, and caustic ingestions, neck masses, and facial trauma.

I want to offer my heartfelt congratulations to Dr. Wetmore and the authors for providing us with this outstanding and useful volume in **The Requisites in Pediatrics** series. We hope you enjoy *Pediatric Otolaryngology*.

Louis M. Bell, MD
Patrick S. Pasquariello, Jr. Chair in General Pediatrics
Professor of Pediatrics
University of Pennsylvania School of Medicine
Chief, Division of General Pediatrics
Attending Physician, General Pediatrics
and Infectious Diseases
The Children's Hospital of Philadelphia
Philadelphia, Pennsylvania

Preface

When I entered the field of pediatric otolaryngology, more than 25 years ago, the subspecialty was still well in its infancy with perhaps no more than fifty practitioners who devoted a majority of their time to its practice. Currently the American Society of Pediatric Otolaryngology (ASPO) numbers more than 300 members whose practice is limited exclusively to pediatric otolaryngology. As the subspecialty of pediatric otolaryngology has grown in numbers, it has also expanded as a field. Traditionally, all the members of my surgical group practiced all aspects of pediatric otolaryngology. That is no longer true. Currently only two members manage all the children who require airway reconstruction—that is, children with compromise of either the structure and/or function of the upper airway, specifically the larynx and trachea. Likewise, two other members of our group work with a multidisciplinary team to provide cochlear implants to profoundly deaf children. These same two members also perform any surgery that involves the pediatric skull base. Because their practice involves unique skills to care for a small number of patients, these four surgeons have become "super-specialists" within pediatric otolaryngology. The remainder of our surgical group practices general pediatric otolaryngology, although each of us has our own favorite group of patients, be it those with chronic ear disease, sinus disease, or even pediatric voice disorders. I have called upon the expertise of this group of super-specialists and generalists within the field of pediatric otolaryngology to develop the major sections of this book.

The detail and scope of this volume is intended to appeal to a wide audience of practitioners in pediatrics, otolaryngology, hearing and speech disorders, and other assorted specialties that care for children. As with the other volumes in The Requisites series, this book was originally targeted toward primary care practitioners, residents, and nursing and medical students, but the expertise and interests of the authors have been utilized so that the detail of some topics approaches that of much more comprehensive textbooks in pediatric otolaryngology. It was not the intent of the editor to include every subject within the field of pediatric otolaryngology; instead, this volume includes topics that would be of interest to most readers.

I would like to thank all the authors for their contributions. I asked each of them to discuss a broad topic, but then gave them license as to what detail they should include in their chapter. All have performed an outstanding job of providing enough information to satisfy nearly all readers without having the book become a truly encyclopedic reference. I would also like to thank the editorial staff of Elsevier for their assistance in the preparation of this volume. As is often the case, the authors never really see the hard work and time that a good editorial staff must devote in order to create an outstanding finished product such as this textbook. Finally, I would like to dedicate this book to all physicians, nurses, and ancillary practitioners who devote their practice to the care of children with otolaryngological disorders.

Ralph F. Wetmore, MD

Contents

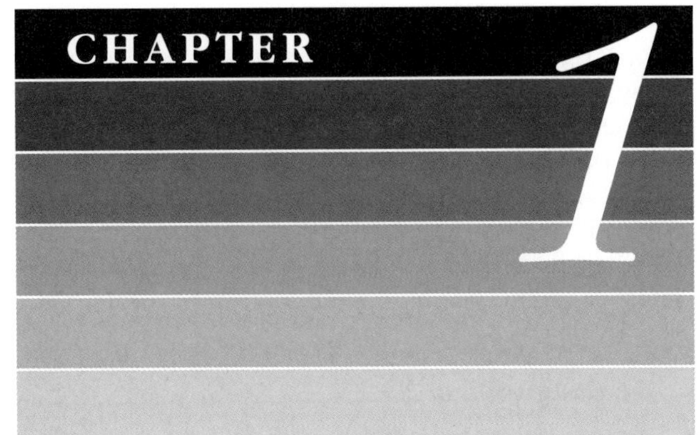

Congenital Malformations of the Head and Neck

KEN KAZAHAYA, MD, MBA
DAVINDER J. SINGH, MD

HEMATOLOGIC AND LYMPHATIC MALFORMATIONS

Vascular anomalies are among the most common congenital and neonatal abnormalities. Most of these lesions are located in the head and neck. Vascular anomalies have an incredibly diverse presentation, ranging from a seemingly benign discoloration (Fig. 1-1A) to the other extreme of severe abnormality (Fig. 1-1B). Even though these vascular anomalies have been well identified and classified, we still see children with disfiguring anomalies who have been misdiagnosed and consequently mismanaged. The key in treating these anomalies is in the physician's diagnosis and understanding of the disease process.

There are four major classification schemes for vascular lesions. The descriptive classification is not helpful in developing a therapeutic plan, because lesions that look alike often vary greatly in cause, prognosis, and treatment. The anatomic-physiologic system is more accurate, but is of little value to a clinician because it is a microscopic description. The embryologic classification system also lacks clinical applicability. In the early 1900s, investigators began defining the biologic behavior of these lesions.

The landmark paper that provided a turning point in the history of diagnosing and classifying vascular anomalies was published by Mulliken and Glowacki in 1982.[1] In this paper, they simplified the nomenclature of vascular anomalies by classifying them based on cellular features. This classification system is extremely useful in

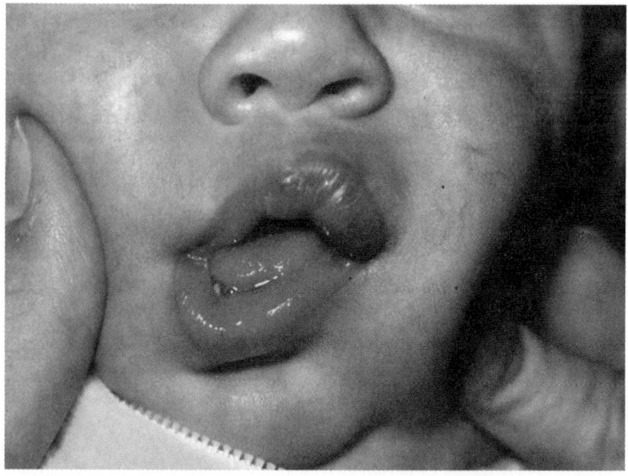

A

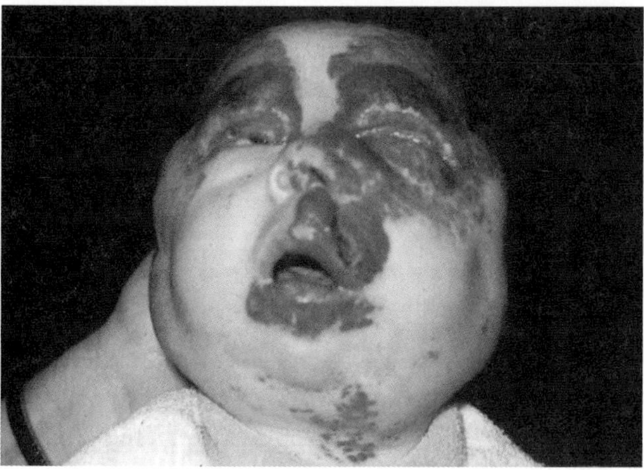

B

Figure 1-1.

the diagnosis, management, and prognosis of these lesions. Hemangiomas are defined as tumors that enlarge by rapid endothelial proliferation, and vascular malformations as structural abnormalities that are subcategorized based on channel type (e.g., capillary, venous, arterial, lymphatic, and combinations).[1] Imaging is useful in the diagnosis and differentiation of vascular anomalies, including magnetic resonance imaging (MRI) (Fig. 1-2), ultrasonography, and computed tomography (CT).

Hemangiomas

Hemangiomas are the most common tumors of infancy and have an incidence of 1% to 2.6% at birth and 10% to 12% by 1 year of age. Of all hemangiomas, 80% are noted in the first month of life and the female-to-male ratio is 3:1. Approximately 14% to 20% of affected infants have more than one hemangioma, and 60% of hemangiomas occur in the head and neck region. They have a rapid postnatal proliferation (proliferative phase, first 8 to 12 months of life) and a slow involution (involution phase, slow regression, typically over 5 to 8 years). The deeper lesions appear with a bluish hue and the superficial lesions are bright red or crimson. They usually have a firm doughy consistency. Vascular malformations are present at birth but may not be evident. Their growth is proportionate with the child and the female-to-male ratio is 1:1. Venous or arterial malformations often have a bluish hue and are typically compressible or cystic (Fig. 1-3).[2]

The diagnosis of vascular anomalies can present a challenge; a thorough history and physical examination is often revealing but imaging studies are needed for some cases. A proliferating hemangioma appears as a uniformly enhancing soft tissue mass by MRI, whereas an involuted

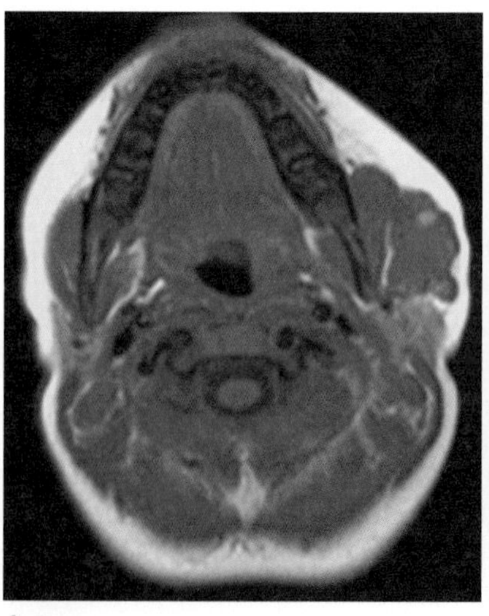

A

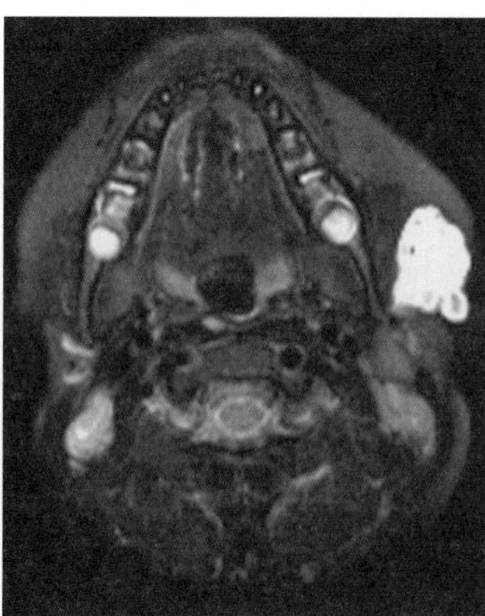

B

Figure 1-2. Magnetic resonance imaging scans (**A**, T1-weighted; **B**, T2-weighted) of a venolymphatic malformation.

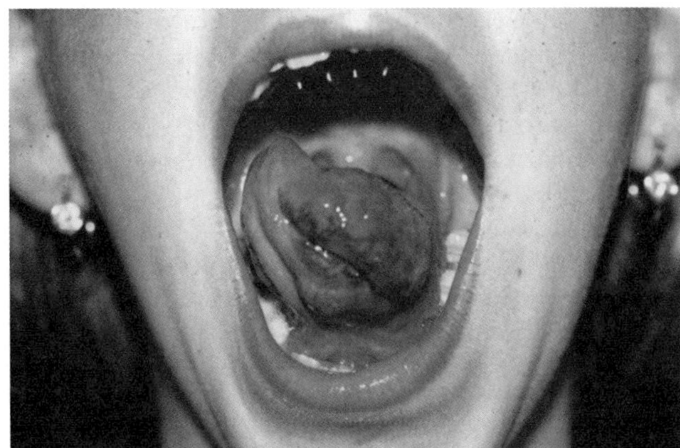

Figure 1-3.

hemangioma does not enhance with contrast and exhibits fibrofatty deposition.[3]

Although it is psychologically stressing to the parents for a child to have any degree of abnormality, there are certain complications that can guide the physician's management of the child and dictate intervention. Complications during the proliferative phase include bleeding, ulceration, infection, high-risk anatomic sites, and obstruction of the visual axis, auditory canal, or nasopharyngeal airway. There are certain absolute indications for intervention; the relative indications then depend on the parent-physician rapport and the psychological state of the child. Absolute indications for intervention include any obstruction of the visual axis, airway, or auditory canal (Fig. 1-4).[4]

Patients are most susceptible during the first year of life to amblyopia ex anopsia, in which abnormalities of the optics of the eye impair its normal use in early childhood by preventing the formation of a clear image on the retina.

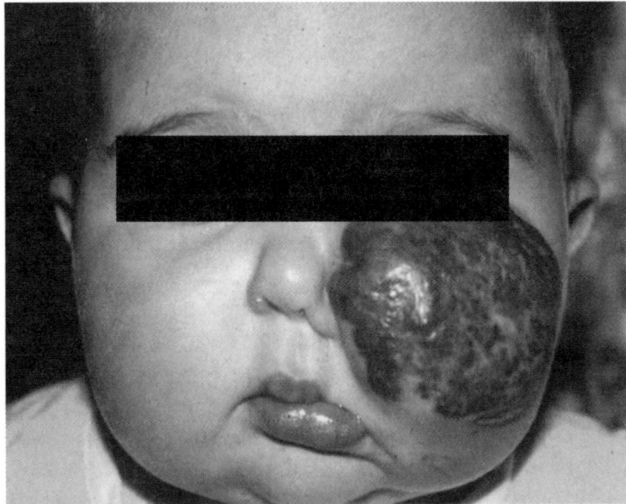

Figure 1-4.

Anisometropia is a condition in which the power of refraction in one eye differs markedly from that in the other, which prevents development of binocular vision. Any compression within the periorbital region resulting in strabismus, ocular proptosis, optic atrophy, or corneal distortion is also an absolute indication for intervention.[4]

Other indications for intervention include large ulcerated lesions with hemorrhage or infection, affected regions that are prone to long-term cosmetic deformities, and lesions that are a source of psychosocial trauma to the child. Nasal hemangiomas, although not a functional problem unless there is intranasal extension, pose a significant cosmetic problem both immediately and in the long term, and may be very psychologically stressful to the parents. Final appearance after involution is usually a fibrofatty residuum with epidermal atrophy, redundant skin, and telangiectasias.[4]

Noninvasive treatment of hemangiomas includes systemic steroids, intralesional steroids, interferon alfa-2a, sclerosing agents, and radiotherapy. The most commonly used therapy is systemic steroids, and 50% to 90% of hemangiomas respond to this. Systemic steroids are used for obstruction of functional structures, extensive facial lesions, or facial lesions at risk for cosmetic deformity. Side effects of systemic steroids include irritability, crying, and interference with growth. Intralesional steroid injections often require multiple treatments at 6- to 8-week intervals and have a response rate similar to that of systemic steroids. Periocular lesions should not be injected because of the risk for central retinal artery occlusion. Interferon alfa-2a is an angiostatic agent that is indicated if steroids are ineffective, if there is recurrence after steroid withdrawal, or when observation of the lesion is not an option. Side effects of interferon are substantial, and it should be used only if absolutely necessary. Radiotherapy is no longer used because its complications far outweigh its benefits.[4]

Invasive treatment includes surgical excision, selective embolization, laser photocoagulation, and combination therapy. Early excision has a risk of recurrent or persistent disease due to an evolving zone of surrounding diseased tissue, which may not be excised if performed early. With observation, there is less chance of leaving abnormal tissue behind and minimizing the excision. Indications for early surgical excision include functional ocular obstruction or airway compromise, when eventual resection is inevitable, or when early debulking may prevent continued derangement of local tissues while awaiting involution of large pedunculated lesions. Also, if the length of scar is not anticipated to change significantly with delayed surgery, it is psychologically beneficial for the family to proceed with excision.[4]

Indications for laser photocoagulation include symptomatic hemangiomas that demonstrate ulceration, bleeding, and obstruction of function and rapidly proliferating hemangiomas. Pulsed dye and argon lasers are commonly used. The goal of laser therapy is to allow the child to appear normal by the time he or she is of school age. Ulcerated lesions are successfully treated with the argon laser. The pulsed dye laser may be effective in eliminating the superficial component of hemangiomas, but it has limited influence on the deeper component of the hemangioma. Another laser that has been used is the neodymium:yttrium-aluminum-garnet (Nd:YAG) laser. Its wavelength penetrates deeper into the dermis, but there is a higher incidence of scarring and tissue slough.[4]

Vascular Malformations

Although hemangiomas are the most common pediatric head and neck anomalies, vascular malformations are important in the differential diagnosis because they are managed differently. Vascular malformations are present at birth, and their clinical behavior is characterized by growth proportionate to that of the child without regression. The malformations may expand rapidly as a result of infection, trauma, hormonal changes, or embolic or surgical intervention. Unlike with hemangiomas, there is no evidence of cellular proliferation; instead, there is an abnormal progressive dilation of vessels and abnormal structures. They do not invade adjacent tissue or bone, but cause distortion from mass effect.[3]

Classification of vascular malformations is based on channel abnormalities determining flow characteristics—capillary, arterial, venous, and lymphatic. Combined forms, such as arteriovenous and capillary-venous-lymphatic, are often seen.

The most frequently seen vascular malformation is the port wine stain, which is histologically a capillary malformation (Fig. 1-5).[3] These malformations consist of abnormally dilated capillaries or venule-sized vessels in the superficial dermis. They should be treated early in life, before the child enters school. Capillary malformations are best treated with the flashlamp-pumped pulsed dye laser with a wavelength of 585 nm.

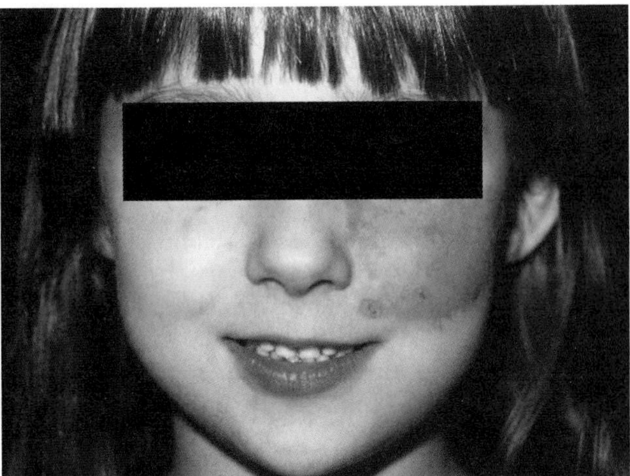

Figure 1-5. Capillary vascular malformation—port wine stain.

Venous malformations are low-flow lesions, which may present in isolation or combined as a capillary-venous or venolymphatic malformation. They have dilated or ectatic vascular channels lined with normal epithelium. Thrombosis and calcifications may be revealed on clinical and radiologic examination. These lesions are common in the skin and subcutaneous tissues of the head and neck. Typically, they are soft and nonpulsatile, with rapid refilling. The lesions may expand with occlusion of the jugular vein, a Valsalva maneuver, or the dependent position of the head. These lesions may be treated by observation, sclerosing agents, argon or Nd:YAG laser, or excision. Complete surgical resection of these lesions is usually impossible; however, subtotal resection may be considered to normalize contours, relieve pain, or improve function.[5]

Lymphatic malformations are most often located in the neck, although they can be present in the tongue, cheek, or floor of mouth. They are frequently combined with venous malformations and do not regress spontaneously. They are low-flow lesions. Lymphatic malformations are congenital and are obvious at birth or may be detected before the child is 2 years old. They may increase or decrease in size with the flow of lymphatic fluid or with inflammation, infection, or intraluminal bleeding. These lesions consist of dilated lymphatic channels lined with a flattened layer of endothelium. Macrocystic lesions, formerly referred to as cystic hygromas, typically affect the neck and are less infiltrative of surrounding tissues. Microcystic lymphatic malformations are more severe and extensively infiltrate tissues, causing significant deformities.

Surgical resection is the typical treatment of choice, and multiple resections may be necessary. Because lymphatic malformations are benign, complete resection of the lesion is not necessary and is sometimes not possible. Lesions below the mylohyoid muscle (type I) are ideally removed in one procedure, which can usually be carried out at approximately 9 to 12 months of age. Lesions above the mylohyoid muscle (type II) are typically microcystic and are more difficult to manage. Type II lesions are not curable and complete resection is almost impossible. Surgical intervention for type II lesions should be considered before 5 to 6 years of age. Surgical morbidity is high, with prolonged drainage, slow wound healing, recurrence, and risk of nerve damage.[5]

High-flow vascular malformations of the head and neck are arteriovenous malformations (AVMs) or, less commonly, arteriovenous fistulas. These high-flow lesions are less common than the slow-flow lesions described earlier. Histologically, AVMs are arteriovenous shunts with dysmorphic arteries of irregular caliber and with thick walls. AVMs typically present during late childhood, adolescence, or early adulthood. Signs and symptoms may include elevated skin temperature, palpable pulsations and/or thrill, throbbing pain, pulsatile tinnitus, and audible bruit. Shunting of blood may cause skin ulceration, tissue necrosis, and bleeding. Slow destruction of facial bones may occur and patients typically seek treatment for swelling, pain, or hemorrhage. Various methods of ligation, embolization, and resection have been tried, but treatment of these lesions in the head and neck region has a low success rate. Positive resection margins probably result in recurrence.[2] Superselective preoperative embolization may be useful before surgical extirpation to help reduce blood loss. Embolization must be directed at the epicenter or nidus of the AVM.[5]

EAR ABNORMALITIES

The ear has a complex embryologic development because it forms in three anatomic divisions—inner, middle, and external. A full discussion of embryologic development of the ear is beyond the scope of this chapter.

Embryology

Inner ear development begins early in the fourth week of gestation, with the formation of the otic placode, a thickening in the surface ectoderm. The otic placode invaginates into the surrounding mesenchyme, forming an otic pit. The edges of the pit come together and pinch it off to form the otic vesicle, or otocyst. The otic vesicle loses its connection to the surface epithelium and a diverticulum elongates out to form the endolymphatic duct and sac. Two regions of the otic vesicle become distinct, the dorsal utricle portion and the ventral saccular portion. The utricle portion becomes the utricle, semicircular ducts, and endolymphatic duct. The saccular portion develops into the saccule and cochlear ducts. The cochlear duct is a tubular diverticulum that grows out of the ventral saccular portion; it elongates and coils to form the cochlea. The spiral organ of Corti develops from the wall of the cochlear duct, whereas the ganglion cells of the eighth cranial nerve migrate into the coils and become the spiral ganglion.

The mesenchyme around the otic capsule becomes a cartilaginous capsule and, as the membranous labyrinth develops, spaces appear in the cartilaginous otic capsule that eventually develop into the perilymphatic space—the scala tympani and scala vestibuli. The remainder of the cartilaginous otic capsule ossifies to form the bony labyrinth of the inner ear. The inner ear develops into its adult size and shape by 20 to 22 weeks of gestation.

The middle ear is a derivative of the first branchial arch. The tubotympanic recess forms from the first pharyngeal pouch; the distal end enlarges to become the tympanic cavity and the mastoid antrum, and the proximal end becomes the eustachian tube. The dorsal end of the first arch cartilage, Meckel's cartilage, ossifies to become the malleus and incus. The stapes crus develops from the dorsal end of the second branchial arch cartilage, Reichert's cartilage.

The external auditory meatus develops from the dorsal end of the first branchial groove. The first branchial membrane separates the first branchial groove (ectoderm) from the dorsal end of the first pharyngeal pouch (endoderm). Mesenchyme from the first and second branchial arches grows into the branchial membrane to form the middle layer of the tympanic membrane.

The ectodermal cells at the base of the first branchial groove proliferate and fill in the groove with a meatal plug. Late in fetal life, the meatal plug degenerates to form a cavity that will become the internal part of the external auditory canal.

The auricle develops from six auricular hillocks, which arise around the margin of the first branchial groove. At about 6 weeks of gestation, three hillocks develop from the first branchial arch mesenchyme and three from the second branchial arch mesenchyme. The hillocks fuse at about week 8 and, as the auricle develops, the proportional contribution of the first arch mesenchyme diminishes.

Congenital Hearing Loss

Sensorineural hearing loss is the most common form of congenital hearing loss. Approximately 3 to 5 children in 1000 are born with some form of hearing loss. The incidence of severe to profound hearing loss is about 1 in 1000 live births.[6,7] Because the inner ear develops independently from the middle and external ears, hearing problems may be conductive as a result of abnormalities of the external canal or middle ear structures, or may be sensorineural as a result of cochlear anomalies. Newborn hearing screening programs in the United States have improved the average age at confirmation of a hearing loss from 24 to 30 months to 2 to 3 months. Almost 93% of all newborn infants now undergo audiologic screening.[8]

Approximately 50% of all cases of hearing loss have a genetic basis.[9] In about 15% to 30% of cases, hereditary hearing loss may involve other organ systems and may occur as a syndrome.[10] There are more than 200 different syndromes associated with hearing impairment. Identification of syndromic causes of hearing loss may allow for proper management and prediction of future issues. A complete medical and perinatal history, family history, physical examination, and audiologic testing are imperative for the thorough evaluation of congenital hearing loss. Additional radiologic and laboratory studies, as well as evaluations by other specialists, including an otolaryngologist, ophthalmologist, and geneticist, are also important.

Congenital Malformations of the External Ear

In newborns, there are various auricular malformations that may occur as a result of abnormal fetal development or malpositioning of the fetus. One study from Japan showed that about 50% of these deformities resolve spontaneously within the first month of life.[9]

Prominotia

Prominent auricles (Fig. 1-6) may be the result of a lack of development of the antihelical fold, an excessively deep or large conchal cavum or conchal bowl, and/or lobule protrusion. The top of the helical rim is normally 16 to 21 mm from the tympanomastoid surface of the skull to the point of maximal protuberance, and the cephaloauricular angle is about 30 degrees.[11] The incidence of prominotia actually increases from about 0.4% at birth to 5.5% at 1 year.[12]

Lop ears are present in about 38% of babies at birth but, by 1 year of age, only 6% of infants still have a lop ear. In this condition, the superior portion of the auricle is flattened and folded over. Newborns with lop ears can potentially have the ear re-formed if intervention is begun within the first 2 weeks of life. If a newborn with a folded auricle or prominotia is identified, an otolaryngologic consultation can be sought.

There is evidence that the malposition of auricles may be corrected by splinting of the auricle within the first few days after birth.[13,14] A form made of dental wax or some other malleable material can be placed within the helical rim to push the helix into a more normal position. A gentle pressure dressing is applied and changed daily for 4 to 6 weeks.

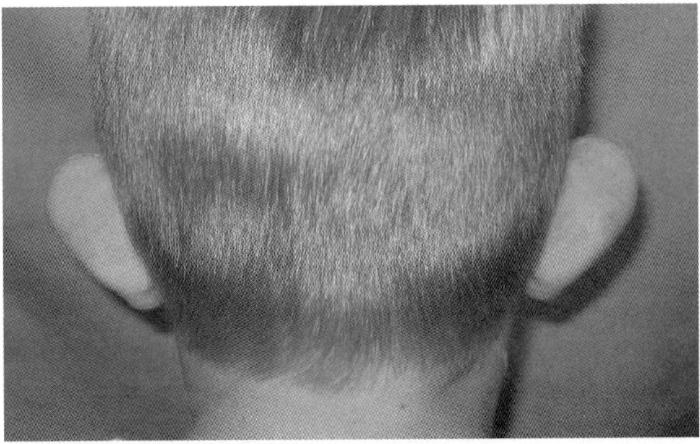

Figure 1-6. Prominotia.

Otoplasty for the repair of prominotia may be considered once a child is 5 to 6 years of age. Various techniques are available to correct the deformity. An otolaryngologist or plastic surgeon may be consulted for the repair. Postoperatively, a compressive dressing is applied. After this dressing is removed, a headband-like dressing is used to help hold the auricles medially during the healing process.

Cup ear deformity presents with a protruding ear that results from an excessively deep concha cavum or conchal bowl. There may also be a forward cupping of the lobule and a deformity of the helical margin. This may be remedied by shaving of the conchal cartilage or excising a rim of the bowl, with or without conchal setback sutures. The lobule that is protruding forward is more challenging to correct; however, it may be repositioned with appropriately placed sutures and/or amputation of an appendage of cartilage at the base of the concha.

Microtia and Atresia

Absence or maldevelopment of the auricle results in an obvious cosmetic deformity (Fig. 1-7). However, an abnormal external ear does not mean abnormal formation of the middle or inner ear. Hearing assessment should be performed at some point to determine inner ear function and whether there is only a conductive hearing loss or whether there is a sensorineural component. Moderate to severe forms of congenital aural atresia are estimated to occur with an incidence of 1 to 5 in 20,000 live births.

Rarely are both auricles visualized at the same time. If the auricles are asymmetrical, no intervention may be necessary. If an auricle is significantly malformed, reconstruction may be considered. A plastic surgery or otolaryngology consultation should be obtained. Reconstruction of the auricle is usually considered during

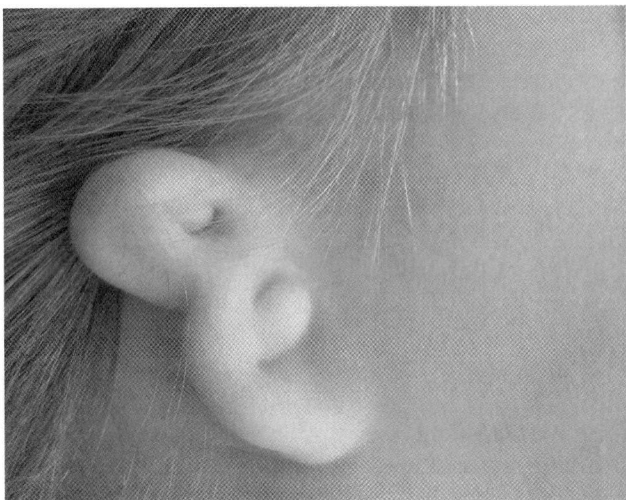

Figure 1-7. Microtia.

the middle of the first decade of life. Of patients with microtia, 85% are unilaterally affected. Bilateral microtia is present in 50% of syndromic cases but in only 12% of nonsyndromic cases.

Patients with microtia should also be evaluated for congenital heart anomalies and other system defects. Some associated defects include cleft palate, esophageal atresia, vertebral defects, and renal anomalies. In most cases of microtia, the external canal also fails to develop.[15]

Reconstruction of the external ear is generally undertaken by the reconstructive surgeon when the child is in the middle of the first decade of life. Typically, rib cartilage is harvested to reconstruct the auricle. A multistaged procedure is required to reconstruct and mature the ear into its final form. Other options include a prosthetic ear, which may be created and fixed to the head with osseointegrated implants.

Ear Canal Stenosis and Atresia

Atretic ear canals are associated with moderate to severe conductive hearing loss. In children with canal atresia, including unilateral cases, hearing in the ear with the normal external structures cannot be assumed to be normal. Both ears need to be screened for hearing. Otoacoustic emissions may be used for an ear with normal canal and middle ear structures; however, patients with bilateral microtia and canal atresia need to be screened with auditory brainstem response (ABR) testing. Screening should be performed in the newborn nursery; with confirmation of any hearing impairment before 3 months of age, the infant should be appropriately fitted with an amplification device by 3 months of age. Bone conduction oscillators may be used to stimulate the cochlea through the skull bone.

If a child has unilateral atresia and normal hearing on the contralateral side, he or she should have periodic evaluations for normal speech and language development and routine hearing screening to ensure continued normal hearing on the contralateral side. Once the child reaches school age, preferential seating and consideration for a frequency-modulated (FM) system should be pursued. Once a child with unilateral aural atresia reaches 5 years of age, consideration and evaluation for possible reconstructive surgery can be considered. CT scanning of the temporal bones will allow for an assessment of prognostic indicators for auditory rehabilitation and help decide whether external auditory canal reconstruction should be considered (Fig. 1-8). External ear reconstruction is undertaken first and reconstruction of the canal may proceed after completion of the external ear reconstruction. However, in a recent study, it has been shown that hearing rehabilitation can be achieved with reduced risk (compared with an external auditory reconstruction) by using an osseointegrated bone conduction implant system, such as the BAHA (Entific, Cochlear Americas, Englewood, Colo).[16]

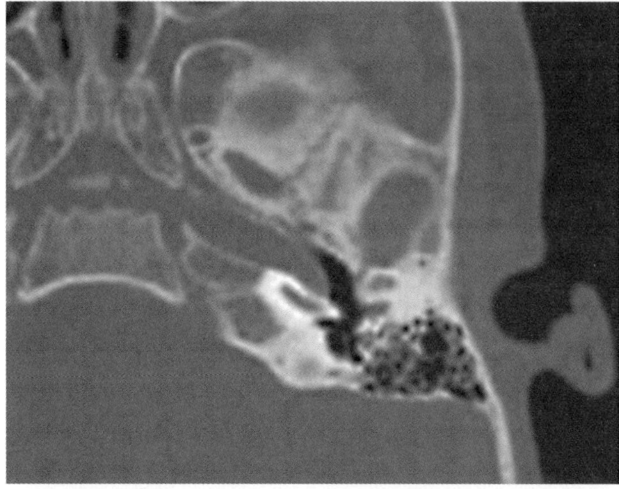

A

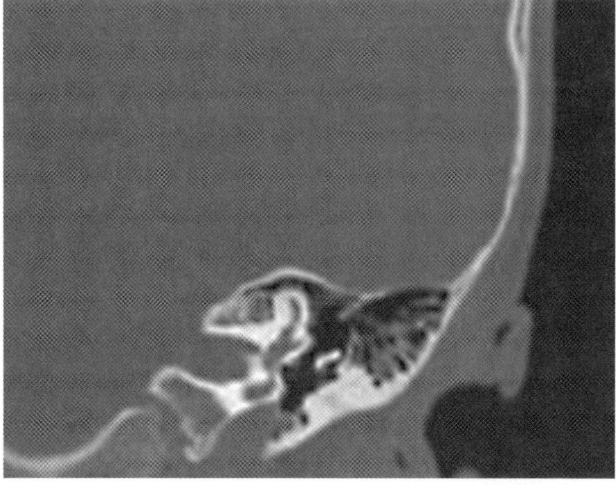

B

Figure 1-8. Computed tomography scans showing external auditory canal atresia.

Aural atresias may be associated with malformations or syndromes such as Crouzon's disease, Treacher Collins syndrome, and other craniofacial or mandibulofacial dysostoses.

Periauricular Pits and Cysts

Auricular appendages or skin tags are common and are the result of abnormal development of accessory auricular hillocks. Skin tags usually consist of skin and subcutaneous tissues, but may also contain cartilage. Usually, they occur unilaterally appear anterior to the auricle.

Incomplete or abnormal fusion of the auricular hillocks may result in the formation of a pit or epithelium-lined tract. If the tract is not in communication with the surface, it may result in a cyst. The cyst may enlarge and become infected. If the tract connects to the surface, it may produce drainage and/or become infected. Preauricular pits (Fig. 1-9) that do not have drainage or

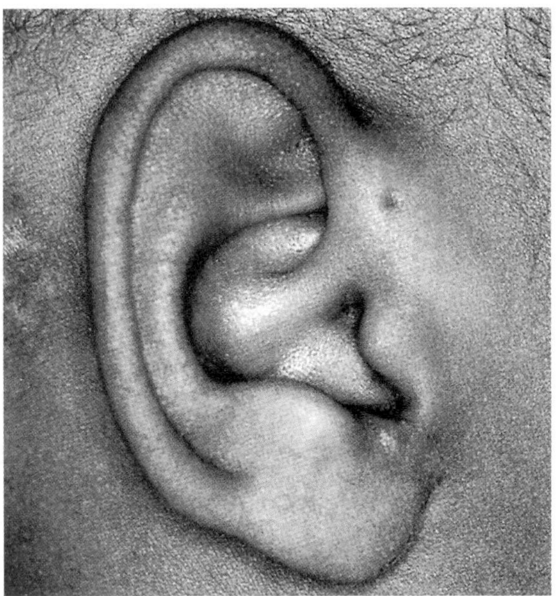

Figure 1-9. Preauricular pit.

swelling may be observed conservatively. Management of preauricular tracts or cysts involves complete surgical excision. Excision may involve a portion of adjacent cartilage and surrounding tissues to ensure removal of potential offshoots from the cyst or tract. Cysts or tracts may recur, which can require more radical resection.

Middle Ear Abnormalities

Congenital Cholesteatomas

A cholesteatoma is composed of keratinizing squamous epithelium that grows within the temporal bone. It will proliferate and expand erosively, and can be extremely destructive if not identified and resected completely. Cholesteatomas do not have linear growth patterns and may lie dormant for some time or have accelerated growth spurts.

The existence of congenital cholesteatomas as an entity has been debated for some time, but this lesion is now an accepted pathologic process. Congenital cholesteatomas are assumed to be present since birth, but some may not be diagnosed until the child is 4 to 5 years old (average). Boys are affected three times more often than girls.[13] The most current accepted criteria for congenital cholesteatomas were described in 1986 by Levenson and associates,[17] and include an intact tympanic membrane, with no history of previous perforation or otorrhea, and no prior otologic surgery.

A number of theories have speculated about the causes of congenital cholesteatomas. The favored theory is the embryonic or epidermoid cell rest, whereby congenital middle ear cholesteatomas arise from the persistence and growth of the epidermoid formation in the anterosuperior quadrant. Epidermoid rests may be traced back to early fetal life and the ectoderm of the first branchial groove. After 33 weeks of gestation, the epidermoid rest usually regresses.[18] However, a study by Potsic and colleagues[19] noted that a subset of their congenital cholesteatomas arose from the posterosuperior quadrant; this conclusion is in conflict with the epidermoid rest cell theory and may indicate that there is a different pathogenesis or a multifactorial process. Other theories include metaplasia of the middle ear mucosa[20] and epithelial migration.[21]

Anterosuperior cholesteatomas (Fig. 1-10) tend to be discovered in younger patients, whereas posterosuperior quadrant cholesteatomas tend to be found across a broader age range. Potsic and associates[19] noted that 13% of their congenital cholesteatomas were found at the time of myringotomy for otitis media with effusion. Evacuation of the middle ear fluid and the increased magnification and brighter illumination under an operating microscope may make diagnosis easier.

CT scanning of the temporal bone is a useful tool to help determine the bony anatomy and extent of the cholesteatoma (Fig. 1-11). For an isolated middle ear congenital cholesteatoma that is well encapsulated and restricted to a single quadrant, a tympanoplasty without mastoidectomy may be sufficient for complete resection of the lesion (Fig. 1-12). More extensive lesions may require a tympanomastoidectomy, with an intact posterior canal wall, or a modified mastoidectomy procedure, with creation of a mastoid bowl and a large external meatus for débridement. If the cholesteatoma has broken out of its cyst, a second-look operation may be required.

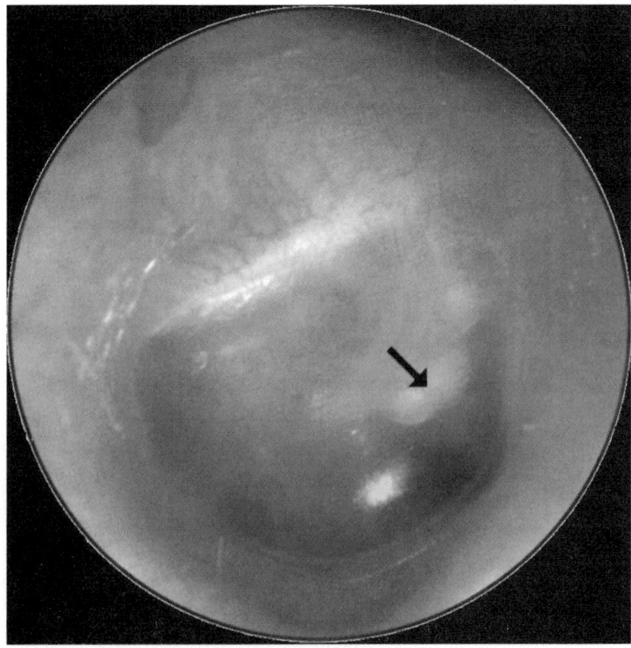

Figure 1-10. Congenital cholesteatoma.

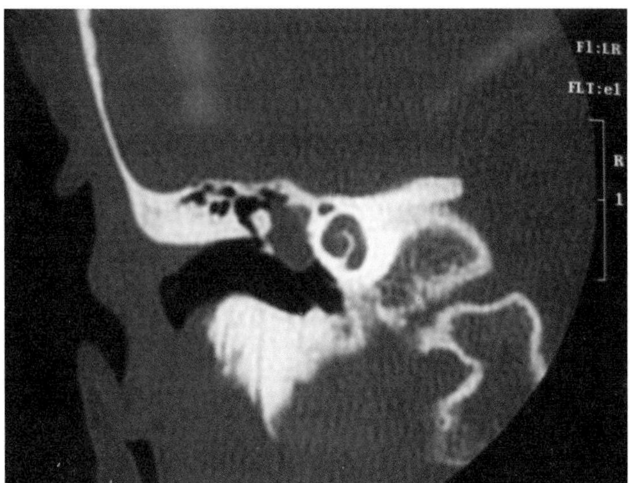

Figure 1-11. Computed tomography scan of congenital cholesteatoma.

Less commonly, cholesteatomas may be found in other areas of the temporal bones, such as in the petrous apex. The cause of these cholesteatomas is unclear. Cholesteatomas of the petrous apex typically grow insidiously and may become rather large before they present with symptoms. Initial symptoms and signs may include headaches, hearing loss, facial nerve paresis, and spasms. Patients may not present until they are teenagers or young adults. Surgical resection is required; however, because of its location, access to this region may prove challenging. If there is no hearing in that ear, a transcochlear approach may be considered. If hearing is still present, the lesion may be approached through the middle cranial fossa.

Ossicular Anomalies

Ossicular anomalies may be present with or without external ear abnormalities. Ossicular anomalies include the following: malleolar abnormalities, such as abnormal formation or absence of the malleus; incudal abnormalities, such as abnormal formation or absence of the incus; stapes anomalies, such as absence of an anterior or posterior crura or the entire superstructure; abnormal stapes footplate; and a fusion defect between the malleus, incus, and stapes and the round window and promontory. Ossicular anomalies may also be associated with an aberrant facial nerve or facial nerve anomalies and absence of the stapedial muscle. In cases of congenital stapes footplate fixation, there may be a patent cochlear aqueduct, which may result in a perilymphatic or CSF "gusher" at the time of mobilization or stapedectomy. With cochlear abnormalities, there may be a malformation of the stapes footplate and the crura, which may result in a spontaneous perilymphatic fistula.

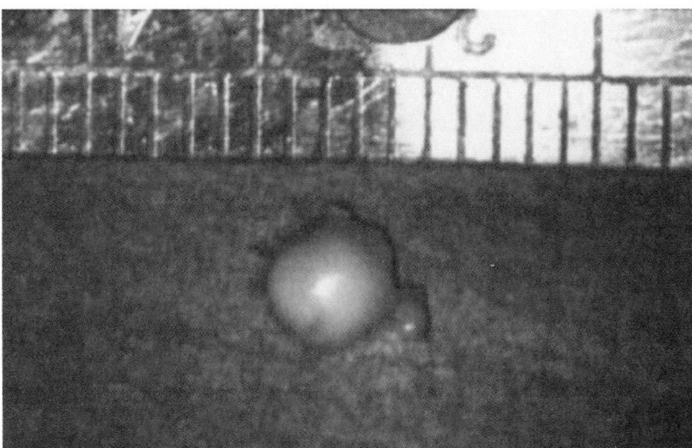

Figure 1-12. Congenital cholesteatoma pearl after resection.

Aberrant Carotid Artery

On inspection of the tympanic membrane, a vascular mass may be seen anteriorly or inferiorly within the middle ear space. This may represent an aberrant carotid artery. The vessel may pass up through the hypotympanum and turn anteriorly just below the stapes and toward the eustachian tube. The artery may not be encased in a bony canal. Patients may report a pulsatile tinnitus, or a bruit may be heard at the external meatus. An aberrant carotid artery may be confused with an aneurysm or glomus tumor. The presence of an aberrant carotid artery is a relative contraindication for myringotomy, with or without tube placement (Figs. 1-13 and 1-14).

Inner Ear Abnormalities

Inner ear malformations are a result of a defect in development and typically occur in the first trimester of

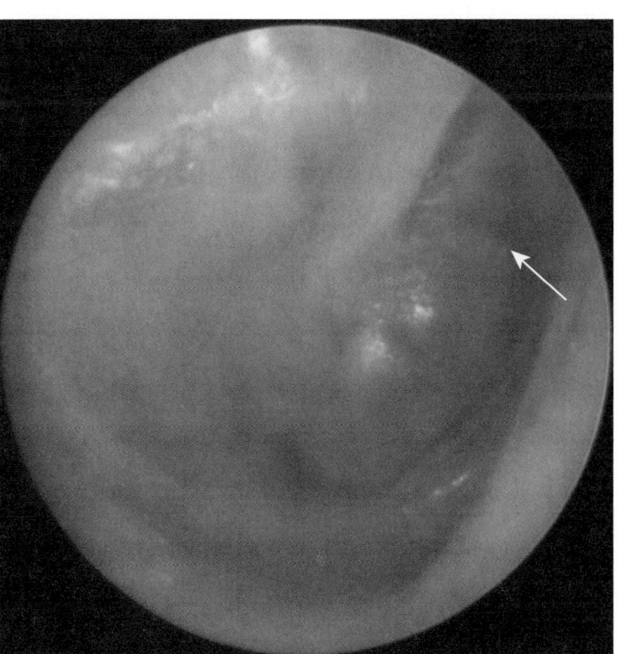

Figure 1-13. Aberrant carotid artery (arrow).

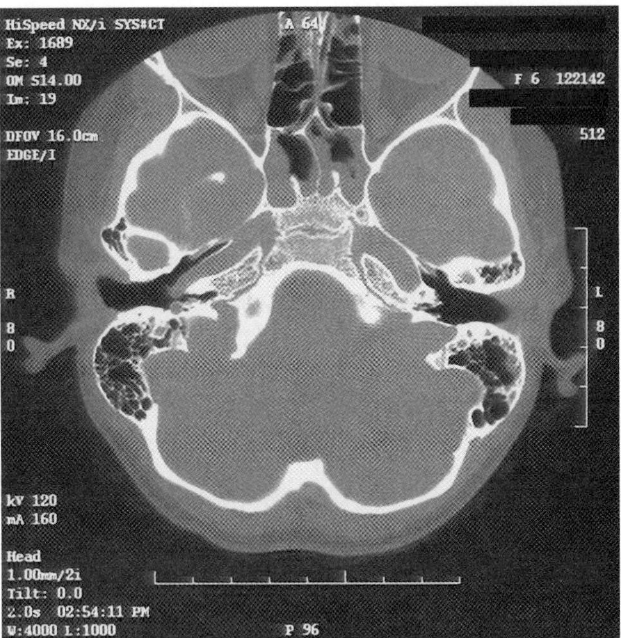

Figure 1-14. Computed tomography scan of aberrant carotid artery.

pregnancy, during the formation of the membranous labyrinth. At about the fourth week of gestation, the otocyst develops branches and coils to form the labyrinth. Cartilage and the osseous labyrinth form during the second trimester and usually development of the inner ear is complete by the 26th week of gestation. Inner ear anomalies are generally associated with sensorineural hearing loss (Fig. 1-15).

A full discussion of cochlear and labyrinthine developmental anomalies is beyond the scope of this chapter. However, a child with hearing loss should have temporal bone imaging for visualization of the anatomy of the inner ear to determine whether there are any developmental anomalies that may be associated with the hearing loss or may be predictive of progression. Additionally, in children with profound sensorineural hearing loss, imaging is important as part of the evaluation to determine whether the child is a candidate for cochlear implantation; cochlear aplasia, a complete lack of development of the cochlea, and absence of the eighth cranial nerve are both contraindications for implantation.

In children with sensorineural hearing loss, imaging of the temporal bone is also important to help rule out an enlarged vestibular aqueduct (EVA). The vestibular aqueduct is usually a narrow bony canal that contains the endolymphatic duct. The duct connects the endolymphatic sac to the vestibule. The endolymphatic sac lies adjacent to the dura, acts as a reservoir for endolymph, and has an active exchange between the CSF and endolymph. The vestibular aqueduct is considered enlarged if it measures larger than 1.5 mm in width, although there are some variations in what is considered the upper limit of normal.[22,23] Jackler and De La Cruz[22] also described EVA as the most commonly radiographically detectable anomaly of the inner ear (Figs. 1-16 and 1-17). Cochlear and vestibular anomalies are also associated with EVA and are commonly seen in conjunction with Mondini malformations (see Fig. 1-15).

Jackler and De La Cruz[22] have reported that there is a slight female preponderance, approximately 94% of the cases of EVA are bilateral, and almost 65% of patients with EVA have progression of sensorineural hearing loss with head trauma (11% have progression of hearing loss

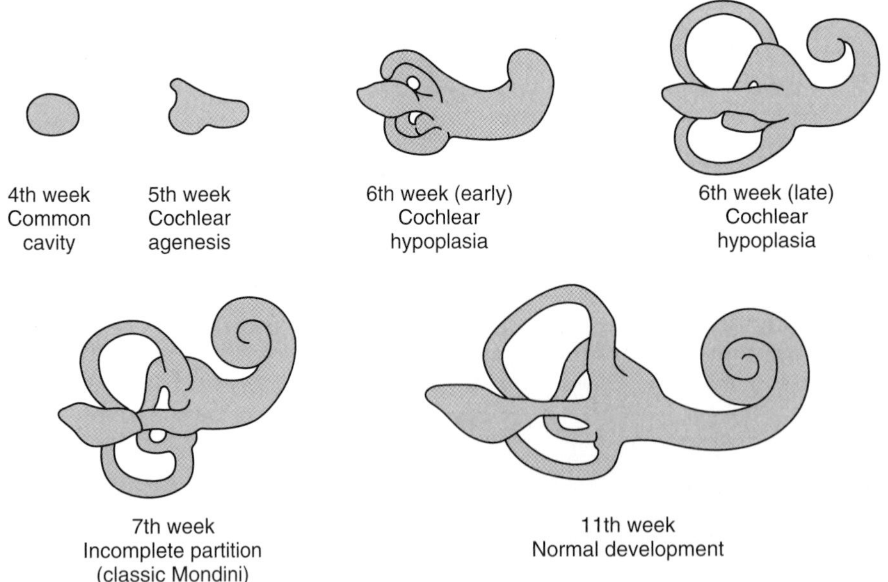

Figure 1-15. Cochlear abnormalities.

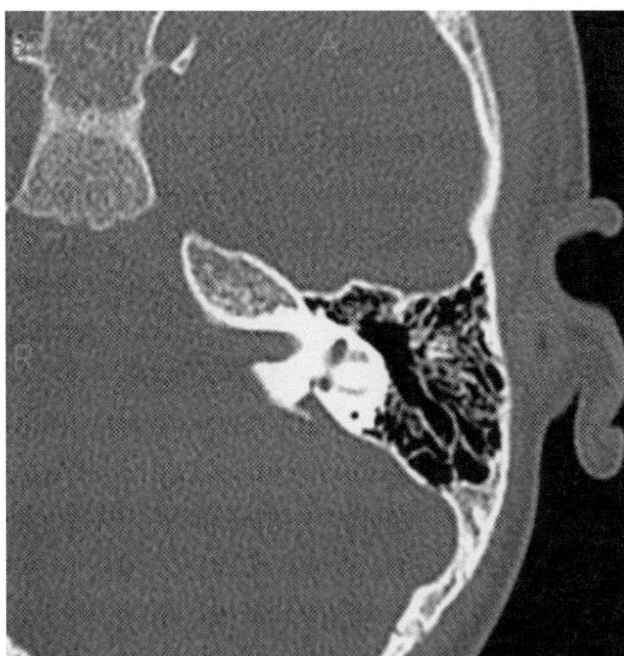

Figure 1-16. Computed tomography scan showing left enlarged vestibular aqueduct.

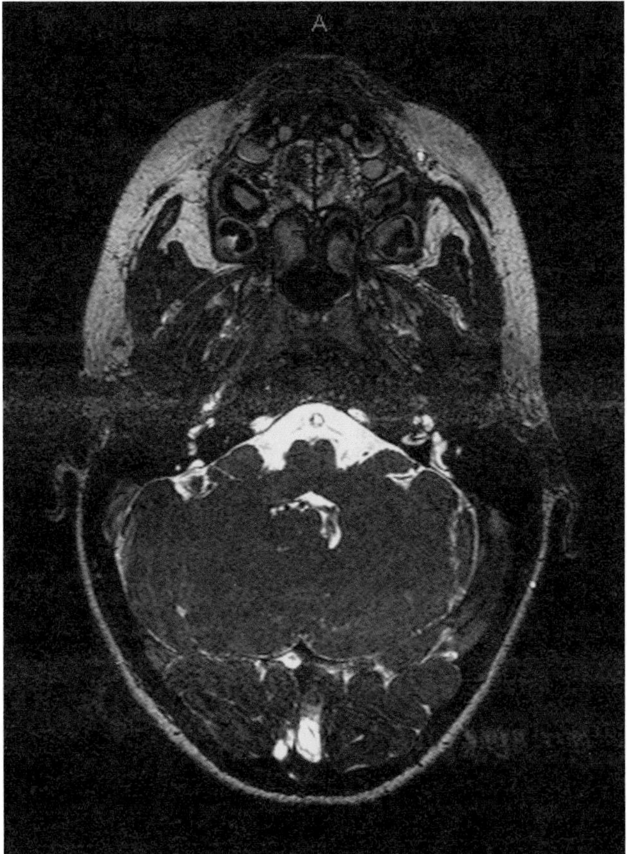

Figure 1-17. Magnetic resonance imaging scan showing left enlarged vestibular aqueduct.

with relatively minor head trauma). Patients with normal hearing may have EVA, but definitive evidence is lacking that they may be predisposed to hearing loss. Sudden and fluctuating hearing loss may be associated with EVA. It should be recommended to parents of a child with EVA that they try to avoid the child's participation in activities that might increase the chances of head trauma or jarring, such as football, soccer, and riding in roller coasters, because such activities could elicit a sudden sensorineural hearing loss. For similar reasons, activities such as skydiving or scuba diving, in which sudden pressure changes might occur, should also be avoided. Children with EVA should also have their hearing monitored and appropriate and timely intervention instituted if the hearing loss progresses.

CONGENITAL FACIAL NERVE PARALYSIS

Congenital facial nerve paralysis has been estimated to have an incidence of 0.8 per 1000 to 1.8 per 1000 births and can be broken down into traumatic and developmental causes.[24,25] Traumatic causes relate to intrauterine positioning or delivery; developmental causes relate to faulty embryogenesis. Traumatic congenital paralysis may resolve spontaneously in about 90% of cases; however, developmental facial paralysis does not resolve with time. Traumatic cases may require surgical intervention. Neonates with facial palsy may undergo electrophysiologic testing to help discriminate between traumatic and developmental paralysis. Traumatic congenital facial palsy typically is unilateral and involves the entire nerve and its branches on the affected side. In cases of traumatic congenital facial palsy, there may also be evidence of trauma, such as a hemotympanum or external ecchymosis.

Developmental facial paralysis may occur in association with other anomalies or with a facial diplegia or isolated palsy of a segment of the nerve, rather than a complete unilateral paresis. Developmental paralysis may also be associated with abnormalities in the facial musculature that are innervated by the anomalous nerve branches. Most cases of developmental facial paralysis are associated with Möbius' syndrome,[26] the oculoauriculovertebral spectrum, and congenital unilateral lower lip palsy. True congenital palsy is a fixed deformity that neither worsens nor improves.

Möbius' syndrome is a rare congenital anomaly characterized by a unilateral or bilateral facial paralysis that usually spares the lower half of the face. There is also a coexisting abducens nerve palsy. Other comorbid conditions may include the absence of pectoral musculature, anomalies of the extremities, and involvement of other cranial nerves. The cause remains unknown.

The oculoauriculovertebral spectrum includes Goldenhar's syndrome and hemifacial microsomia and involves the unilateral malformation of the first and second branchial arch derivatives. Affected children typically manifest hypoplasia of the maxilla and mandible, microtia, and microstomia. Of children with these disorders, 10% to 20% present with facial palsy.[27]

Congenital unilateral lower lip palsy (CULLP) is sometimes referred to asymmetrical crying facies. It is one of the more common causes of congenital facial paralysis. CULLP is a weakness in the lower lip depressors and is typically seen in the eyes, where one side of the lower lip fails to depress with crying. It has been postulated that there is a deficiency of the depressor anguli oris muscle, with an associated brainstem abnormality. CULLP may be associated with other defects, including cardiac anomalies, which are present in up to 10% of affected children; this is referred to as cardiofacial syndrome.[28]

As with any facial paralysis, evaluation of the eye for proper corneal protection and lubrication must be performed. An ophthalmologic consultation for corneal abrasions or exposure keratitis should be sought if there is any evidence of weakness in the facial nerve involving closure of the eyelids. Fortunately, infants usually have adequate passive eyelid closure to protect the cornea. Facial reanimation is performed from the age of 5 to 7 years with various techniques, including cross-facial nerve grafting and free muscle transfer, masseter and temporalis muscle transfers, and, infrequently, static sling procedures.[26]

EYELID AND OCULAR ABNORMALITIES

The critical period for development of the head and face is the fourth through eighth weeks of gestation. By 8 weeks, most of the embryonic face is complete. Most of the facial structure is derived from ectodermal neural crest tissue. Eyelid formation is more closely related to the development of the eye than the face. As eye development proceeds from the diverticula of the forebrain early in the fourth week of gestation, the optic cup gives rise to the lens and cornea. During its sixth week, small folds of ectoderm form to become the upper and lower eyelids. The lids grow toward each other and fuse between weeks 8 and 10. They remain fused until the fifth to seventh gestational months, at which time they separate. During this time, the orbicularis oculi muscle forms. Normal orbital development depends on normal eye development.[29]

The anatomy of the eyelids and adnexa is complex and is summarized here only briefly to mention the various structures that provide vision and protection of the visual system. The eyelids can be divided into the anterior and posterior lamellae, separated by the septum. They are composed of four layers—skin, orbicularis oculi muscle, tarsus, and conjunctiva. Approximately 10 mm above the upper lid crease, the eyelid includes the orbital septum, orbital fat, levator aponeurosis, and Müller's muscle. The orbicularis oculi muscle is critical in blinking and closure of the eyelids, as well as providing the pumping mechanism for the lacrimal sac. The tarsus and canthal tendons provide structure to the eyelid. Medially and laterally, the tarsal plates are attached to the orbital rims by the canthal tendons. The conjunctiva lines the inner aspects of the lids and surface of the eye. The orbital septum originates from the periosteum of the orbital rims and is the anterior barrier of the orbit. Deep to the septum is the orbital fat, and deep to the fat pads is the levator muscle, which is critical in lid opening. Müller's muscle travels along the posterior surface of the levator aponeurosis and inserts onto the tarsus. It is a sympathetic muscle that also contributes to lid elevation. The lacrimal drainage system includes the puncta of each lid medially, the canaliculi, and the lacrimal sac. The sac opens into the nasolacrimal duct. The globe, optic nerve, and extraocular muscles are the final critical components of the anatomy and serve as the main impetus for growth and development of the orbit and surrounding structures.[30]

Colobomas

Colobomas of the eyelids occur when there is a disruption of the eyelid margin. A failure of migration of the ectoderm or mesoderm may cause this abnormality, as can mechanical forces such as those due to amniotic bands. Colobomas may be isolated, occur in conjunction with other clefting phenomena, or may be seen in craniofacial syndromes. True colobomas can be distinguished from pseudocolobomas by documenting a discontinuity of the eyelid margin. Pseudocolobomas are seen in Treacher Collins syndrome. Management involves protection of the ocular surface with lubrication and occlusive dressings, if necessary. Because amblyopia may result, this must be done judiciously with a plan for repair at 6 to 12 months of age.[31]

Ptosis

Ptosis results in incomplete opening of the upper eyelid in children and is one of the most common ocular disorders. It has various causes, which may be myogenic, aponeurotic, neurogenic, mechanical, or traumatic. It is critical to define the cause and also determine the need for and timing of correction. If severe, it must be corrected early to avoid development of amblyopia. If there is no risk of amblyopia, correction can be deferred until 6 to 12 months, when anesthetic risks are lower.[32]

Other Eyelid Malformations

The most common medial canthal variation is epicanthal folds, which are excess folds of tissue in the medial canthal region. They may be a normal ethnic finding, an isolated developmental anomaly, or part of a craniofacial syndrome. Epicanthal folds are primarily a cosmetic issue although, in severe cases, vision can be blocked medially.

Lateral canthal malposition is rarely an isolated finding. It is most often associated with conditions such as Treacher Collins or Apert's syndrome.[33]

Epiblepharon and entropion describe the eyelid malpositions when the lash line is rolled inward toward the globe. In epiblepharon, the rotation is caused by the mechanical effect of a fold of skin running across the lower lid margin, whereas entropion entails a true turning inward of the lid margin. In many situations, the entropion or epiblepharon may be asymptomatic and not require treatment. However, signs and symptoms such as chronic discharge and corneal irritation will lead to surgical intervention. Congenital ectropion is often a result of an inflammatory reaction in the conjunctiva, which leads to a mechanical eversion of the lower lid.[33]

Microphthalmos and Anophthalmos

Microphthalmos and anophthalmos are congenital ocular malformations. Anophthalmos is extremely rare and refers to a complete absence of ocular tissue, whereas microphthalmos refers to a smaller, more rudimentary ocular remnant. The growth of the orbit and lids is proportionately affected, related to the degree of underdevelopment of the ocular tissue. Because of a deficiency in ocular tissue, the growth of the orbital bones and lids is also stunted, resulting in a smaller palpebral fissure and adnexal structures, hypoplastic maxilla, and lateral and superior orbital rims.[33]

NASAL ANOMALIES

The face begins its fetal development at about 3 to 4 weeks of gestation; its most critical period is until about 12 weeks of gestation. The facial process develops by the end of the fourth week as a result of development of the matrix of the neural tubules and cellular differentiation. The head at this point is a large bulge at the cephalic end of the embryo. Two small, horseshoe-shaped bulges develop above the stomadeum to form the nasal placodes, each with a medial and a lateral nasal process.[34]

During the sixth week, the maxillary process of the first branchial arch from each side develops along with the medial nasal process, and the maxillary processes migrate medially to fuse in the midline to form the upper lips, philtrum, and columella. Over the next 2 weeks, the nasal pits deepen and form the nasobuccal membrane. This membrane later ruptures to create the nasal cavity, with a primitive choana. The palatine processes of the maxilla proliferate and grow medially to fuse at the midline and with the septum to form the palate.[35]

Nasal Dermoids, Nasal Gliomas, and Encephaloceles

Nasal dermoids are midline subcutaneous epithelial cysts that may have a sinus tract opening to the skin and/or a connection intracranially with the dura. Nasal gliomas and anterior encephaloceles are theorized to result from a similar embryologic defect. Nasal gliomas, encephaloceles, and nasal dermoids are commonly grouped as congenital midline nasal masses, which occur in approximately 1 per 20,000 to 40,000 live births.[36]

During embryogenesis, the space between the forming nasal and frontal bones is usually filled with a firm membrane called the fonticulus frontalis. There is also a space between the developing septal cartilage and the nasal bones called the prenasal space. From the cranial side, a herniation of dura passes down through the foramen cecum and prenasal space, continuous with the periosteum of the nasal bones and eventually coming into contact with the skin. During normal development, bony ingrowth obliterates the foramen cecum and fonticulus frontalis. Their incomplete closure may provide a path for herniation. As the foramen cecum closes, the dura detaches from the overlying skin by the ingrowth of mesenchyme. If the dura does not detach and retract, it may carry ectoderm into the prenasal space, including intracranially, to form a dermoid cyst or nasal dermal sinus. If the dural tract fails to detach and does not retract, there may be herniated brain tissue trapped as the foramen cecum closes, forming a nasal glioma.[33] Nasal gliomas may be located extranasally (60%), intranasally (30%), or both.[37] Encephaloceles may develop if there is failure in the closure of the foramen cecum, fonticulus frontalis, or roof of the nose.

Nasal dermoids and extranasal gliomas may present as a firm swelling at the root of the nose. Nasal dermoids may also have a sinus tract that opens to the skin and may have hairs protruding from the pit (Fig. 1-18). The pit may be located anywhere from the columella to the glabella. Encephaloceles usually appear as bluish compressible lesions that may transilluminate and may be pulsatile as a result of communication with CSF. Encephaloceles in the nasal region are categorized as sincipital or basal. Sincipital encephaloceles have an external mass located around the nasal dorsum, orbits, and forehead and result from failure of closure of the foramen cecum (Fig. 1-19). The less common basal encephaloceles present within the nasal cavity, nasopharynx, or posterior part of the orbit and are formed from a defect in the cribriform plate or body of the sphenoid. Encephaloceles may be divided by their contents—meningoceles contain

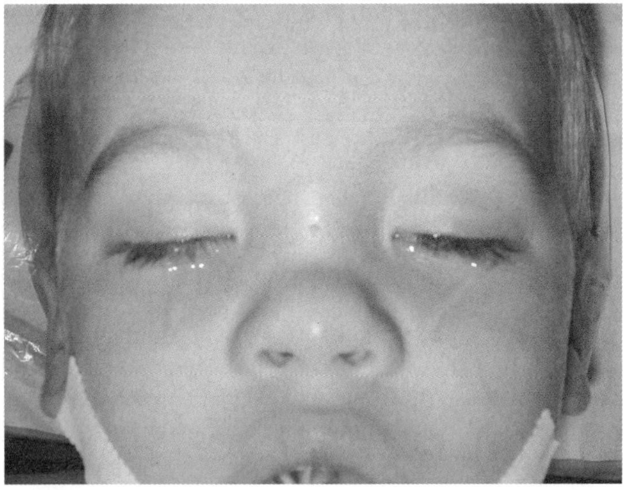

Figure 1-18. Nasal dermoid with pit on dorsum of nose.

only meninges, encephalomeningoceles contain brain tissue and meninges, and encephalomeningocystoceles contain brain, meninges, and part of the ventricular system.

Both CT and MRI are necessary to evaluate these deformities. Both studies allow for the evaluation of the bony vault and paranasal areas, delineation of the contents of the cyst or sac (brain, CSF, or other soft tissue), and determination of intracranial extent, including involvement of the dura and subdural space.

Neurosurgery and otolaryngologic consultations should be obtained for the evaluation and management of these lesions. Nasal dermoids and gliomas that have not been infected and are not growing rapidly may be observed until the child is 1 year of age, at which point surgical resection should be considered. Complete resection of the cyst and sinus tract is required to avoid recurrence. A frontal craniotomy may be required if the lesion extends through the foramen cecum and has an intracranial component. Children with nasal encephaloceles should be evaluated for hydrocephalus and may require shunt placement prior to repair of the encephalocele. Early intervention is recommended to avoid the increased risk of meningitis. As part of the repair, the skull base defect may need to be repaired, along with any CSF leak.

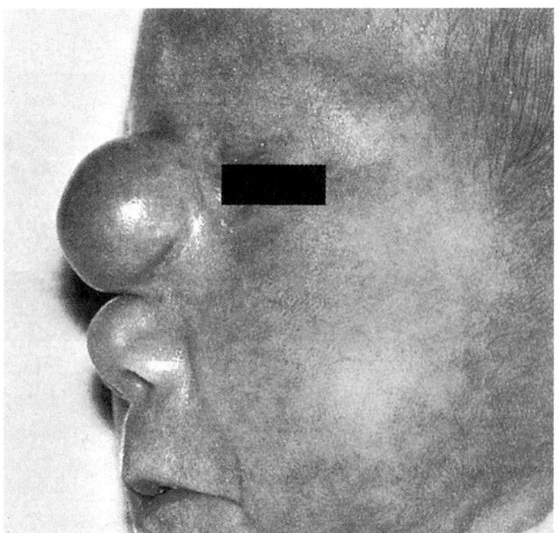

Figure 1-19. Frontal encephalocele.

Median Nasal Cleft

Median nasal clefts may range in severity from a simple median scar on the nasal dorsum to a bifid nose, which is a completely split nose with independent medial walls of the nares. The nasal patency and airway are usually adequate. A complete multidisciplinary evaluation should be performed prior to repair to exclude syndromes and associated anomalies, as well as to identify other deformities such as nasal dermoids or encephaloceles. Craniofacial surgery will be required to repair a median nasal cleft and the associated craniofacial anomalies.

Choanal Atresia

Choanal atresia has a reported incidence that varies from 1 in 5000 to 1 in 7000 live births. There is an equal female-to-male predilection, and unilateral cases may be twice as likely to occur as bilateral cases. Major congenital anomalies have been described in approximately 47% of children with choanal atresia.[35] Syndromes associated with choanal atresia include the CHARGE association, Apert's syndrome, DiGeorge syndrome, trisomy 18, Treacher Collins syndrome, and camptomelic dysplasia.

Embryologically, if the nasobuccal membrane does not thin appropriately and persists, choanal atresia results. During normal development, the rupture of the nasobuccal membrane occurs at about the sixth week of gestation; the palatine shelves fuse in the midline to create the secondary palate and bony floor of the nose during the seventh week. The septum descends inferiorly and fuses with the palate during the ninth week. The soft palate separates the nasopharynx from the oral cavity by the 12th week.

There are some typical anatomic variations that occur with choanal atresia, including the medial displacement of the posterior part of the lateral nasal walls, an accentuated arch of the hard palate, and a shortened nasopharyngeal space. Choanal atresia may consist of a complete bony plate or may be combined with bony and membranous components. Choanal stenosis may also appear as a patent but extremely narrowed posterior choana.

Bilateral choanal atresia is usually evident at birth or shortly thereafter, with respiratory distress. Because neonates are obligate nasal breathers, cyanosis at rest, which resolves with crying, may be observed. An oral airway or intubation may be required to maintain ventilation.

Unilateral choanal atresia rarely causes acute respiratory distress and may actually remain undiagnosed until later in infancy or thereafter. The presence of unilateral choanal atresia may be noted by the inability to pass a 6 French nasal suction through one side of the nose into the oropharynx or by the presence of persistent unilateral nasal discharge. It may sometimes be misdiagnosed as a unilateral nasal foreign body and/or unilateral chronic rhinosinusitis. Choanal stenosis may present as the inability to pass a 6 French catheter, but it is usually asymptomatic and does not require surgical intervention.

Choanal atresia or stenosis may be diagnosed by nasal endoscopy, which may be safely performed using a flexible pediatric nasopharyngoscope. A simple test for nasal patency is to hold a dental mirror at each naris to see if fogging occurs. A CT scan is essential for describing the atretic plate and posterior nasal anatomy and to aid in preoperative planning.

Intervention for choanal atresia depends on the infant's symptomatology and type of atresia. Neonates with bilateral atresia generally require immediate intervention for management of ventilation. Once the airway has been stabilized, feeding may be instituted via an oral gastric tube and imaging studies performed. Otolaryngologic consultation should be obtained for evaluation and management of choanal atresia. Endoscopic nasal surgery and powered instrumentation have enabled surgeons to attempt repair of choanal atresia by a transnasal-transseptal route rather than by a transpalatal repair, which has a higher incidence of morbidity. Following surgical repair, intranasal stents are placed for up to 3 weeks.[38]

Children with unilateral atresia usually present later and may undergo surgical repair when diagnosed. As noted earlier, choanal stenosis rarely requires intervention.

Pyriform Aperture Stenosis

Congenital nasal pyriform aperture stenosis has been theorized to develop as a result of excessive medial displacement of the maxillary prominences, with overgrowth of ossification in the area of the pyriform aperture.[39] Typically, children present with a poor nasal airway, difficulty with feeding, mouth breathing, apneic episodes, and inability to pass a suction or flexible endoscope through the nares. The nasal valve reveals a narrowing to about 1 to 2 mm, which is caused by the medial protrusion of the lateral aspects of the pyriform aperture. CT scans are useful to confirm the diagnosis (Fig. 1-20). Congenital nasal pyriform aperture stenosis may also be associated with a maxillary megaincisor; if a

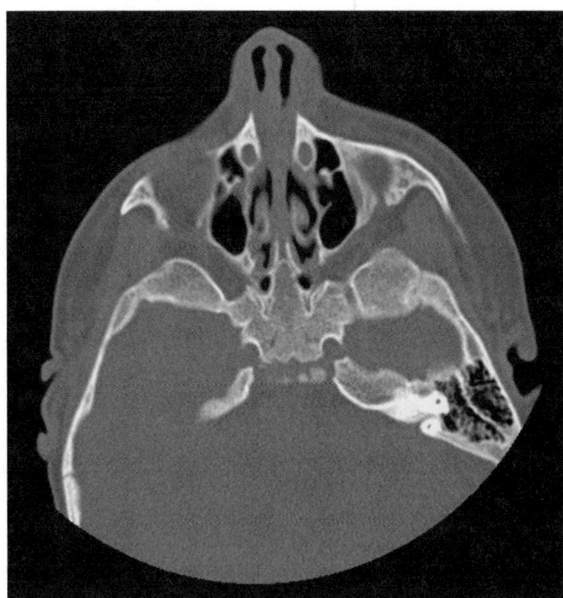

Figure 1-20. Pyriform aperture stenosis.

megaincisor erupts, it is recommended that chromosomal analysis and evaluation of the central nervous system, especially the hypopituitary-pituitary-thyroid axis, be performed.[40]

As with bilateral choanal atresia, an oral airway may be useful in management. Failure to thrive, inability to obtain adequate nutrition, or continued respiratory distress may necessitate surgical intervention. Surgical intervention may be accomplished through a sublabial approach, with the lateral bony edges of the pyriform aperture being removed submucosally. Care must be taken to preserve the nasolacrimal ducts laterally and avoid the tooth buds inferiorly. If the nasolacrimal ducts are too medial, a dacryocystorhinostomy may need to be performed. Intranasal stents are usually placed for 2 weeks. Care must be taken to avoid nasal alar pressure necrosis while the stents are in place.[41]

ORAL ANOMALIES

The development of the face begins in the third week of gestation with the formation of the branchial arches and growth of the frontonasal prominence. The first and second branchial arches become the maxilla and mandible, respectively. The neural crest cells are responsible for the fusion of the facial prominences. The frontonasal prominence contributes to the philtrum and primary palate by fusing with the maxillary prominences, which are responsible for the lateral upper lip, maxilla, and secondary palate. This growth and fusion process is complete by week 12 of gestation.[34]

Various disorders of the oral cavity and surrounding structures may cause functional and appearance concerns. Many of these disorders lead to problems with the airway and feeding.

Cleft Lip and Cleft Palate

Cleft lip and/or cleft palate constitute the second most frequently occurring of the major congenital anomalies, resulting from a failure of mesenchymal penetration and fusion of the nasofrontal and lateral facial processes during weeks 4 through 7 of gestation. Clefts may be unilateral or bilateral, and the degree of severity is variable (Fig. 1-21). Early considerations for treating affected infants are feeding, maintenance of an airway, middle ear disease, and the association with other abnormalities. A complete cleft involves the lip and alveolus in addition to affecting the position of the nasal ala. A cleft lip can be repaired at any time after birth in otherwise healthy infants, but most centers wait until the infant is 3 months of age because of anesthesia safety concerns.[42] Cleft palate may involve only the soft palate or the soft and hard palates. Repair is usually performed in conjunction with ear tube placement at approximately 9 months; the timing is dictated by the child's overall health. Proper dental, orthodontic, otolaryngologic, and speech evaluations and follow-up are all critical for these children. Bone grafting of the alveolar cleft is done during the stage of mixed dentition, in some cases later in the first decade. Approximately 25% of patients require orthognathic surgery for maxillary retrusion secondary to the clefting process.[43]

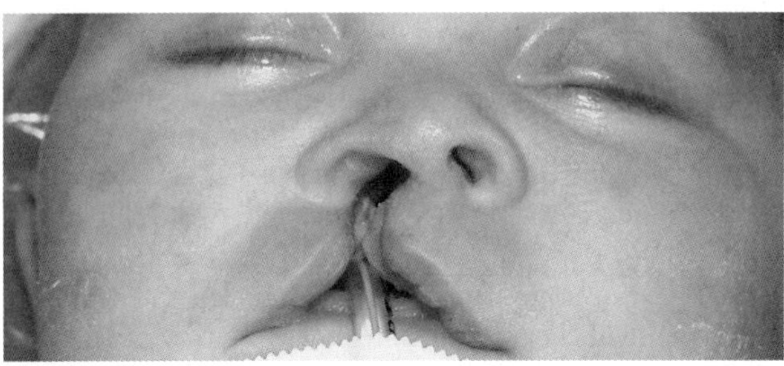

A

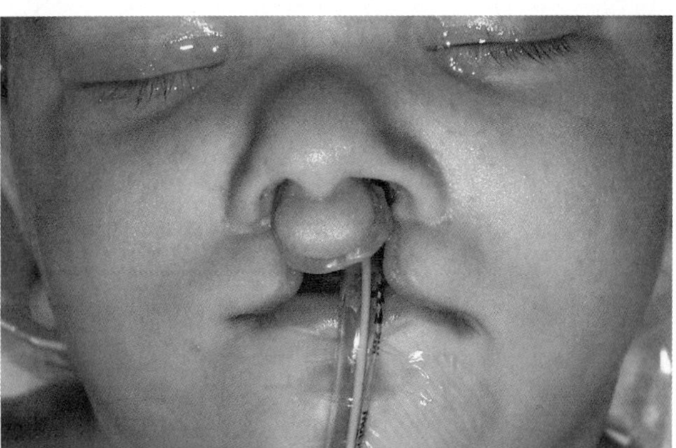

B

Figure 1-21.

Pierre Robin Sequence

Pierre Robin sequence involves micrognathia-retrognathia, glossoptosis, and airway obstruction, with or without a cleft palate. The primary concern with these children is the patency of their airway. Although some neonates are responsive to prone positioning, many have difficulty while feeding and require procedures to facilitate breathing.[41] Depending on the severity of the micrognathia-retrognathia, techniques such as tongue-lip adhesion and mandibular distraction have been used to improve the airway. In severe cases, tracheostomy may be required.[44]

Isolated micrognathia is uncommon, because it is usually associated with syndromes such as Treacher Collins and bifacial microsomia. As in Pierre Robin sequence, the primary concerns are with the airway and feeding.

Macroglossia

Macroglossia is rare as an isolated finding, and is usually associated with Beckwith-Wiedemann or Down syndrome. It can also result from lymphatic or mixed channel malformations. The size can contribute to airway obstruction, but generally these children have an open-mouthed posture, with a protuberant tongue.

Macrostomia

Macrostomia is typically a result of lateral facial clefting, which may be unilateral or bilateral. Tessier[45] has classified this lateral oral cleft as a rare craniofacial cleft (no. 7), in which there is a cleft of the red lip, orbicularis oris, and mucosa. This cleft may extend to involve the bony maxilla. These clefts are frequently seen in conjunction with hemifacial or bifacial microsomia and Treacher Collins syndrome.[45]

Temporomandibular Joint Ankylosis

Temporomandibular joint (TMJ) ankylosis may be a result of soft tissue and/or bony ankylosis and limits the opening of the mouth. It may be congenital or posttraumatic. If it is congenital, airway and feeding issues may prove to be critical for the neonate. Growth of the mandible may be disturbed, because the condyle is a major growth center. As the child matures, oral hygiene becomes more of a challenge, as does feeding. Surgical release of the ankylosed TMJ often leads to disappointing results if the child is not old enough to be compliant with postoperative oral therapy to maintain the opening.[46]

CRANIOFACIAL SYNDROMES

A craniofacial syndrome is a set of deformities that occur together, with some involving the cranial vault and face. Gorlin and associates have described numerous craniofacial syndromes that may be classified by certain predominant features.[47]

Craniosynostosis

The craniosynostosis syndromes involve premature closure of one or more cranial vault sutures, in addition to other facial, limb, and organ findings. Apert's syndrome is also known as acrocephalosyndactyly; it involves bicoronal synostosis and syndactyly involving all four extremities. The cranial base is foreshortened and results in midface hypoplasia, with abnormal crowding and impaction of the dentition (Fig. 1-22). Crouzon's syndrome involves synostosis, midfacial hypoplasia, and exophthalmos. The clinical expression is variable, with two or more sutures involved, and a variable degree of midfacial hypoplasia. With more severe hypoplasia of the maxilla, a more significant exorbitism results and places the globes at risk. Pfeiffer syndrome, described in 1964, consists of craniosynostosis, broad thumbs and great toes, and occasional partial soft tissue syndactyly. Saethre-Chotzen syndrome is also characterized by craniosynostosis, shallow orbits, low-set hairline, and partial syndactyly.

In general, treatment of all craniosynostosis syndromes involves cranial vault expansion and reshaping within the first year of life to prevent development of elevated intracranial pressure. Many of these patients require repeat cranial vault surgeries in addition to midfacial advancement to improve airway and facial esthetics.[48]

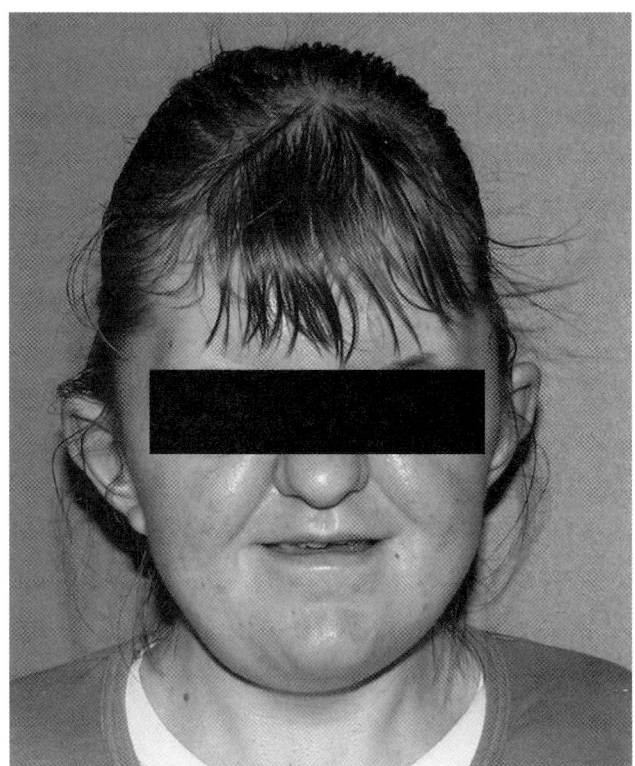

Figure 1-22.

Hemifacial Microsomia

Hemifacial microsomia is also known as the first and second branchial arch syndrome, otomandibular dysostosis, craniofacial microsomia, and lateral facial dysplasia. Affected patients have unilateral microtia and hypoplasia of variable degree of the mandibular ramus and condyle (Fig. 1-23). These patients may also have macrostomia associated with lateral facial clefting. The mandibular deformity is the earliest skeletal manifestation and seems to play a role in the progressive distortion of ipsilateral and contralateral structures, with deviation toward the affected side. The orbit, zygoma, temporal bone, maxilla, and nose may also be involved. In addition to the skeletal deformities, the facial soft tissue on the

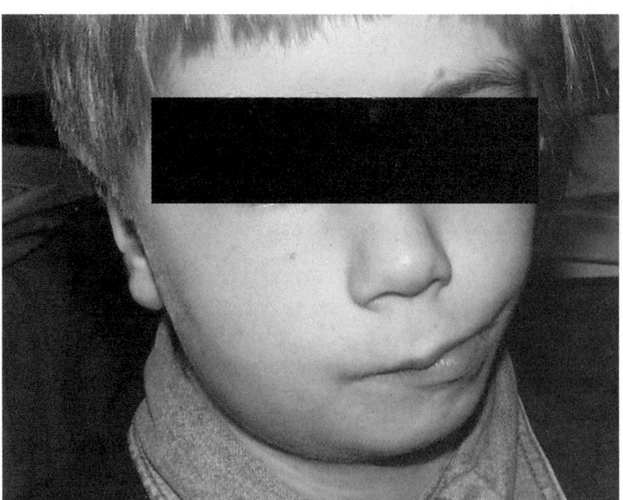

Figure 1-23.

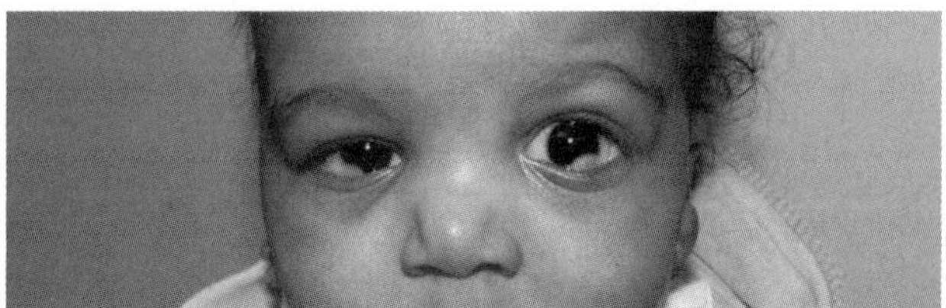

Figure 1-24.

affected side varies from normal to severely deficient. The skin, subcutaneous tissue, and facial muscles of expression may all be affected. Goldenhar's variant is hemifacial microsomia with epibulbar ocular dermoids and vertebral anomalies (Fig. 1-24). Approximately 5% of hemifacial microsomia cases are identified as a Goldenhar's variant. The severity of the asymmetry dictates the timing of surgical intervention. In general, if the child does not have any airway compromise, the ear reconstruction is performed at age 7 to 8 years, and the mandible is addressed based on its severity. The more hypoplastic the mandible, the earlier an intervention is needed to prevent progressive growth restriction of surrounding facial structures.[49,50]

Treacher Collins Syndrome

Treacher Collins is also known as Franceschetti syndrome (in the French literature) and as mandibulofacial dysostosis. The following malformations are observed: notching between the lateral and middle thirds of the lower eyelid, with absent eyelashes; colobomas of the upper lids; inferiorly displaced lateral canthus, with a horizontally short palpebral fissure; mild hypoplasia to severe agenesis of the zygoma; microtia; condylar hypoplasia; short mandibular rami, with prominent antegonial notching; and a retrusive chin. [51] Operative correction is directed at reconstructing the missing or deficient elements of the facial skeleton and soft tissue; it must be done in multiple stages until growth is complete.[52]

Parry-Romberg Syndrome

Parry-Romberg syndrome, or progressive hemifacial atrophy, is characterized by a progressive loss of skin, soft tissue, and sometimes bone in half of the face. This loss usually commences during the first 2 decades of life (average age, 8.8 years) and culminates within 2 to 15 years. The cause of this syndrome is unknown, because most cases are sporadic. In 35% to 40% of patients, ocular changes secondary to atrophy of periorbital fat result in enophthalmos. The atrophy begins with the soft tissue of the midface but, in severe cases, can involve the bone of the orbit, maxilla, and mandible. Approximately 85% of patients with bony involvement have onset before 9 years of age. The deformity is usually self-limiting and stabilizes within 2 to 15 years (average, 9 years) from time of onset. Treatment is delayed until the atrophy has stabilized. Depending on the degree of severity, various reconstructive procedures, including fat grafting, microvascular tissue transfer, and alloplastic implants, are used.[53]

Möbius' Syndrome

Möbius' syndrome is characterized by a congenital paralysis of cranial nerve VII and is usually bilateral, with or without other cranial nerve palsies and limb anomalies. Most cases are sporadic and of unknown cause. This syndrome is usually diagnosed at birth, because the infant sleeps with open eyelids and is void of facial expressions. Atrophy and limited mobility of the tongue may be present secondary to poor hypoglossal innervation. Limb deformities vary in presentation but often involve absence of muscles, such as the deltoid or pectoralis, or of bones, such as the radius or phalanges. Treatment involves facial reanimation.[54]

Hypertelorism

Hypertelorism is a finding characterized by lateralization of the orbital position (Fig. 1-25).[55] This anatomic condition may be associated with an array of congenital anomalies, including frontonasal dysplasia, midline encephaloceles, orbitofacial clefts, and craniosynostosis disorders such as

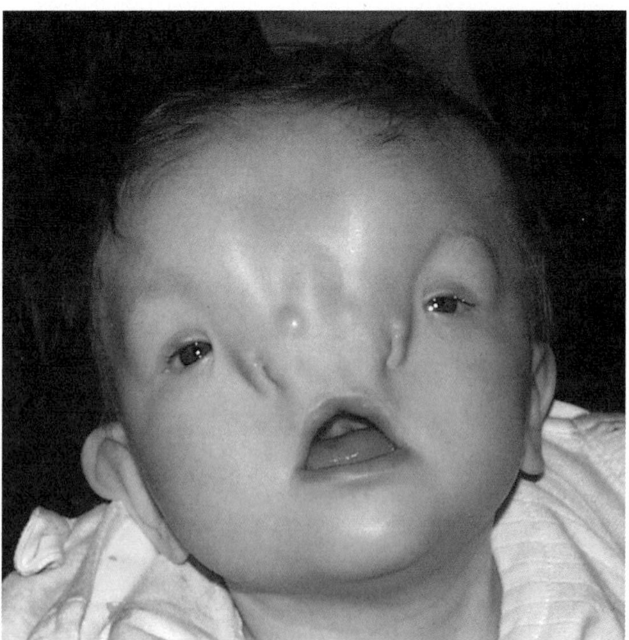

Figure 1-25.

Apert's, Crouzon's, and Pfeiffer syndromes. In severe cases, binocular vision may fail to develop. Hypertelorism is typically not corrected until age 6 or 7 years, at which time the permanent dentition erupts, so that osteotomies around the orbits can allow movement.[56]

TUMORS AND ABNORMAL GROWTHS

Teratomas

Teratomas are rare congenital tumors that present in the midline of the neck. Radiographs may demonstrate calcification or tooth remnants and evidence of rapid growth (Fig. 1-26). Malignant teratomas, although rare, have been reported in the neck, pharynx, nasopharynx, orbit, and paranasal sinuses. Most of these lesions are present at birth and may cause respiratory distress. Treatment is surgical excision. Multidrug chemotherapy may also be used for malignant lesions.[57]

Neurofibromatosis

Neurofibromatosis (NF) can have heterogeneous causes and includes types 1 through 9, although two types, neurofibromatosis type 1 (NF1) and neurofibromatosis type 2 (NF2), are the most frequently encountered in the head and neck region. NF1, or the von Recklinghausen type, is the most frequently occurring form and includes six or more café au lait spots, cutaneous neurofibromas, and Lisch nodules. Cutaneous lesions appear around the onset of puberty and increase in number throughout life. The plexiform neurofibroma involving the orbit, eyelid, and temporal region may extend intracranially and result in buphthalmos, pulsatile exophthalmos, and skeletal deformity. NF2, or the acoustic type, involves bilateral acoustic neuromas that cause pressure on the vestibulocochlear and facial nerve complexes. Café au lait spots and cutaneous neurofibromas are also present, but less frequently than in NF1.[58]

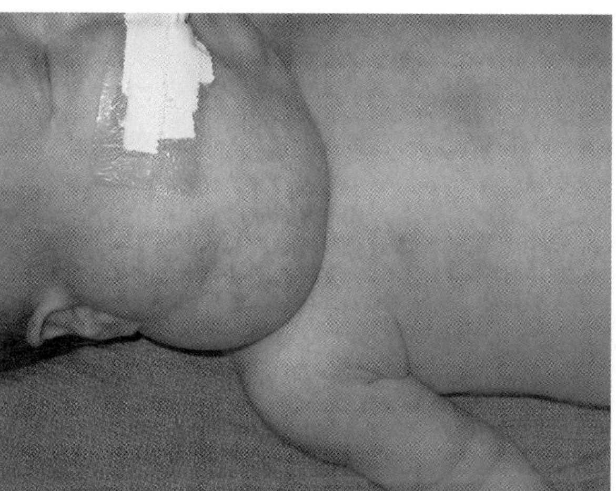

A

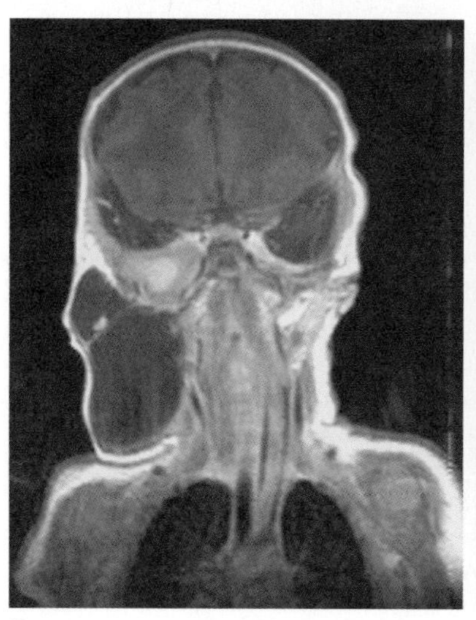

B

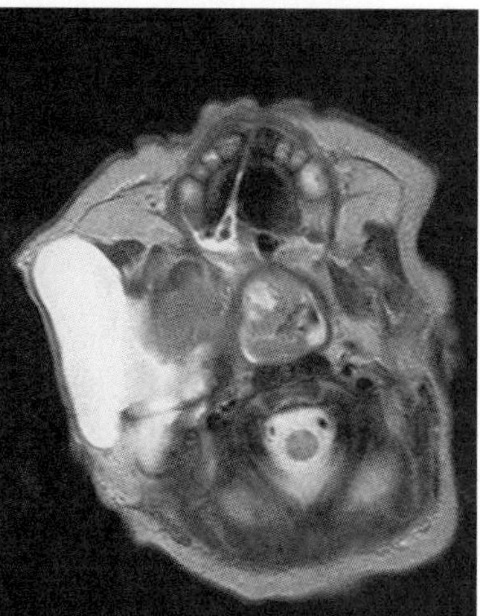

C

Figure 1-26 **A,** Teratoma. **B, C,** Magnetic resonance imaging scans of teratoma.

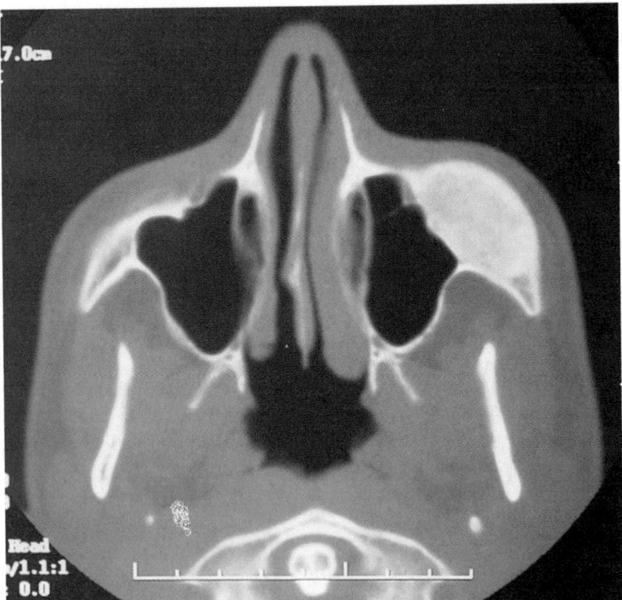

Figure 1-27.

Approximately 3 to 5 in 1000 children are born with some form of hearing loss. Early identification of hearing loss is crucial so that interventions may be initiated early to optimize language acquisition and development.

Congenital cholesteatomas should be suspected with any white mass medial to the tympanic membrane; otolaryngologic consultation should be obtained for evaluation of any lesion of concern, because early intervention is optimal.

Nasal dermoids may present as a pit along the nasal dorsum. Intranasal masses or lesions in infants and children should be evaluated as possible encephaloceles or gliomas.

Bilateral choanal atresia usually presents in a newborn with respiratory distress, which may be remedied with crying or an oral airway. Unilateral choanal atresia may not be diagnosed at birth, but should be suspected in children with chronic unilateral rhinorrhea without evidence of an intranasal foreign body.

Fibrous Dysplasia

Fibrous dysplasia may be monostotic or polyostotic and affects the membranous facial bones of younger patients. It usually becomes quiescent with maturity. Patients present with an increasing firm mass, usually of the maxilla or mandible, but also potentially involving the frontal and orbital bones and extending to the orbital apex.[59] The radiographic appearance is characteristic (Fig. 1-27). Treatment is usually palliative, because it is difficult to resect all involved tissue completely. For lesions involving the orbital bones, there must be close ophthalmologic follow-up for early detection of optic nerve compression.

MAJOR POINTS

Vascular anomalies are categorized as hemangiomas or vascular malformations.

Hemangiomas are tumors that have a proliferative phase and an involution phase. Hemangiomas will usually involute in 5 to 8 years.

Hemangiomas typically can be treated with conservative management unless there are functional issues, such as obstruction of the eyes, or ulceration or bleeding.

Vascular malformations are low-flow or high-flow lesions. Capillary, venous, and lymphatic malformations are low-flow lesions. Arteriovenous malformations are high-flow lesions.

REFERENCES

1. Mulliken JB, Glowacki J: Hemangiomas and vascular malformations in infants and children: A classification based on endothelial characteristics. Plast Reconstr Surg 1982;69: 412-422.
2. Kohout MP, Hansen M, Pribaz JJ, Mulliken JB: Arteriovenous malformations of the head and neck: Natural history and management. Plast Reconst Surg. 1998; 102:643-654.
3. Burrows PE, Mulliken JB, Fellows KE, Strand RD: Childhood hemangiomas and vascular malformations: Angiographic differentiation. AJR Am J Roentgenol 1983;141:483-488.
4. Achauer BM, Chang CJ, Vander Kam VM: Management of hemangioma of infancy: Review of 245 patients. Plast Reconstr Surg 1997;99:1301-1308.
5. McGill TJ: Vascular anomalies of the head and neck. In Wetmore RF, Muntz HR, McGill TJ (eds): Pediatric Otolaryngology: Principles and Practice Pathways. New York, Thieme, 2000, pp 87-102.
6. Grundfast KM, Lalwani AK: Practical approach to diagnosis and management of hereditary hearing impairment. Ear Nose Throat J 1992;71:497-493.
7. Steele KP: Progress in progressive hearing loss. Science 1998;279:1870-1871.
8. Morton CC, Nance WE: Newborn hearing screening—a silent revolution. N Engl J Med 2006;354:2151-2164.
9. Cohen MM, Gorlin RJ: Epidemiology, etiology, and genetic patterns. In Gorlin RJ, Torriello HV, Cohen MM (eds): Hereditary Hearing Loss and Its Syndromes. New York, Oxford University Press, 1995, pp 9-21.

10. Satoh R, Hirose T, Matsuo K, et al: Morphology of the auricles. Jpn J Plast Reconstr Surg 1986;29:560-567.

11. Adamson JE, Horton CE, Crawford HH: Growth patterns of the external ear. Plast Reconstr Surg 1965;36:466-470.

12. Matsuo K, Hayashi R, Kiyono M, et al: Nonsurgical correction of congenital auricular deformities. Clin Plast Surg 1990;17:383-395.

13. McGill TJ, Merchant S, Healy GB, Friedman EM: Congenital cholesteatoma of the middle ear in children: A clinical and histopathological report. Laryngoscope 1991;101:606-613.

14. Millay DJ, Larrabee WF, Dion FR: Nonsurgical correction of auricular deformities. Laryngoscope 1990;100:910-913.

15. Melnick M: The etiology of external ear malformations and its relation to abnormalities of the middle ear, inner ear, and other organ systems. Birth Defects: Orig Article Series 1980;16:303-331.

16. Evans AK, Kazahaya K: Canal atresia: Surgery or implantable hearing devices? The expert's question is revisited. Int J Pediatr Otol (in press).

17. Levenson MJ, Parisier SC, Chute P, et al: A review of twenty congenital cholesteatomas of the middle ear in children. Otolaryngol Head Neck Surg 1986;15:169-174.

18. Michaels L: An epidermoid formation in the developing middle ear: Possible source of cholesteatomas. J Otolaryngol 1986;15:169-174.

19. Potsic WP, Korman SB, Samadi DS, Wetmore RF: Congenital cholesteatoma: 20 years' experience at the Children's Hospital of Philadelphia. Otolaryngol Head Neck Surg 2002;126:409-414.

20. Sade J, Baiacki A, Pinkus G: The metaplastic and congenital origin of cholesteatoma. Acta Otolaryngol 1983;96:119-129.

21. Aimi K: Role for the tympanic ring in the pathogenesis of congenital cholesteatoma. Laryngoscope 1983;93: 1140-1146.

22. Jackler RK, De La Cruz A: The large vestibular aqueduct syndrome. Laryngoscope 1989;99:1238-1241.

23. Pappas DG, Simpson LC, McKenzie RA, Royal S: High-resolution computed tomography: Determination of the cause of pediatric sensorineural hearing loss. Laryngoscope 1990;100:564-569.

24. Falko NA, Erickson E: Facial nerve palsy in the newborn: Incidence and outcome. Plast Reconstr Surg 1990; 85:1-4.

25. Smith JD, Crumley R, Harker L: Facial nerve paralysis in the newborn. Otolaryngol Head Neck Surg 1981;89:1021-1024.

26. Harris JP, Davidson TM, May M, Fria T: Evaluation and treatment of congenital facial paralysis. Arch Otolaryngol 1983;109:145-151.

27. Bergstrom L, Baker BB: Syndromes associated with congenital facial paralysis. Otolaryngol Head Neck Surg 1981;89:336-342.

28. Pape KE, Pickering D: Asymmetric crying facies: An index of other congenital anomalies. J Pediatr 1972;81:21-30.

29. Moore KL, Persaud TVN: The Developing Human, 5th ed. Philadelphia, WB Saunders, 1993.

30. Lemke BN: Anatomy of the ocular adnexa and orbit. In Smith BC, Della Rocca RC, Nesi FA, Lisman RD (eds): Ophthalmic Plastic and Reconstructive Surgery. St. Louis, CV Mosby, 1987, pp 3-74.

31. Foster JA, Katowitz JA: Developmental eyelid abnormalities. In Katowitz JA (ed): Pediatric Oculoplastic Surgery. New York, Springer Verlag, 2002, pp 177-215.

32. Heher KL. Katowitz JA:. Pediatric ptosis. In Katowitz JA (ed): Pediatric Oculoplastic Surgery. New York, Springer Verlag, 2002, pp 253-288.

33. Pratt LW: Midline cysts of the nasal dorsum: Embryologic origin and treatment. Laryngoscope 1965;75:968-980.

34. Smith JD, Bumsted RM (eds): Pediatric Facial Plastic and Reconstructive Surgery. New York, Raven Press, 1993.

35. Harris J, Robert E, Kallen B: Epidemiology of choanal atresia with special reference to CHARGE association. Pediatrics 1997;99:363-367.

36. Hughes GB, Sharpino G, Hunt W, Tucker H: Management of the congenital midline nasal mass: A review. Head Neck Surg 1980;2:222-233.

37. Younas M, Coode PE: Nasal glioma and encephalocele: Two separate entities. J Neurosurg 1986;64:516-519.

38. Stankiewicz JA: The endoscopic repair of choanal atresia. Otolaryngol Head Neck Surg 1990;103:931-937.

39. Brown OE, Myer CM, Manning SC: Congenital nasal pyriform aperture stenosis. Laryngoscope 1989;99:86-91.

40. Arlis H, Ward RF: Congenital nasal pyriform aperture stenosis: Isolated anomaly vs. developmental field defect. Arch Otolaryngol Head Neck Surg 1992;118:989-991.

41. Singh DJ, Bartlett SP: Congenital mandibular hypoplasia: Analysis and classification. J Craniofac Surg 2005;16:291-300.

42. LaRossa D: Unilateral cleft lip repair. In Bentz ML (ed): Pediatric Plastic Surgery. Stamford, Conn, Appleton & Lange, 1998, pp 47-62.

43. Furlow LT: Cleft palate repair by double opposing Z-plasty. Plast Reconstr Surg 1986;78:724-738.

44. Kirschner RE, Low DW, Randall P, et al: Surgical airway management in Pierre Robin sequence: Is there a role for tongue-lip adhesion? Cleft Palate Craniofac J 2003;40:13-18.

45. Tessier P: Anatomical classification of facial, craniofacial and latero-facial clefts. J Maxillofac Surg 1976;4:69-92.

46. Posnick JC, Goldstein JA: Surgical management of temporomandibular joint ankylosis in the pediatric population. Plast Reconstr Surg 1973;91:791-798.

47. Gorlin RJ, Cohen MM, Levin LS: Syndromes of the Head and Neck. New York, Oxford University Press, 1990.

48. Fink SC, Hardesty RA: Craniofacial syndromes. In Bentz ML (ed): Pediatric Plastic Surgery. Stamford, Conn, Appleton & Lange, 1998, pp 1-18.

49. Gorlin RJ, Jue KL, Jacobsen U, et al: Oculoauriculovertebral dysplasia. J Pediatr 1963;63:991-999.

50. Cousley RR, Calvert ML: Current concepts in the understanding and management of hemifacial microsomia. Br J Plast Surg 1997;50:536-551.

51. Franceschetti A, Klein D: The mandibulofacial dysostosis: A new hereditary syndrome. Acta Ophthalmol 1949;27: 143-224.

52. Treacher Collins E: Cases with symmetrical congenital notches in the outer part of each lid and defective development of the malar bones. Trans Ophthalmol Soc UK 1960;20:190-192.

53. Fink SC, Hardesty RA: Craniofacial syndromes. In Bentz ML (ed): Pediatric Plastic Surgery. Stamford, Conn, Appleton & Lange, 1998, pp 18-22.

54. Abramson DL, Cohen MM Jr, Mulliken JB: Mobius syndrome: Classification and grading system. Plast Reconstr Surg 1998;102:961-967.

55. Grieg DM: Hypertelorism: A hitherto undifferentiated congenital craniofacial deformity. Edinburgh Med J 1924;31: 560-593.

56. Tessier P: Orbital hypertelorism: I. Successive surgical attempts, material and methods. Causes and mechanisms. Scand J Plast Reconstr Surg 1972;6:135-155.

57. Grosfeld JL, Billmire DF: Teratomas in infancy and childhood. Curr Probl Cancer 1985;9:1-53.

58. Posnick JC: Other frequently seen craniofacial syndromes. In Posnick JC (ed): Craniofacial and Maxillofacial Surgery in Children and Young Adults. Philadelphia, WB Saunders, 2000.

59. Hunt JA, Hobar PC: Common craniofacial anomalies: Conditions of craniofacial atrophy/hypoplasia and neoplasia. Plast Reconstr Surg 2003;111:1497-1508.

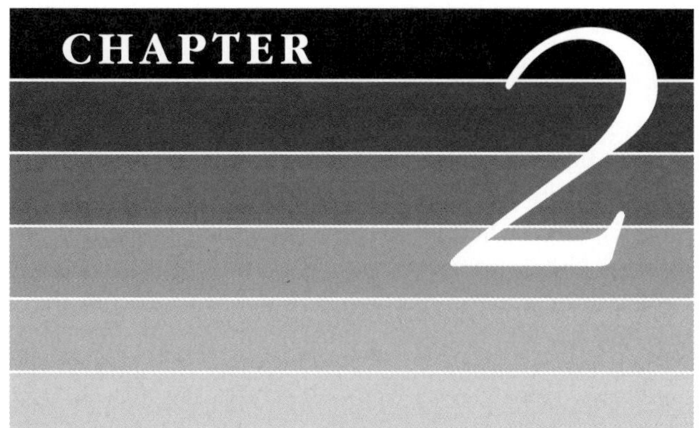

Diseases of the External Ear

JEFFREY L. KELLER, MD

INTRODUCTION

The auricle and external auditory canal serve important functions, both in sound transmission and in protection of the middle and inner ear structures.

Adnexal structures such as the cerumen- and sebum-producing glands line the outer portion of the external canal. These structures create an important protective barrier that helps prevent infection and trauma but can also be the source of various pathologic processes. Obstruction of the ear canal from excess cerumen, local trauma, or cyst formation not only decreases sound transmission but also leads to inflammation and exquisite discomfort. Early recognition of the common disease processes of the external ear will improve the effectiveness of treatment and decrease the morbidity and pain often associated with them.

NORMAL ANATOMY AND FUNCTION

The external ear consists of the auricle or pinna, external auditory canal, and tympanic membrane. The pinna is composed of elastic cartilage covered by skin. It is subdivided into the helix, antihelix, tragus anteriorly, and lobule inferiorly.

The external auditory canal is an S-shaped structure lined by stratified squamous epithelium, with the lateral third consisting of fibrocartilage and the medial two thirds consisting of bone. The external canal skin is unique in that its cells are continually migrating laterally, moving cerumen and debris, making it a self-cleansing system. Pulling the auricle upward and back straightens the cartilaginous external canal and facilitates visualization of the tympanic membrane. The skin that covers the lateral third or cartilaginous portion of the external canal contains adnexal structures, including hair follicles and ceruminous and sebaceous glands. However, the skin covering the bony external canal is devoid of adnexal structures and is tightly adherent to the underlying periosteum. Therefore, cerumen is produced in the outer portion of the ear canal. The thin, tightly adherent skin of the medial two thirds of the ear canal makes it especially vulnerable to trauma during attempts to clean the ear canal.

The auricle is innervated by contributions from the fifth, seventh, ninth, and tenth cranial nerves, making the ear exquisitely sensitive to inflammation and trauma.

COMMON CONDITIONS

Cerumen Impaction

Cerumen is a mixture of desquamated skin and secretions produced by sebaceous and ceruminous glands located in the lateral external canal. Cerumen is hydrophobic and antibacterial, forming a protective layer that helps prevent infection and trauma.[1] Racial differences exist in the lipid, lysozyme, and immunoglobulin composition of cerumen, with whites having a "wet" cerumen (higher lipid content) and Asians having a "dry" cerumen (higher protein content). The use of cotton-tipped swabs to clean the external canal should be discouraged, because this practice often pushes cerumen medially with resultant impaction and irritation, thereby interfering with the self-cleansing property of the canal. The impacted cerumen can trap moisture, cause temporary hearing loss, and predispose to otitis externa.

Although various commercially available preparations are available for cerumen removal, their improved efficacy over peroxide or water irrigation of the external canal has not been established. Caution is advised in using irrigation to remove cerumen if a tympanic membrane perforation is suspected. Cerumen can generally be removed in the office by an experienced practitioner using a cerumen loop or a Frazier suction tip and headlight. Occasionally, general anesthesia may be required to remove severely impacted cerumen or foreign bodies, especially when adjacent to the tympanic membrane.

Foreign Bodies

Foreign bodies in the lateral external ear canal (Fig. 2-1) can often be removed easily with a cerumen loop, alligator forceps, or right-angle hook. Objects in the medial external ear canal can present a challenge, even with appropriate instrumentation and experience. A Frazier suction tip may be helpful in this setting. Irrigation with water or placement of drops may sometimes facilitate foreign body removal. One exception is organic foreign bodies, such as seeds or vegetable matter, which frequently swell when exposed to moisture. Miniature batteries in the ear canal need to be removed expeditiously because the erosive chemicals that can leak from them may cause inflammation and ulceration of the canal and/or tympanic membrane. Live insects found in the canal should first be immobilized by instilling oil or alcohol prior to their removal. When foreign bodies are severely impacted or are adjacent to the tympanic membrane, a short-acting general anesthetic may be used to avoid unnecessary pain and additional trauma.

Trauma

The prominent and exposed location of the auricle makes it vulnerable to trauma, including lacerations and blunt trauma. Lacerations can usually be managed using local anesthesia, with careful approximation of the perichondrium and skin using standard surgical techniques. The lateral auricle is especially vulnerable to hematoma formation. Blood or serous fluid can accumulate between the cartilage and perichondrium, thereby depriving the cartilage of some of its blood supply (Fig. 2-2). If this occurs on both the medial and lateral

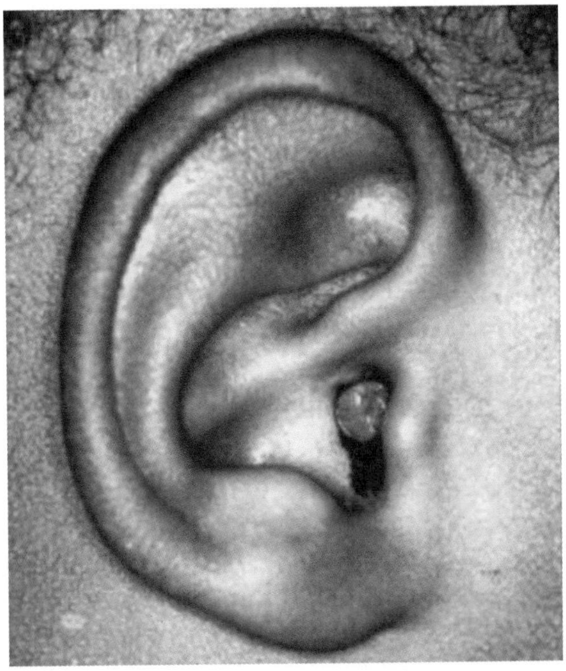

Figure 2-1. A foreign body in the lateral external canal is visible to inspection.

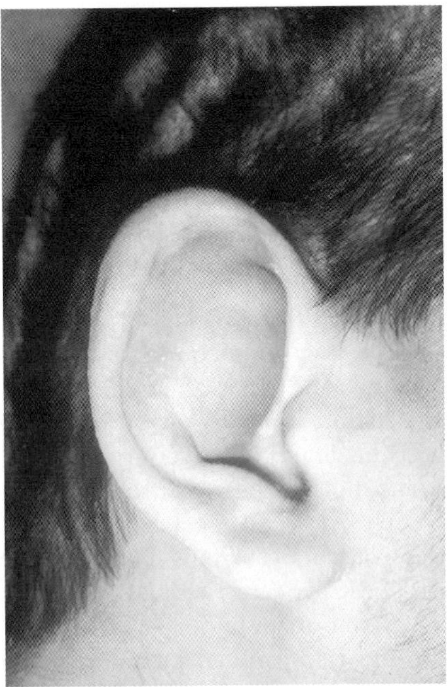

Figure 2-2. Auricular hematoma. Trauma to the pinna may result in a collection of blood between the auricular cartilage and overlying perichondrium. Infection of this fluid may destroy the underlying cartilage, resulting in a permanent deformity.

surfaces, cartilage necrosis can occur, resulting in a "cauliflower ear."[2] This complication can be avoided by removing the fluid within the first 24 to 48 hours. In children, incision and drainage of an auricular hematoma usually require general anesthesia. Cotton bolsters are placed on the medial and lateral surfaces and sutured into position for 3 to 4 days to prevent reaccumulation of blood.

Otitis Externa

The external auditory canal is normally a warm, humid environment with variable amounts of exfoliated skin and cerumen. Increased moisture in the external ear canal, especially during the warm summer months, produces an ideal environment for bacterial growth. Pathogens often gain entry into the skin through minor abrasions or irritation. Although approximately 80% of cases of otitis externa are bacterial, fungal and viral agents, along with dermatologic conditions, may also play a role. The most common bacterial pathogens are *Pseudomonas aeruginosa* and *Staphylococcus aureus.* Fungal infections cause less than 3% of otitis externa cases, with *Candida albicans* and *Aspergillus fumigatus* representing the major pathogens.[3] The most important viral cause is herpes zoster, which results in herpes zoster oticus, or Ramsay Hunt syndrome. Facial paralysis, hearing loss, and vertigo, along with vesicular eruptions of the external canal, are characteristic of this herpes zoster infection.

Diagnosis

The clinical presentation of otitis externa is distinct and allows for prompt diagnosis and treatment. The hallmark symptoms and signs include pain, especially with manipulation of the auricle, decreased hearing, and ear discharge. Physical examination reveals swelling and erythema of the external canal, variable amounts of debris within the canal, and periauricular lymphadenopathy (Fig. 2-3). Removal of external canal debris allows for visualization of the tympanic membrane to determine whether a perforation or acute otitis media is also present. A white mucoid discharge is typical in bacterial infections, although fungal infections may present with white or black debris, with overlying hyphae. Cultures of the external canal can confirm the pathogen, but this is usually reserved for patients who do not respond to initial treatment.

Treatment

Removal of debris from the external canal is an important initial step in the treatment of all forms of otitis externa. This is best accomplished with gentle suctioning of the ear canal. An alternative technique is dry mopping the ear canal, in which a rolled-up tissue is gently placed into the external canal to absorb as much debris and moisture as possible. The use of cotton-tipped swabs should be avoided, because this frequently causes additional irritation, swelling, and pain.

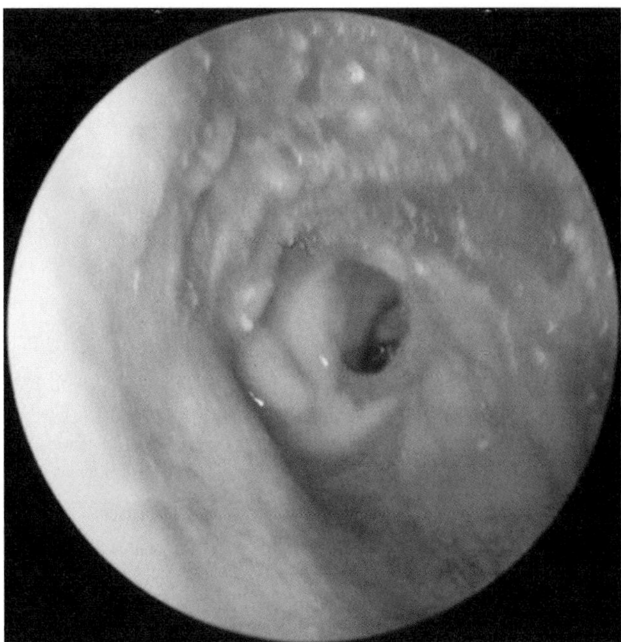

Figure 2-3. In this view of the ear canal of a child with severe external otitis, the external canal is swollen, and pus and crusts nearly fill the remaining lumen. In patients in whom the canal is completely occluded, a wick of sponge or gauze may be necessary to allow ototopical drops to reach the infected region.

Topical antibiotic eardrops are the mainstay of treatment for bacterial otitis externa. If the ear canal is swollen, thereby preventing the entry of eardrops, a wick (expandable sponge) should be placed into the external auditory canal to facilitate instillation. There is no evidence that systemic antibiotics alone or combined with topical preparations improve treatment outcome compared with topical antibiotics alone. If otitis externa is present in the setting of a tympanic membrane perforation or a patent tympanostomy tube, caution should be used in regard to using potentially ototoxic medications such as neomycin, gentamicin, or tobramycin.[4] Quinolone drops offer superior safety and efficacy in this setting and have not been shown to cause sensorineural hearing loss.[5] Another study has suggested that the addition of steroids to ototopical medications further improves the effectiveness of these preparations (Table 2-1).[6] Because topical medications are delivered directly to the infected site, a high antibiotic concentration is achieved locally, eradicating bacterial overgrowth and reducing the risk of antibiotic resistance. In addition, the localized target site of the medication lessens the risk of systemic side effects more commonly found with oral antibiotics.[7] Children with infection unresponsive to ototopical preparations alone may have developed an antibiotic-resistant bacterial infection or a

Table 2-1 Ototopical Preparations

Drug Class	Examples
Antiseptic (acidifying agent)	Acetic acid, boric acid, salicylic acid, *m*-cresyl acetate/ chlorobutanol/alcohol (Cresylate), hydrogen peroxide
Antibiotic	Colistin, polymyxin B, neomycin, gentamicin, tobramycin, ofloxacin (Floxin Otic), ciprofloxacin/ dexamethasone (Ciprodex)
Corticosteroid	Hydrocortisone (VõSol HC Otic)
Antifungal	*m*-Cresyl acetate/chlorobutanol/ alcohol, Sulzberger's Powder, clotrimazole, amphotericin B, oxytetracycline-polymyxin

Modified from Wetmore RF, Muntz HR, McGill TJ (eds): Pediatric Otolaryngology: Principles and Practice Pathways. New York, Thieme, 2000, p 256.

secondary fungal infection. If fungal spores are visualized, a topical antifungal medication should be used instead, or bacterial and fungal culture and sensitivity testing should be carried out to clarify the cause. In severe cases of otitis externa or when there is an associated periauricular cellulitis, systemic antibiotics may be necessary.

Dry ear precautions should be encouraged until the inflammation and pain have resolved. Otitis externa is frequently painful and appropriate analgesics should be used until the swelling and discomfort have resolved.

Dermatitis

Various dermatologic conditions can affect the external ear, including atopic, contact, and seborrheic dermatitis. Symptoms often include itching and pain and physical examination reveals erythema, edema, and flaking and fissuring of the skin, especially of the lateral external canal. Metal sensitivity from nickel is a common cause of chronic dermatitis affecting the ear in patients who wear earrings. Stainless steel or other metal alloys that are gold- or silver-plated can release nickel, causing chronic dermatitis. Shampoos or other hair preparations may also contribute to the problem. Treatment includes elimination of the offending agent, local cleansing, and application of topical steroids and drying agents.

Furunculosis

A furuncle is an inflammatory skin lesion that results from obstruction of an apocrine or sebaceous gland. Symptoms include pain, itching, and occasionally decreased hearing (if the lesion is obstructing the canal). Physical examination reveals localized swelling, erythema of the overlying skin, and tenderness on palpation of the ear. Topical and oral antibiotics, along with warm compresses, are frequently curative. In patients in whom large abscesses are found or if initial treatment fails, incision and drainage of the abscess or excision of the cyst may be required.

Malignant External Otitis

Malignant external otitis represents a progressive, debilitating, and sometimes fatal osteomyelitis of the external auditory canal, surrounding tissues, and skull base. Fortunately, this is an uncommon infection in children but can occur in immunosuppressed or diabetic patients. *Pseudomonas* species are the causative organisms, and the exotoxins and neurotoxins they elaborate are responsible for the invasive nature of this infection. The infection most commonly begins at the bony-cartilaginous junction of the external canal and can spread through Santorini's fissures into the periauricular tissues, including the parotid gland, temporomandibular space, and skull base. Facial paralysis or other cranial nerve involvement is an ominous sign and is associated with a high mortality rate.

Diagnosis

Progressive otitis externa that is unresponsive to topical antibiotics in an immunosuppressed or diabetic child should raise the suspicion of malignant external otitis. Physical examination reveals an intact tympanic membrane, with granulation tissue at the junction of the cartilaginous and bony portions of the external auditory canal. Cultures are most frequently positive for *Pseudomonas aeruginosa.*

Gallium and technetium bone scans are the most sensitive methods for determining both the presence of malignant external otitis and extent of disease. Although technetium scans tend to remain positive after the osteomyelitis clears, a gallium scan is useful for following progression and resolution of the infection. Conventional radiography and computed tomography (CT) are not particularly useful in confirming the diagnosis or in following the progression and resolution of malignant otitis externa. Magnetic resonance imaging (MRI) may be a useful adjunct to the bone scan to determine the extent of soft tissue involvement at the skull base.

Treatment

Intravenous and topical anti-*Pseudomonas* antibiotics, along with local débridement of necrotic debris and granulation tissue, are the mainstays of treatment. Hyberbaric oxygen can also be used as an adjunctive treatment for patients who do not respond to antibiotics or débridement. The duration of treatment is based on clinical improvement and sequential gallium scans.

Perichondritis

Perichondritis is an infection of the tissues surrounding the auricular cartilage and is often caused by local trauma or irritation. Blood or serous fluid may collect between the conchal cartilage and skin, depriving the cartilage of some of its blood supply and further exacerbating the problem. The fluid trapped in this space can become infected, often with *Pseudomonas* or gram-positive bacteria. Treatment requires incision and drainage if significant fluid is present. Mild infections may respond to oral antibiotics with anti-*Pseudomonas* and gram-positive coverage (e.g., ciprofloxacin) but in unresponsive or severe cases, IV antibiotics may be required If necrotic cartilage is present because of prolonged infection or inadequate blood supply from hematoma or seroma, cartilage débridement may be required as well.

Keratosis Obturans

Accumulation of squamous epithelium and ceruminous debris in the bony external canal can result in local inflammation and destruction. This rare entity, known as keratosis obturans, is probably a result of faulty migration of desquamated skin cells from the tympanic membrane and medial portion of the external ear canal. Ear pain, minimal otorrhea, and conductive hearing loss are the typical presenting manifestations. Physical examination reveals a pearly white mass located in the medial external canal, similar in appearance to a cholesteatoma in the middle ear (Fig. 2-4). Treatment requires periodic removal of accumulated squamous debris. If the lesion is extensive, débridement may require general anesthesia. Although the association of keratosis obturans with bronchiectasis and sinusitis has been well documented, the cause of this association is uncertain.[8]

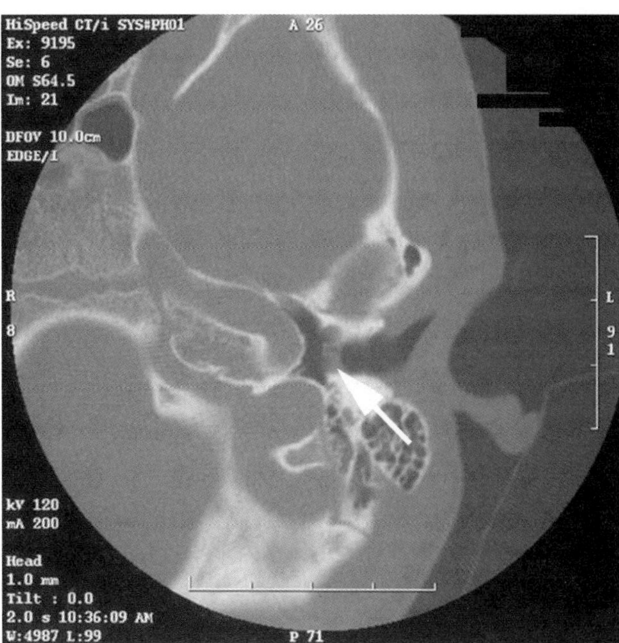

Figure 2-4. Computed tomography scan of the temporal bone illustrates an accumulation of squamous debris in the medial canal, keratosis obturans.

Relapsing Polychondritis

Relapsing polychondritis is an episodic inflammatory disease that affects adults more frequently than children. It most commonly presents with inflammation of the cartilage of the ears, nasal septum, or larynx, but may also affect the trachea, resulting in upper airway obstruction. Progressive necrosis and destruction of cartilage may result in a saddle nose deformity, cauliflower ear, or airway collapse, depending on the site(s) involved. Rheumatoid arthritis, lymphoma, and infectious perichondritis are part of the differential diagnosis. Diagnosis can often be confirmed by biopsy of the affected area. The cause is probably autoimmune. Treatment consists of nonsteroidal antiinflammatory drugs and systemic corticosteroids to control the acute attack and to suppress recurrences. Resistant cases my require dapsone, cyclophosphamide, or azathioprine.

SUMMARY

The anatomy of the external canal maximizes its function for sound transmission and protection of the middle and inner ear structures. These same qualities make it vulnerable to infection and trauma, problems that are common in clinical practice. In addition, less common systemic diseases can present with symptoms that may initially be localized to the auricle and temporal bone.

MAJOR POINTS

The location of the auricle makes it vulnerable to blunt trauma, which can result in hematoma formation, cartilage necrosis, and the development of a cauliflower ear. Early recognition and drainage of the hematoma can avoid these complications.

Epithelium lining the external auditory canal is unique in that its cells are continually migrating laterally, moving cerumen and debris along with it. Obstruction of the canal from excess cerumen, trauma, or a foreign body can block this self-cleansing system, trap moisture, and lead to otitis externa.

Meticulous and repeated cleansing of the ear canal is the cornerstone of effective treatment for otitis externa. Topical antibiotics in conjunction with ear cleansing are curative in most cases; systemic antibiotics are reserved for patients with periauricular cellulitis or suspected malignant otitis externa.

Repeated infection and inflammation of the auricle may represent systemic disease, such as relapsing polychondritis, and should be considered in the differential diagnosis.

Early recognition and treatment of these entities can minimize morbidity and discomfort.

REFERENCES

1. Kelly KE, Mohs DC: The external auditory canal. Otolaryngol Clin North Am 1996;29:725-739.
2. Ohlsen L, Skoog TL, Sohn SA: The pathogenesis of cauliflower ear. Scand J Plast Reconstr Surg 1975;9:34-39.
3. Roland PS, Stroman DW: Microbiology of acute otitis externa. Laryngoscope 2002;112:1166-1177.
4. Welling DB, Forrest LA, Goll F: Safety of ototopical antibiotics. Laryngoscope 1995;105:472-474.
5. Hannley MT, Denneny JC 3rd, Holzer SS: Use of ototopical antibiotics in treating 3 common ear diseases. Otolaryngol Head Neck Surg 2000;122:934-940.
6. Aslan A, Altuntas A, Titiz A, et al: A new dosage regimen for topical application of ciprofloxacin in the management of chronic suppurative otitis media. Otolaryngol Head Neck Surg 1998;118:883-885.
7. Langford JH, Benrimoj SI: Clinical rationale for topical antimicrobial preparations. J Antimicrob Chemother 1996;37:399-402.
8. Morrison AW: Keratosis obturans. J Laryngol Otol 1956;70:317-321.

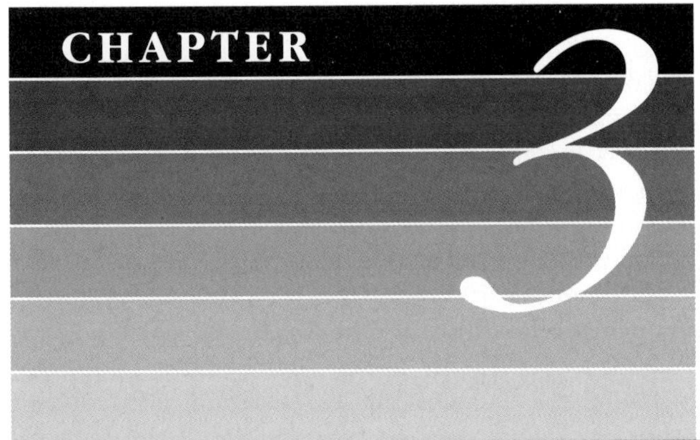

Pediatric Communication Disorders

JUDITH S. GRAVEL, PhD
JENNIFER R. BURSTEIN, MA
JOSEPH G. DONAHER, MA
KEVIN H. FRANCK, PhD, MBA
CAROL KNIGHTLY, AuD
CYNTHIA SOLOT, MA
AMY WHITE, AuD

Arguably, communication is the most significant aspect of child development, because the development of language allows the child to interact meaningfully with others in his or her environment. In the first few months of life, an infant can discriminate between speech sounds of any spoken language. However, by age 6 months, infants are able to discriminate vowels of their native language with greater accuracy then those of a non-native language.[1] By 10 months of age, canonical (reduplicated) babbling has been established. This stage of communication development is a precursor to spoken language[2] and is such a critical milestone of communication that lack of canonical babbling is a high-risk indicator for hearing loss or other communication or developmental disorders.[3,4] By 1 year of age, first words emerge, although the infant's receptive vocabulary is considerably larger than the expressive.[5] The acquisition of language is dramatic during the first 3 years of life. Typically, developing toddlers (24 to 25 months) from supportive homes with numerous opportunities for language learning have vocabularies that average 180 words.[6] By the time a child enters the formal education system at age 5 to 6 years of age, she or he is speaking in complete, syntactically complex sentences and speech is readily intelligible to a stranger. Language and reading abilities in childhood and adolescence are related to early lexical development.[7,8]

For children with communication disorders, this typical pattern has been disrupted by a sensory, cognitive, motor, or neurologic disorder that alone or in combination has affected the development of communication to various degrees. The child with a communication disorder has multiple limitations that affect knowledge acquisition, social-emotional development, self-esteem, and future vocational opportunities. This chapter describes various types of childhood communication disorders—specifically, hearing, speech, and language disorders that compromise the child's acquisition or use of the most fundamental of human abilities. We hope that the information contained in this chapter will be useful to pediatric practitioners' understanding of early identification, comprehensive assessment, and timely and appropriate intervention for children with various forms of communication disorders.

The chapter is organized according to three major areas of communication: hearing, language, and speech. Each section describes communication disorders that are congenital, familial, or acquired. Methods are presented that can be used to screen for communication disorders in settings that include the pediatrician's office, and the comprehensive assessments used by audiologists and speech-language pathologists to delineate a condition are discussed. In addition, recommendations regarding intervention and follow-up at the local and state levels are made in the context of currently available programs and resources available to support families of children with communication disorders.

We present the approach to communication disorders in childhood as practiced at the Center for Childhood Communication (CCC) at The Children's Hospital of Philadelphia. The CCC provides a multidisciplinary team approach to assessment and intervention that includes the professions of audiology, speech-language pathology, social work, education, and behavioral health and family wellness, along with medical and allied health providers in pediatric otolaryngology, pediatrics, genetics, developmental pediatrics, occupational therapy, physical therapy, and psychology.

A multidisciplinary team approach is critical to early identification efforts, comprehensive assessment, and appropriate intervention for children with communication disorders. This chapter is focused on specific aspects of hearing, language, and speech disorders approached in the context of an interdisciplinary team that adheres to a family-centered approach to service delivery. The evaluation of childhood communication disorders requires a developmental approach that offers continued support to the child and family throughout childhood.

Finally, although the skills, methods, and technologies discussed in this chapter are available to all professionals, we believe that those who have particular expertise working with children and their families are in a unique position to deliver the services discussed. That is, addressing communication disorders in childhood is best done by professionals who have the background, requisite training, and experience to work with infants and children and their families most efficiently and effectively.

CHILDHOOD HEARING LOSS

The advent of newborn hearing screening indicates that the incidence of significant (>40-dB hearing level [HL], moderate to profound) bilateral permanent congenital or neonatal onset hearing loss is estimated at approximately 1/1000.[9] More recent studies have suggested a rate of about 2.5/1000 when mild (>20- to <40-dB HL) permanent forms of hearing loss in one or both ears are included.[10] When the incidence of hearing loss in infants cared for in the neonatal intensive care unit is compared with that for infants in well baby units, the rate of hearing loss is nearly 10 times as great.[11] Before universal newborn hearing screening and current physiologic screening technologies (see later), this significant difference between high-risk and regular nurseries was why efforts at early identification were focused only on infants at greatest risk.[12]

Evidence from large ascertainment studies in England,[13] metropolitan Atlanta,[14] and the Third National Health and Nutrition Evaluation Survey (NHANES-III)[15] has suggested that prevalence rates for permanent hearing loss increase with age. Estimating the prevalence of hearing loss in children is highly dependent on the definition of hearing loss used and the methods used to conduct the prevalence estimate (e.g., records review versus direct hearing assessment). When mild and high-frequency hearing loss in one (unilateral) or both (bilateral) ears and evidence of noise-induced hearing loss are included, the incidence of permanent hearing loss in school-age children has been reported at between 5.4/100[16] and 12.5/100.[17]

The effects of hearing loss on the individual, family, and society are generally far-reaching. Children with hearing loss generally have poorer linguistic, reading, and academic achievement scores than their normally hearing peers, which can affect social, emotional, and, ultimately, occupational status.[18] Clearly, children with the most severe and profound hearing loss are at the greatest disadvantage for the development of spoken language. However, some children with mild degrees of permanent bilateral hearing loss, as well as those with unilateral hearing loss, require grade repetition or educational support services.[16,19] An increasing number of studies have suggested that for children with congenital and early-onset hearing loss who are learning spoken language for the first time, no amount of permanent hearing loss can be considered insignificant or inconsequential. This is particularly true for those children with hearing loss and one or more additional disabilities.[20]

Classification

Hearing loss is typically described according to the features presented in Table 3-1. These descriptions are based on the audiologic assessment using technologies and methods that are described in more detail in the following sections. Broadly, the type, degree, and configuration of the hearing loss can be described based on the results of the audiometric evaluation, whereas the stability of the hearing loss is described by examining the audiometric results of two or more assessments over time.

The audiogram is most commonly used to display and store audiometric results. Data may also be stored in tabular form, providing an efficient means of examining the stability of the hearing thresholds. Figure 3-1 presents an audiogram that depicts frequency in hertz (Hz) (perceptually, pitch) on the abscissa (*x* axis) and hearing level in decibels (dB HL) (perceptually, loudness) on the ordinate (*y* axis). The audiogram displays the range of frequencies in human speech (octave and half-octave intervals from 125 to 8000 Hz) as a function of the HL at which a sound (typically a pure tone) is just detectable

Table 3-1 Features Used to Describe Childhood Hearing Loss

Type	Degree	Configuration	Stability	Laterality	Symmetry
Conductive	Minimal	Flat	Stable	Bilateral	Symmetrical
Sensory	Mild	Sloping	Progressive	Unilateral	Asymmetrical
Neural	Moderate	Precipitous	Fluctuant		
Mixed	Severe	Reverse slope, rising	Permanent		
Central	Profound	Trough, U-shaped	Transient		

(0-dB HL) to the point at which a sound is very uncomfortable (120-dB HL). Signals may be detected at −10 or −5-dB HL; thus, 0-dB HL does not mean the absence of sound, but merely designates the threshold of normal hearing, with some listeners actually hearing between 5 to 10 dB better than average.

Figure 3-2 displays an audiogram that represents normal hearing and the ranges that are usually used to describe minimal, mild, moderate, severe, and profound degrees of hearing loss across frequencies for children. The range of normal hearing for infants and children (−10 to 15 dB HL) is more stringent than that typically considered as normal hearing for adults (0- to 20- or 25-dB HL).[21] This is because infants and young children who are learning language need access to all of the sounds in speech, whereas adults who have acquired language and later experience hearing loss can fill in sounds in speech based on their years of normal auditory experiences.

The type of hearing loss is determined using signals that are conducted by air and bone. Air-conducted signals are delivered to each ear through earphones (circumaural or, more commonly, insert-type earphones) or through a loudspeaker (wherein the test signal is detected by the better-hearing ear). Bone-conducted signals are delivered via an oscillator or vibrator that is placed on the mastoid, just behind one pinna. Differences in thresholds for air-conducted versus bone-conducted signals at each frequency are used to determine whether the loss is sensorineural (air- and bone-conducted responses are the same or differ by no more than 10 dB), conductive (bone conduction thresholds are within the normal range and more than 10 dB better than air-conduction thresholds), or mixed (a hearing loss for both air- and bone- conducted signals, with bone-conducted thresholds more than 10 dB better than air-conducted thresholds).

The types of hearing loss (conductive, sensorineural, and mixed) described are those that most commonly occur in children and are represented routinely on the pure-tone audiogram. Conductive hearing loss in children may be temporary (commonly associated with otitis media with effusion) or permanent (e.g., caused by a middle ear malformation). There are many causes of permanent sensorineural hearing loss; these are comprehensively reviewed elsewhere in this text (Chapter 4).

Hearing loss may occur in one ear only (unilateral hearing loss) or in both ears (bilateral hearing loss).

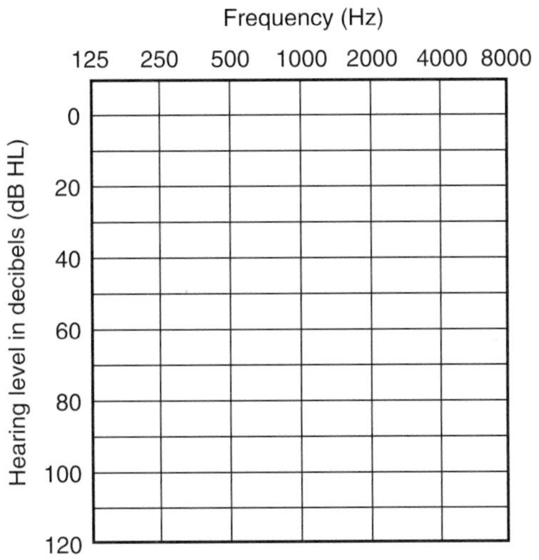

Figure 3-1. Audiogram displaying frequency (Hz) as a function of decibels hearing level (dB HL).

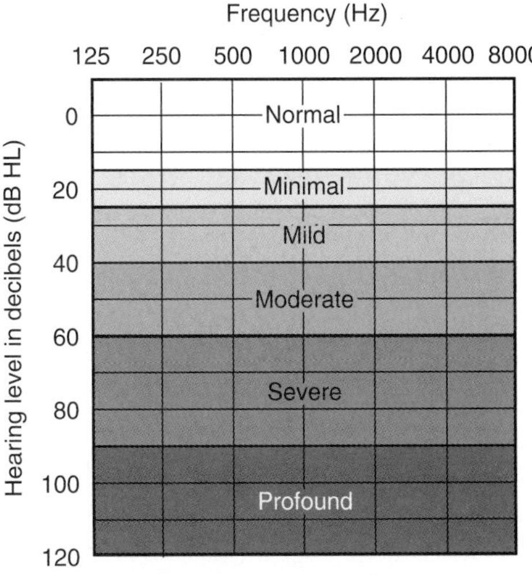

Figure 3-2. Audiogram depicting ranges for normal hearing and minimal, mild, moderate, severe, and profound degrees of hearing loss in children.

In cases of bilateral hearing loss, the impairment can be the same in both ears (symmetrical) or differ between ears (asymmetrical; thresholds between ears differ by 15 dB or more). Figure 3-3 depicts examples of various configurations of hearing loss, including those that are frequently described as flat, sloping, precipitously sloping, rising, notched, corner, and trough-shaped (the latter is also termed *U-shaped* or *cookie bite*) in configuration.

Based on all the audiometric information obtained and the results of the otologic evaluation, hearing loss is typically described according to its symmetry, degree, configuration, and type. Thus, in the report of the audiologic evaluation, a child's hearing loss may be described as (1) bilateral, mild, flat conductive hearing loss; (2) bilateral, moderate, sloping, high-frequency sensorineural hearing loss; (3) bilateral, moderate to severe flat mixed hearing loss; (4) unilateral, severe sensorineural hearing loss; or (5) bilateral, profound, corner sensorineural hearing loss.

Figure 3-4 depicts an audiogram with individual speech sounds displayed on it. This audiogram emphasizes the importance of hearing for the detection of individual speech sounds (phonemes), which are the basis of auditory-based language development. This type of audiogram display is particularly helpful to parents for understanding the implications of any hearing loss that their child may have for the perception of speech.

There are two other forms of hearing loss other than sensory, conductive, or mixed that are receiving increased attention by audiologists and parents. The first is auditory processing disorder (APD), formerly known as central auditory processing disorder (CAPD). APD is applied to children with normal peripheral hearing who have various listening problems that are manifested when the child enters the formal academic environment. These include difficulties listening in noisy environments, inability to maintain attention to auditory-based tasks, and difficulties in speech perception (confusion of similar-sounding words). There are advocates of various approaches to the diagnosis of APD; these involve traditional audiologic testing as well as tests of listening in noise, dichotic speech perception, tonal pattern perception, and others. As yet, psychoacoustic testing of basic auditory abilities, as well as electrophysiologic measures of auditory system integrity, is not regularly used in the audiologic evaluation. The differential diagnosis also involves evaluation by speech-language pathologists, who generally provide information regarding speech and language abilities, and psychologists, who examine children for cognitive and attention-behavioral deficits and performance in academic areas such as reading and mathematics. Regardless of the approach to diagnosis, the interventions recommended for children with APD often include the use of sound field frequency modulation (FM) amplification systems (see later, "Interventions").

The differentiation of neural from sensory hearing loss, referred to as sensorineural hearing loss, has been made possible by the availability and application of otoacoustic emissions (OAE) and auditory brainstem response (ABR) testing in each child suspected of having hearing loss. Technology now allows audiologists the unique opportunity to assess sensory and neural function separately. In sensory hearing loss, OAEs are usually absent whereas, given a sufficient stimulus level, an ABR can be recorded, except in the case of children with profound sensory hearing loss. In cases of neural hearing loss, OAEs are recorded, but the ABR is absent or highly abnormal. This condition has been termed *auditory neuropathy* (AN) or *auditory dyssynchrony* (AD). The terminology used for this disorder is controversial, because the specific site of pathology in the auditory system often cannot be delineated using current technologies (see Rapin and Gravel[22] for a review). Problems in the encoding or transmission of the auditory signal in the peripheral, neural, and central pathways frequently result in some deficit, from mild to severe, in speech understanding, particularly in background noise. This is because of the reduced ability of the listener to perceive rapid temporal changes in the speech signal accurately. The pure-tone audiogram, however, may indicate behavioral thresholds ranging from normal to profound in degree. Therefore, the traditional audiogram is not an accurate representation of global hearing ability. In children, increased risk for nonsyndromic neural (AN-AD) hearing loss has been reported for neonatal intensive care unit (NICU) graduates, those who had hyperbilirubinemia, and those with a family history of childhood hearing loss.[20]

Early Identification

Screening for hearing loss and monitoring for communication development are recommended across childhood.[23] For example, the American Speech-Language-Hearing Association (ASHA) has provided hearing screening guidelines for children from the newborn period through school age.[24] Programs and test methods used to screen hearing differ, depending on the age of the child. However, following identification by hearing screening, the recommendations for follow-up are similar and include a comprehensive audiologic evaluation.

Newborn Hearing Screening

Universal newborn hearing screening (UNHS) has received a significant amount of attention in recent years, and the number of hospitals that have instituted

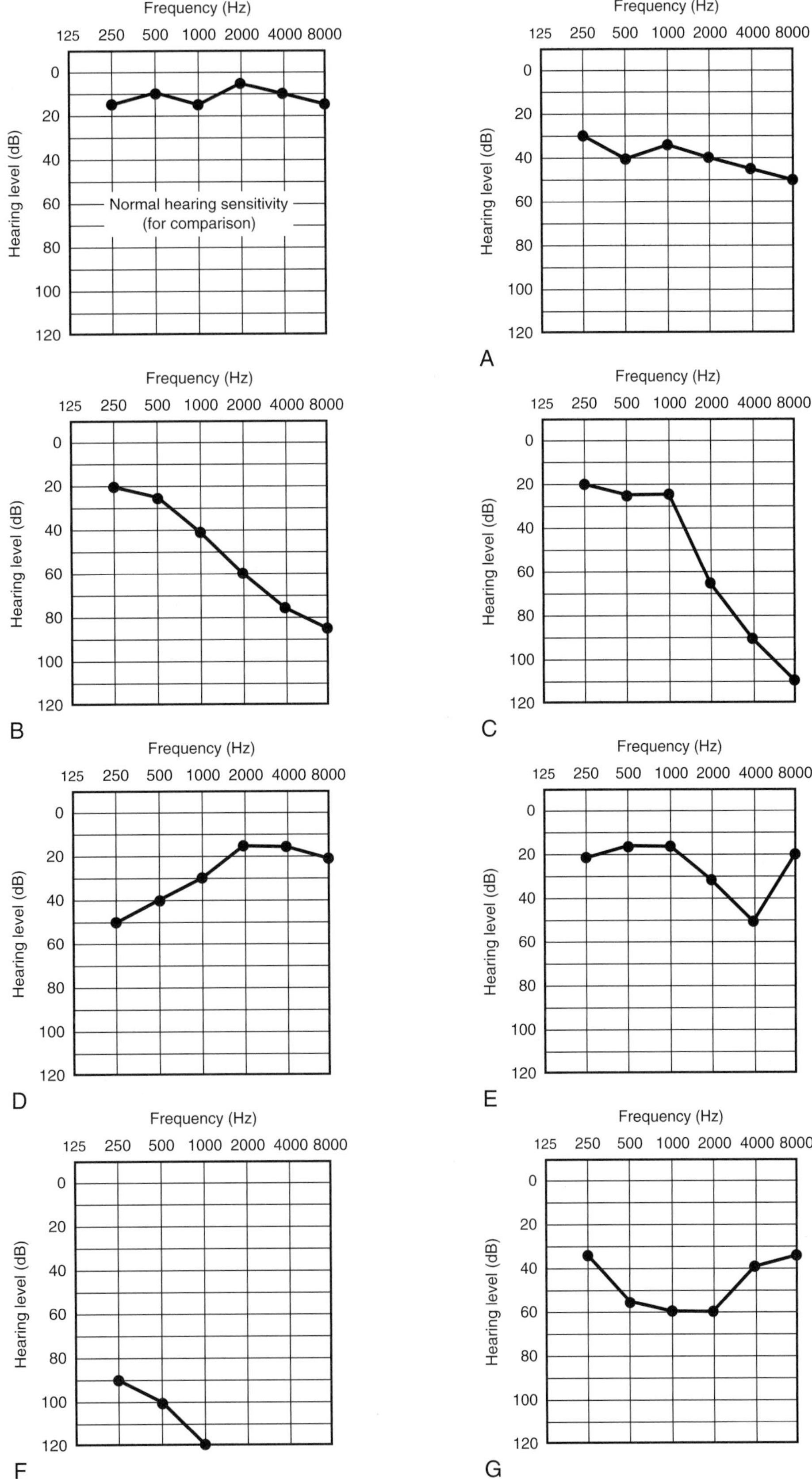

Figure 3-3. Configurations of hearing loss. **A,** Flat. **B,** Sloping. **C,** Precipitously sloping. **D,** Rising. **E,** Notched. **F,** Corner. **G,** Trough-shaped.

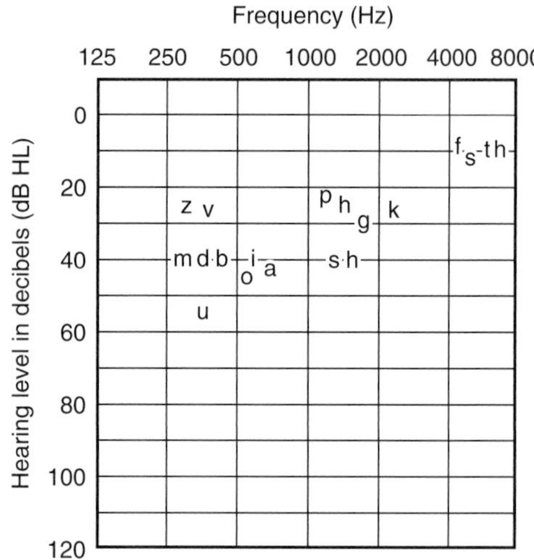

Figure 3-4. Audiogram with individual speech sounds displayed (as a function of frequency region and intensity). (Modified from Northern J, Downs M: Hearing in Children, 5th ed. Baltimore, Williams & Wilkins, 2002.)

UNHS has grown exponentially over the last 10 years.[25] The National Center for Hearing Assessment and Management (NCHAM) reported that in 2005 there were 37 states (plus the District of Columbia and Puerto Rico) with statutes related to UNHS.[26] Currently, nearly 93% of newborns in the United States receive hearing screening before hospital discharge (www.infanthearing.org); hearing loss in this birth population is the most prevalent of all newborn disabilities, more common than phenylketonuria (PKU), galactosemia, and hypothyroid disease combined—metabolic disorders for which routine newborn screening is commonly performed.[25] When carrying out UNHS based on the accepted principles for screening, efforts aimed at identifying permanent hearing loss at birth meet the criteria for mass screening.[27]

The position statements and guidelines developed by the Joint Committee on Infant Hearing (JCIH*) have served as the basis for early hearing detection and intervention (EHDI) programs since the publication of the first JCIH position statement in 1971 and through its most recent update in 2000.[20] It is expected that a new JCIH position statement will be published near the end of 2006. Past and current JCIH position statements and guidelines can be found at www.jcih.org.

*Member organizations: Alexander Graham Bell Association for the Deaf and Hard of Hearing, American Academy of Audiology, American Academy of Pediatrics, American Academy of Otolaryngology-Head and Neck Surgery, American Speech-Language-Hearing Association, Council on the Education of the Deaf, Directors of Speech and Hearing Programs in State Health and Welfare Agencies.

Prior to the advent of UNHS, only babies with known risk indicators for hearing loss received hearing screening. However, studies have indicated[25] that only about 50% of children with hearing loss have any known risk factors. Stated differently, testing only newborns and young infants who have one or more risk indicator(s) for hearing loss will miss 50% of those with congenital or early-onset hearing loss. Dependency on the presence of risk indicators has resulted in a late age of identification for most young children with hearing loss, whereas UNHS has reduced the age of identification to well below 6 months of age.[28]

Objective physiologic methods are the only effective and valid test procedures for screening for hearing loss in newborns and infants younger than 6 months of age.[20] Hearing loss in newborns and young infants cannot be detected reliably through observation—that is, methods that require an overt response or change in behavior in response to sound.

Fortunately, two different types of noninvasive, painless, physiologic technologies are now available for hearing screening in this population, OAEs and ABR. Based on a large multicenter clinical investigation supported by the National Institute on Deafness and Other Communication Disorders (NIDCD), both OAEs and ABR technologies have been shown to have good sensitivity and specificity in newborn hearing screening programs for the detection of congenital and neonatal-onset permanent hearing loss.[29]

OAEs are faint sounds (several decibels to as much as 20 dB) produced in the cochlea; they occur spontaneously as a by-product of healthy outer hair cells. However, OAEs are most useful clinically when they are produced in response to auditory stimulation (i.e., evoked), such as clicks or tones. Hence, OAE screening assesses cochlear function, specifically—outer hair cell function. Evoked OAEs can be most reliably recorded in the frequency range of 1500 to 6000 Hz. However, OAEs do not provide any information relative to the eighth cranial nerve or brainstem pathway. Individuals with hearing sensitivity better than about 30-dB HL have recordable evoked OAEs. OAEs are sensitive to outer and middle ear obstruction (e.g., vernix in the ear canal or middle ear effusion), in which case OAEs may be absent, producing a "refer" result on the screening when cochlear function is actually normal. Therefore, it is recommended that a second screening be performed when an initial screening produces a refer result. OAEs are measured by placing a flexible probe tip into the infant's ear canal to seal the opening of the canal. The probe tip contains one or more receivers and a microphone. The receivers transmit frequency-specific tones or clicks into the ear canal. The microphone records the cochlear emission produced in response.

Whereas OAEs reflect only cochlear function (and, to a degree, outer and middle ear status), the ABR is an auditory evoked potential that reflects the status of the cochlea, auditory nerve, and brainstem auditory pathways. Manually controlled ABR testing is rarely performed as a screening measure because of the complexity of the test procedure. Automated ABR (A-ABR) devices permit screening by nurses, technicians, or trained volunteers, if desired, to help control costs. A-ABR measures can detect hearing loss associated with middle ear, cochlear, auditory nerve, or brainstem pathway dysfunction. Thus, the A-ABR fail result may be the result of conductive, sensory, or neural hearing loss (the last is commonly referred to as auditory neuropathy or auditory dyssynchrony; see earlier).

A-ABR screening is performed by placing disposable earphones on the infant and attaching a set of three electrodes. The electrodes are usually placed at the high forehead, nape of the neck, and shoulder, although electrode placement differs depending on the manufacturer of the equipment. The electrodes record the change in electrical potential along the auditory pathway produced by the acoustic stimulation; a computer averages the response. Multiple presentations of click (broadband) stimuli are delivered through the earphone at a suprathreshold level, usually, 35-dB nHL, referenced to a behavioral threshold for the stimulus in normally hearing adults. Most screening units do not display an averaged response (waveform) but instead produce a result of pass or refer, based on the manufacturer's screening algorithm.

OAE screening is sometimes considered less expensive and faster to perform than A-ABR screening, primarily because of the cost of the disposable equipment associated with performing A-ABR screening. Because ABR screening is less affected by outer and middle ear conditions, many programs screen first using OAE and, if the infant fails, rescreening is done immediately using A-ABR (two-technology, two-stage screening).[9] This practice has significantly improved the overall refer rate from newborn hearing screening.[30] It is advantageous to use A-ABR screening as the first-stage screening for NICU babies. These infants are at higher risk for sensory and neural hearing loss, the latter of which can only be detected using ABR.[20] OAE and ABR screening are best carried out when the baby is resting quietly, preferably sleeping.

Any baby who refers on a second hearing screening should receive a comprehensive evaluation by an audiologist by 3 months of age. The audiologic battery should include a visual and otoscopic examination of the outer ear, an assessment of middle ear status (e.g., tympanometry), and diagnostic OAE and ABR testing. Depending on the results of the diagnostic evaluation, the infant may be referred for a medical evaluation by an otolaryngologist and/or other medical professionals (e.g., ophthalmologist, geneticist). Together, these evaluations will determine the type, degree, configuration, and, when possible, the cause of the hearing loss. The evaluations will also help in ruling out other disabilities and determining the options for treatment (see later, "Audiologic Assessment").

Infants with hearing loss are referred for early intervention services. The Individuals with Disabilities Education Act (IDEA) requires states to implement a system of early intervention services for infants and young children. Most states have state Early Hearing Detection and Intervention (EHDI) coordinators and pediatricians who have been designated as state American Academy of Pediatrics (AAP) chapter champions. They lead state and local early identification efforts and are advocates for the early identification of hearing loss in newborns. The list of state EHDI coordinators and AAP chapter champions can be found on the website of the NCHAM (www.infanthearing.org), along with other information relevant to early identification of hearing loss.

The goal of EHDI programs is to begin intervention as soon as possible after confirmation of hearing loss to facilitate the acquisition of age-appropriate auditory and spoken language skills. Any child referred for early intervention services will receive interdisciplinary evaluations examining cognitive, physical, and emotional development. As discussed later in this chapter, early fitting of hearing aids is initiated within 1 month of the confirmation of hearing loss, preferably by 4 months of age.

EHDI has become a national health care objective.[9,20,31] National EHDI goals have been developed by representatives from states that receive funds to support EHDI systems through two agencies of the U.S. Department of Health and Human Services, the Maternal and Child Bureau (MCHB) and the EHDI Program of the Centers for Disease Control and Prevention (CDC). Figure 3-5 presents the National EHDI Goals, established by the Maternal and Child Health Bureau and the Centers for Disease Control and Prevention; these have been incorporated into the recent position statements and guidelines of the JCIH. These National EHDI Goals form the basis for today's efforts at early identification of and prompt intervention for children with hearing loss using a family-centered approach.

For convenience, the National EHDI Goals are sometimes abbreviated and simply referred to as the 1-3-6 goals:

- Identification by 1 month
- Confirmation by 3 months
- Intervention by 6 months

For interested pediatricians, a training module entitled *Childhood Hearing: A Sound Foundation in the Medical Home*, is available through the American Academy of Pediatrics (www.PediaLink.org).

Beyond Newborn Hearing Screening

It is important to remember that following the hearing screening in the newborn period, there are no other

Goal 1: All newborns will be screened for hearing loss before 1 month of age, preferably before hospital discharge.

Goal 2: All infants who screen positive will have a diagnostic audiologic evaluation before 3 months of age.

Goal 3: All infants identified with hearing loss will receive appropriate early intervention services before 6 months of age (medical, audiologic, and early intervention).

Goal 4: All infants and children with late-onset, progressive, or acquired hearing loss will be identified at the earliest possible time.

Goal 5: All infants with confirmed hearing loss will have a medical home as defined by the American Academy of Pediatrics.

Goal 6: Every state will have a complete EHDI Tracking and Surveillance System that will minimize loss to follow-up.

Goal 7: Every state will have a comprehensive system that monitors and evaluates the progress toward the EHDI Goals and Objectives.

Figure 3-5. National early hearing detection and intervention (EHDI) goals established by the Maternal and Child Health Bureau and the Centers for Disease Control and Prevention. (From National EHDI Goals. Available at http://www.cdc.gov/ncbddd/EHDI/nationalgoals.htm.)

organized hearing screening efforts afforded to all children until enrollment in public school. Moreover, although EHDI programs are achieving near-universal coverage in hospitals and birthing centers in the United States, the U.S. follow-up rates are far below ideal. In some geographic areas, it is estimated that 50% of infants who failed testing or were missed by neonatal hearing screening programs are lost to follow-up. The need for surveillance programs, including the use of high-risk indicators for hearing loss, is critical for the goal of achieving early identification of permanent hearing loss in childhood.

Therefore, it is important for the pediatrician to determine whether a newborn hearing screening has been completed, the result of that screen, whether follow-up has occurred and then, regardless of the outcome of newborn hearing screening, to monitor the auditory, speech, and language development of all children. The monitoring of communication development is accomplished through interviews with caregivers during routine office visits and monitoring of developmental milestones.

Use of high-risk indicators for hearing loss is also useful to the pediatrician in the detection of possible cases of hearing loss of a child who experiences late-onset hearing loss[32,33] or who has hearing loss that was not identified by newborn hearing screening.[10] Box 3-1 presents high-risk indicators for identifying infants at risk for hearing loss who were not identified by neonatal screening or experience late-onset hearing loss.

Box 3-1 High-Risk Indicators for Identifying Infants at Risk for Hearing Loss Not Identified by the Neonatal Screening or Who Experience Late-Onset Hearing Loss

Parental or caregiver concern regarding hearing, speech, language, and/or developmental delay
Family history of permanent childhood hearing loss
An illness or condition requiring admission for 48 hours or longer to a neonatal intensive care unit (NICU)
Stigmata or other findings associated with a syndrome known to include a sensorineural or conductive hearing loss or eustachian tube dysfunction
Craniofacial anomalies, including those associated with morphologic abnormalities of the pinna and ear canal
Postnatal infections associated with sensorineural hearing loss, including bacterial meningitis
In utero infections such as CMV infection, herpes, rubella, syphilis, and toxoplasmosis
Neonatal indicators, specifically hyperbilirubinemia, at a serum level requiring exchange transfusion, persistent pulmonary hypertension of the newborn (PPHN) associated with mechanical ventilation, and conditions requiring the use of extracorporeal membrane oxygenation (ECMO)
Syndromes associated with progressive hearing loss, such as neurofibromatosis, osteopetrosis, and Usher's syndrome
Neurodegenerative disorders, such as Hunter's syndrome, or sensorimotor neuropathies, such as Friedreich's ataxia and Charcot-Marie-Tooth syndrome
Head trauma
Recurrent or persistent otitis media with effusion for at least 3 months

*Adapted from Joint Committee on Infant Hearing: Year 2000 position statement: Principles and guidelines for early hearing detection and intervention programs. Pediatrics 2000;106:798-817. Available at http://www.jcih.org.

Older Infants and Toddlers

Beginning at about 6 months developmental age, behavioral methods (visual reinforcement audiometry, VRA) (see later) can be used reliably for hearing screening. If hearing screening of older infants and toddlers (7 months through 2 years) is undertaken, ASHA recommends pass-refer criteria of 30-dB HL at 1000, 2000, and 4000 Hz.[24] Screening hearing using noncalibrated stimuli, such as noisemakers or rattles, or broadband stimuli, such as music or speech, is not recommended.

Although not widely used currently, it is likely that OAE screening devices may allow primary care providers to screen hearing in infants and young children as part of their routine well-child follow-up.

Preschoolers

Beginning at about 2½ to 3 years of age, hearing screening can be performed using conditioned play audiometry. In this method, the child is conditioned to perform some task in response to auditory stimuli. The task could be something like dropping blocks in a can or placing rings on a peg, and the child is usually reinforced verbally for completing the task. Conventional or insert earphones are used to deliver the stimuli (1000-, 2000-, and 4000-Hz pure tones at 20-dB HL). As with younger children, noncalibrated or broadband stimuli are unacceptable. As with newborns and younger infants, if the older infant or preschooler (3 to 4 years old) does not pass hearing screening using VRA or play audiometry or cannot be screened behaviorally, the child should be referred for a diagnostic audiologic evaluation.

School-age Children

Children in this age range, 5 to 18 years old, are at risk for academic failure, even with a minimal or unilateral hearing loss. Studies have shown that at least 30% to 40% of children with unilateral hearing loss are at risk for academic problems, including grade retention.[19] ASHA has recommended hearing screening for school-age children on initial entry to school and annually from kindergarten through third grade and again in grades 7 and 11. In addition, any child should be screened when special education services are indicated.[24]

The method used to screen hearing in this age range is commonly referred to as a voluntary or conventional test procedure. In response to the stimulus, the child is instructed to raise his or her hand or press a button, which activates an indicator light on the audiometer control panel. The screening is performed using earphones with test signals (1000-, 2000-, and 4000-Hz pure tones) presented at a 20-dB HL. As with younger children, noncalibrated stimuli, such as noisemakers or hand-held devices, or broadband signals, such as speech and music, should not be used for screening purposes.

If the child does not pass the screening, a rescreen is attempted immediately after adjusting the earphones and reinstructing the child. If the child does not pass the rescreening, another screening is scheduled within 1 month to allow for resolution of any transient middle ear disorder. If the child does not pass screening a second time, a referral is made for a comprehensive audiologic evaluation. Currently, a behavioral hearing screening is recommended and the use of a physiologic screen (OAE) alone is not considered sufficient for hearing screening for children in this age range.

Hearing screening programs at school age may also include an educational component about preventive measures to avoid hearing loss. Children at this age are at greater risk from noise exposure resulting from loud music or the use of power tools or guns. Healthy People 2010 has as another of its objectives reducing the incidence of noise-induced hearing loss in children 17 years of age and younger.[31]

Screening for Middle Ear Disorders

Mass screening for middle ear disease is a controversial issue. Whether the effects from chronic otitis media with effusion on speech, language, and academic achievement are long term or resolve over time continues to be debated.[34] However, it is generally accepted that chronic middle ear disease in childhood can have significant medical and developmental consequences for children at risk because of co-occurring developmental or behavioral sequelae.[34] A clinical practice guideline[34] has recommended against mass screening for otitis media with effusion (OME) in children. ASHA has provided guidelines for screening for both outer ear and middle ear disorders as part of a hearing screening program.[24] The criteria for pass-fail vary, although the instrumentation recommended across the age span from birth through 18 years are similar. Box 3-2 lists risk criteria for outer and middle ear disorders of children—that is, children for whom intrinsic and extrinsic factors may put them at risk for the hearing loss associated with OME. The procedures for screening for outer and middle ear disorders include visual inspection of the outer ear and otoscopic examination of the ear canal and tympanic membrane. Standard and screening tympanometers can be used when there are no contraindications (e.g., drainage, foreign bodies, tympanostomy tubes).

Audiologic Assessment

The purpose of the comprehensive audiologic assessment of children is to characterize the type, degree, configuration, and symmetry of the hearing loss. A comprehensive, reliable, and valid test of hearing (for both sensitivity and function) is important for the initiation of early intervention, including the selection and fitting of amplification, as well as for the monitoring of hearing status over time. ASHA has published *Guidelines for the Audiological Assessment of Infants and Young Children from Birth to Five Years*.[35] The approach is consistent with the practice at the Center for Childhood Communication.

The audiometric examination usually begins with a case history or interval history to determine the family's

Box 3-2 Risk Criteria for Outer and Middle Ear Disorders

A first episode of acute otitis media prior to 6 months of age
Bottle feeding in infancy
Craniofacial anomalies, stigmata, or other findings associated with syndromes known to affect the outer and middle ear
Ethnic-related documented increased incidence of outer and middle ear disease (e.g., Native American and Eskimo populations)
Family history of chronic or recurrent otitis media with effusion
Environmental: group day care settings and/or crowded living conditions
Exposure to excessive cigarette smoke
Childhood diagnosis of sensorineural hearing loss, learning disabilities, behavior disorders, or developmental delay and disorders

Adapted from American Speech-Language-Hearing Association: Guidelines for Audiologic Screening, 1996. Available at http://www.asha.org/NR/rdonlyres/A13D0ECC-684B-4E33-BA0E-CAF6681CEDEB/0/v4GLAudScreening.pdf.

overall impression of the child's auditory abilities and to determine the presence of risk factors (see earlier) that may signal concern regarding hearing loss. Once the family has had the opportunity to provide this important information, the actual testing of the child begins.

Tests used for the assessment of hearing can be broadly characterized as behavioral or physiologic. Behavioral tests are often considered subjective measures because they require some sort of a voluntary response (motor or verbal) from the child as an indication of awareness or understanding. Physiologic measures, including acoustic, otoacoustic, and electrophysiologic tests, are considered to be objective in that they require no behavioral response from the child. These measures provide evidence of the integrity of various portions of the auditory pathway, but are not measures of hearing per se. Behavioral measures, such as the pure-tone audiogram or speech recognition testing, are considered the only true measures of hearing in the global sense. As such, in pediatric audiology, the behavioral audiogram is considered the gold standard against which the sensitivity and specificity of screening and diagnostic tests of hearing acuity are examined. This is important, because for very young children, younger than 6 months of age, and for children who are developmentally compromised, physiologic and electrophysiologic measures must be used by audiologists for estimating hearing sensitivity and examining the integrity of the auditory pathway from the periphery through the lower brainstem, beginning at the outer ear. Whereas behavioral tests are considered subjective and electrophysiologic tests are considered objective measures, it is important to remember that the interpretation of objective test results often requires subjective judgments on the part of the audiologist.

Pediatric Audiologic Test Battery

Figure 3-6 illustrates the pediatric test battery and the order in which individual audiologic tests can be administered efficiently for infants younger than 6 months, 6 to 24 months, 24 to 48 months, and those developmentally 5 years and older.[36] For infants younger than 6 months, the primary measures used for audiologic assessment are physiologic; at older ages, behavioral tests are increasingly used in the clinical setting for follow-up. In addition, at each visit, tympanometry and evoked otoacoustic emissions are included in the minimal test battery.

As indicated earlier, a battery of tests that includes behavioral and physiologic measures are used in pediatric audiologic assessment. In the pediatric test battery, behavioral measures are always used to crosscheck the physiologic findings, and behavioral testing alone is not sufficient for the comprehensive assessment of hearing in children. No test is redundant; all are needed to provide information about threshold sensitivity and auditory system integrity.

Physiologic Measures

Multiple acoustic, otoacoustic, and electrophysiologic tests are used to estimate auditory sensitivity and auditory pathway integrity across childhood, beginning during the neonatal period. These measures include tympanometry, evoked otoacoustic emissions, acoustic middle ear muscle reflex threshold testing, and ABR testing, including suprathreshold and threshold, as well as air- and bone-conducted techniques. Although the pediatric audiologic test armamentarium has been bolstered by the availability of such technologies, no single physiologic test is sufficient for use in the assessment of children. Moreover, in pediatric audiologic practice, it is common to support the results of behavioral audiogram with the findings from physiologic and electrophysiologic tests and, conversely, to corroborate physiologic and electrophysiologic outcomes with behavioral audiometric and functional tests of hearing. In this section, we delineate the physiologic tests commonly used in pediatric audiology and the levels of the auditory pathway assessed by each measure.

Tympanometry

Tympanometry (also known as aural acoustic admittance measurement) is a valuable and widely used measure of middle ear function. Tympanometry is similar to pneumatic otoscopy in that the middle ear is examined by varying pressure in the sealed ear canal, at one end bounded by the plastic ear tip of the measurement probe and at the other end by the intact tympanic membrane.

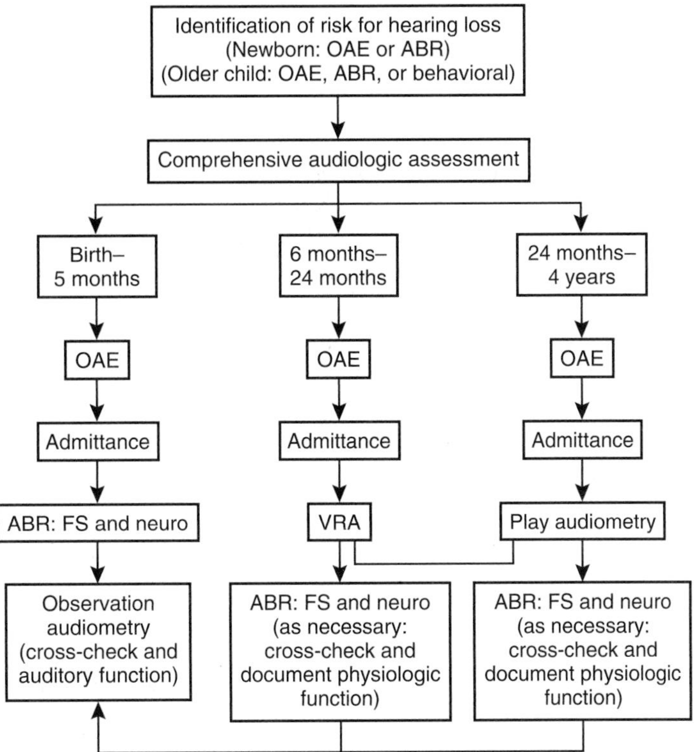

Figure 3-6. Pediatric test battery depicting the order of individual audiologic tests for infants, toddlers, and young children. (Modified from Gravel JS, Hood LJ: Pediatric audiologic assessment. In FE Musiek, WF Rintelmann [eds]: Contemporary Perspective: Hearing Assessment. Boston, Allyn and Bacon, 1999, pp 305-326.)

A single-component (acoustic admittance) tympanogram tracing is recorded by delivering a continuous low-frequency (226 Hz) probe tone of known sound pressure level into the closed ear canal. Air pressure, measured in decapascals, daPa, is varied from +200 to −400 daPa, and change in admittance (or ease in energy flow, the opposite of impedance) is measured in mmho, the reciprocal of ohm. At the peak of the tympanogram, sound energy (in daPa) is optimally transferred through the middle ear system. When peak pressure of the tympanogram is measured at 0 daPa (±50 daPa), this is indicative of normal (atmospheric) pressure within the middle ear space and the finding is consistent with normal eustachian tube function.

Traditionally, tympanograms have been interpreted based on their qualitative pattern or shape. Five tympanogram types, including two subtypes, are commonly referenced when reporting tympanometry findings[37]:

1. Type A, indicating normal middle ear function, with peak compliance at or near normal atmospheric pressure. Two subtypes of the type A tympanogram are also considered: type A_S, indicating normal middle ear pressure but reduced compliance of the tympanic membrane (a stiff middle ear system, consistent with fixed middle ear ossicles or scar tissue); and type A_D, indicating a highly compliant middle ear system, consistent with a flaccid eardrum resulting from a disarticulation of the middle ear ossicles or recently healed tympanic membrane perforation (monomeric eardrum).
2. Type B, or flat tympanogram (no change in compliance with change in pressure), consistent with effusion in the middle ear space.
3. Type C, indicating negative (less than −150 daPa) pressure in the middle ear space and compromised eustachian tube functioning.

Today, when a tympanogram is recorded, measurements of peak admittance (Y_{TM} in mmho), tympanogram peak pressure (TPP in daPa), and width of the tympanogram (TW in daPa) are compared with published normative data for infants and younger and older children to determine whether middle ear effusion is present.[38,39]

Infants younger than 4 months have flaccid ear canals and middle ear systems that are considerably different from those of older infants and children. The standard 226-Hz probe frequency is not valid for estimating middle ear function, in that a normal tympanogram can be recorded from a young infant's ear with middle ear fluid, and an abnormal tympanogram may be recorded from an ear having normal middle ear function. Accordingly, tympanograms are recorded in infants younger than 4 months using a 1000-Hz probe frequency.[40]

Finally, with children, a quantitative measure of equivalent volume of the ear canal (V_{ec} in mL) is useful in determining whether the tympanic membrane is intact or a perforation of the eardrum exists because of trauma or because a patent tympanostomy tube is in place. Both conditions typically yield a flat tympanogram. The measurement of volume helps the clinician determine whether the flat immobile tympanogram is the result of middle ear effusion behind an intact eardrum or a perforation. The perforation and a patent tympanostomy tube both result in atypically high volume measurements. This occurs because the space of the closed ear canal with an intact eardrum at one end is considerably smaller than the combined volume of the ear canal plus the middle ear space, as when a perforation or patent tympanostomy tube is present.

Acoustic Middle Ear Muscle Reflex Thresholds

Acoustic middle ear muscle reflex (AMEMR) threshold testing is an important component of the pediatric audiologic test battery. The same device used for acoustic admittance assessment is used for AMEMR measurement—a probe assembly is fitted to one ear and an insert earphone is fitted to the opposite ear. The AMEMR threshold (in dB HL) is evaluated at the child's tympanometric peak pressure. Stimuli, beginning at 70-dB HL, at the frequencies of 500, 1000, 2000, and 4000 Hz are presented contralaterally and/or ipsilaterally. The stimuli at each test frequency are increased in level in 5-dB steps until a change in acoustic immittance is first recorded: this is the AMEMR threshold. Threshold levels, or the absence of the AMEMR, for ipsilateral and contralateral stimulation are useful in the pediatric audiologic test battery as a cross check or for corroborating other audiologic data regarding the type, degree, and configuration of any hearing loss. Normative values are available for AMEMRs recorded in children with normal middle ear function and normal hearing.

Evoked Otoacoustic Emissions

Otoacoustic emissions (OAEs) evoked by clicks (transient evoked OAEs [TEOAEs]) or tone pairs (distortion product OAEs [DPOAEs]) are useful in pediatric audiology for screening hearing (see earlier) and for audiologic diagnostic purposes. OAEs are the acoustic by-products of healthy outer hair cells (OHCs) of the cochlea. As such, they can be recorded across frequency ranges of interest, such as those within the speech range. Recording OAEs in the external ear canal also requires normal middle ear function for delivering the evoking stimuli and recording the emission from the cochlea. TEAOEs are not usually recorded in the presence of sensory hearing loss greater than about 30-dB HL; similarly, DPOAEs are not recorded with sensory hearing loss exceeding about 60-dB HL.

OAEs are useful in the comprehensive pediatric audiologic test battery.[41] The presence of OAEs indicates that the sensory mechanism and therefore hearing are intact—normative values are available for expected levels of OAEs in infants and children with normal hearing—and that the middle ear system is functioning normally. Minor middle ear involvement may result in the absence of OAEs, so tympanometry is critical for the interpretation of absent OAEs in infants and children. Because OAEs are frequency-specific, they may be useful to audiologists when the audiogram from a young child cannot be obtained at all frequencies. OAE findings can then be used to hypothesize about hearing problems at missing audiometric frequencies. OAEs are also useful in monitoring changes in cochlear status, because they are highly reliable. This is particularly important in the follow-up of children who may be receiving chemotherapeutic drugs known to be ototoxic. Changes in OAE levels can be identified before a change in the behavioral audiogram is detected. Finally, OAEs can be useful for monitoring subtle changes in middle ear status.[41]

The presence of OAE is indicative of the integrity of the peripheral mechanism only, the OHCs of the cochlea and middle ear. Infants and children with neural hearing loss (i.e., auditory neuropathy, auditory dyssynchrony) may have recordable OAEs but mild to profound impairment in understanding speech and a behavioral audiogram indicating hearing loss. Children with milder forms of sensory hearing loss (less than 40-dB HL) may also have recordable OAEs. These losses are important to detect and, for many children, may be deleterious to language development and academic performance. Thus, the presence of OAEs alone does not indicate normal hearing.[42]

Other components of the pediatric audiologic test battery are needed to confirm normal hearing, including the consideration of the child's development of appropriate auditory skills and the achievement of expected speech and language milestones.

Auditory Brainstem Response

The ABR, an electrophysiologic measure, involves the recording of microvolt electrical activity from surface electrodes in a quiet (ideally, sleeping) child. ABR has become one of the most important tests in the pediatric audiologic battery. In particular, it is critical for estimating hearing sensitivity in infants too young or too compromised to provide reliable behavioral hearing thresholds. Accordingly, ABR testing is used as the primary assessment procedure for delineating normal hearing from hearing loss following newborn hearing screening failure.[36]

As with the behavioral audiogram, the ABR can be recorded using air- and bone-conducted stimuli. In addition, frequency-specific (tone burst) stimuli are now used to record the ABR by air and bone conduction. The air- and bone-conducted frequency-specific ABR is now considered the test of choice for estimating the type, degree, and configuration of hearing loss in young infants. The threshold information obtained, at 500, 1000, 2000 and 4000 Hz, is critical to the early selection and fitting of appropriate amplification devices in infants 6 months of age and younger.[35] There is good agreement (±10 to 15 dB) between behavioral thresholds and frequency-specific ABR thresholds in infants and young children. The traditional click stimulus evokes a response in the frequency region between 100 and 8000 Hz. Therefore, a click ABR threshold is not frequency-specific, so a click threshold is insufficient for audiometric purposes when it is critical to estimate hearing sensitivity in each ear.[35,36]

The click-evoked ABR, however, is useful in the examination of neural integrity. Suprathreshold recordings of single-polarity clicks (condensation and rarefaction) are used to determine whether a recorded response is neural or the prolongation of a sensory response (i.e., cochlear microphonic). Because approximately 10% of infants and children with permanent hearing loss have neural as opposed to sensory hearing loss, the click ABR still remains an important component of the pediatric audiologic test battery.[35]

Behavioral Audiometry

Appropriate behavioral tests of hearing are selected based on the developmental and not the chronologic age of the child. Behavioral tests are divided broadly into two categories, unconditioned (overt and reflex responses) and conditioned response procedures. Responses to unconditioned test procedures such as behavioral observation audiometry (BOA) are highly unreliable, depend on the state of the infant or child, habituate rapidly, and are best observed with broadband complex signals, such as white noise or speech, precluding frequency-specific audiologic assessment. Most important, normally hearing infants show wide variability in their responses to sound, precluding a clear criterion for hearing loss. Unconditioned response procedures are not recommended for audiometric purposes, such as determining the presence or absence of hearing loss or adjusting the setting of amplification devices.[35,36]

Conditioned response procedures have become the primary clinical tools in pediatric practice. Fortunately, operant response audiometric test procedures are useful with infants, toddlers, and young children as young as 6 months developmental age. Conditioned response procedures and the use of a specified test algorithm help increase the reliability and validity of audiologic test outcomes and reduce the subjectivity of behavioral audiometry. When infants and children fail to exhibit conditioned responses during audiometric evaluation, this may be because the procedure was inappropriate for the developmental age of the child or because during the conditioning phase of the test procedure, the child did not learn the response contingency.

However, once contingent responding has been established (with VRA, tangible reinforcement operant conditioning audiometry [TROCA], play, or conventional response procedures), behavioral audiometry becomes the most important test in the pediatric test battery. Thresholds for tones and speech can be established by using air- and bone-conducted stimuli. Even at a young age (infants), behavioral thresholds for tonal stimuli are within 10 dB of adult values. Therefore, behavioral audiometric procedures can be used successfully across childhood to determine hearing sensitivity and monitor hearing status (e.g., stability, fluctuation, or progression of any loss of hearing).[35,36]

It is not practical or cost-effective to sedate children for frequency-specific ABR testing each time a measure of sensitivity is required. The importance of reliable and valid methods for the behavioral assessment of infants and young children cannot be overemphasized. Young children with hearing loss require multiple visits to audiologists. Thus, optimizing behavioral audiometry techniques is crucial to the long-term follow-up of children with all forms of hearing loss.[35,36]

Infants and Toddlers

Between about 6 and 24 months developmental age, VRA has been shown to be a reliable and valid method for assessing hearing sensitivity. Standard audiometric air-conducted and bone-conducted frequency-specific test signals and signal delivery (i.e., through insert-type earphones) are used during VRA so that hearing acuity—audiometric thresholds, or minimum response levels—may be delineated in each ear across the range of frequencies important for speech perception (250 to 6000 Hz). VRA allows the audiologist to do the following: (1) determine the symmetry of any hearing loss; (2) establish a baseline for monitoring hearing sensitivity over time; (3) make appropriate referrals for medical and otologic evaluation; and (4) determine the appropriate amplification characteristics for each ear (decibel gain and output sound pressure levels as a function of frequency).[35,36]

In VRA testing, the infant or toddler is seated on the parent's lap or secured into a high chair. A test assistant manipulates quiet attractive toys in front of the child to maintain the infant's gaze at the midline position. A test signal is delivered, which usually results in a head turn in the direction from which the signal was delivered (located 90 degrees to one side). This natural localization, or lateralization, a head turn, is reinforced by the presentation of highly animated, novel visual reinforcement.

Traditionally, visual reinforcement has been in the form of a number of mechanical toys housed in darkly opaque Plexiglas boxes; these are illuminated and activated when the behavioral head turn response occurs during the presentation of a test signal. More recently, visual reinforcement has been provided by the display of appealing animated cartoon clips on a flat screen video monitor (video VRA).[43] The infant is reinforced for responding only during test intervals during which a signal is presented; the behavior (the head turn) is maintained across repeated presentations of the test trials by the novelty of the visual reinforcement. Generally, when a young child achieves the conditioning criterion, which includes demonstrating no response during the presentation of interspersed silent (or control) trials, 30 or more responses to audiometric test signals can be achieved. This number of contingent responses is sufficient to obtain an accurate representation of the audiometric profile for low-, mid-, and high-frequency stimuli in each ear, and often in one test session.[35,36]

The age between about 20 to 30 months can sometimes be challenging, because toddlers habituate rapidly to VRA but are not ready developmentally for play audiometry (see later). One study has indicated that the use of video VRA may support behavioral responding longer than mechanical toys, suggesting that customizing and individualizing the video reinforcement clips to the interests and level of toddlers may result in sustained responding during behavioral audiometry.[43] More data about the benefits and limitations of video VRA are needed.

Other methods that have been traditionally used to obtain responses from toddlers during behavioral audiometry are TROCA and the related VROCA, visual reinforcement operant conditioning audiometry. Instead of a head turn response, as in VRA, the behavioral response, pushing a large face plate or button on a response box, is shaped by pairing the auditory stimulus with a light and teaching the child that each time the light (plus sound) is present, a response will result in tangible (e.g., a piece of cereal) or visual (e.g., activation of a mechanical toy or video) reinforcement. The light is faded and, when the child is responding to the presence of the auditory signal (the operant), the threshold search is initiated.[35] TROCA and VROCA are not as widely used as VRA. However, the availability of video reinforcement may provide more opportunities for modifications of VRA to be implemented clinically.

Computer-controlled VRA and VROCA testing have added a new dimension to behavioral testing and serve to reduce subjectivity and tester bias. Because the test is under computer control, the test algorithm may be specified to conditioning and test trials, a fixed percentage of control trial intervals, interweaved threshold searches at various test frequencies, use of probe (higher level) stimuli to determine attention and motivation of the child during testing, and printing and storage of results. The computer acts as a test assistant; the audiologist interacts with the computer through a hand switch, signaling when the infant is ready for a trial. Through the use of masking (head phones or ear plugs), the audiologist can remain unbiased as to what type of trial is presented, signal or control. The audiologist indicates through a second button when a response has been made by the child. The computer determines whether the infant's response is correct and delivers reinforcement, as appropriate. Computer-assisted procedures are gaining increased use in the clinical setting.[36]

Preschool and School-age Children

At about 3 years of age, children are capable of providing a wider range of voluntary responses to auditory stimuli. Beginning between 24 and 30 months of age, a play task is usually introduced as a behavioral indicator of detection. The child is taught through shaping of the motor act in the conditioning phase to perform a manual play response. This may be the dropping of a block in a bucket or placement of a plastic ring on a stacking pole. Correct performance, completing the play response, is usually rewarded by social praise. However, visual reinforcement for correct responding can also be used to support continued responding over repeated trials.[35]

Usually, at age 5 years, children are ready to respond in a more adult-like manner. Children are asked to raise a hand or push a hand-held button when they detect a tone. Reinforcement by social praise is generally sufficient. Automated audiometry has sometimes been used with a child of this age.[35]

As indicated earlier, the behavioral audiometric procedure is selected based on the developmental age, not the chronologic age, of the child. Therefore, the behavioral pediatric audiologic evaluation of children with developmental, cognitive, and/or physical disabilities must be tailored to meet their individual needs and abilities.

Speech Audiometry

In addition to thresholds for tonal signals, thresholds for speech signals are also included in the pediatric audiologic evaluation. Threshold for speech (e.g., the child's name) can provide information about general sensitivity. However, because the speech signal is broadband, this information is insufficient for monitoring hearing sensitivity or for determining the setting of hearing aids. Individual speech sounds in low- and high-frequency ranges can provide more frequency-specific threshold information. Because speech is intrinsically more appealing to young infants, VRA procedures will often begin by establishing a threshold for speech in each ear and then moving to tonal signals.

As children begin to develop even a simple repertoire of words, speech recognition testing, sometimes called speech discrimination testing, can be undertaken. Speech recognition testing is done at a comfortable level, usually 30 to 40 dB above the child's threshold for speech, to determine how many words (measured in percent) the child recognizes correctly. Toddlers may be asked to identify a word by touching or pointing to a body part, such as the eyes, nose, or mouth. Preschoolers may select one picture among several that sound alike (e.g., socks, from blocks, rocks, clocks). When children have clear speech, they may be asked to repeat words presented to each ear. A percentage correct score (number of correct responses per total items) provides information about the intelligibility of speech. Because of the rapid development of language during the early years, speech recognition testing can be challenging in young children. Speech perception tests that require the child to repeat the word can be problematic in the testing of very young children with normal hearing and in children with hearing loss who have speech articulation errors. When speech recognition tests are at the appropriate developmental and speech levels, they are useful measures for examining the development of functional auditory abilities and speech discrimination skills over time.

Interventions

Interventions for assisting children with hearing loss can include hearing aids and other assistive devices and cochlear implants.

Hearing Aids and Other Assistive Devices

General Considerations

The primary goal of comprehensive audiologic testing is to define the hearing loss as early as possible so that the process of aural rehabilitation can begin. A primary component of this includes fitting for appropriate amplification. Hearing aids, at their most basic level, amplify sound to provide audibility, particularly of speech. Hearing aids come in a wide range of styles, from those that sit outside the ear to tiny devices that fit entirely inside the ear canal. Devices based on other technologies, termed *assistive listening devices*, are used in conjunction with hearing aids to improve signal quality in the presence of background noise or when the speaker is located some distance from the child.

The process of fitting amplification devices to children presents unique challenges in that the audiologist must frequently work with limited auditory information and little feedback from the patient. The audibility of the full range of the speech signal is of utmost importance, because this is the key factor in the development of aural communication—spoken language. At the Center for Childhood Communication, we have adopted an approach to the provision of amplification based on an evidence-based pediatric hearing aid selection and fitting approach developed and validated by Seewald and colleagues at the University of Western Ontario and supported by the findings of Stelmachowicz and co-workers at Boys Town National Research Hospital. These studies and those of others have been reviewed and incorporated into the American Academy of Audiology's Pediatric Amplification Protocol.[44]

Hearing Aids: Selection Considerations

Hearing aids should be fitted as soon as possible on confirmation of permanent hearing loss, which can be sensorineural, conductive, or mixed. Any degree of hearing loss should be considered. Many children with unilateral and minimal hearing losses will benefit from amplification, because these children often experience academic difficulty.[44] Children diagnosed with profound hearing impairment may also benefit from hearing aids and a trial with amplification will be necessary to evaluate aided auditory abilities. If it is not possible to provide sufficient auditory information with hearing aids, cochlear implantation should be considered (see later). Additionally, amplification in the form of FM systems may be appropriate for children who have normal peripheral hearing sensitivity but show evidence of auditory processing disorder.

Age. Hearing aids can be fitted beginning at only a few weeks of age using data from ABR testing. The use of frequency-specific stimuli allows for an adequate base of information. As the child matures, information obtained from behavioral audiometric testing can be used to fine-tune the hearing aid fitting. No age is too young to begin using amplification. With the advent of newborn hearing screening, audiologists are fitting more and more infants with hearing aids, giving them important early access to auditory information.

Style. There are many factors to consider in the hearing aid selection process. The first is the style of the device. For most children, the behind-the-ear (BTE) style of hearing aid is recommended over an in-the-ear (ITE) device. The BTE has the advantages of increased acoustic flexibility and capability of coupling to assistive listening devices. Additionally, the hearing aid itself is kept out of the ear and coupled to a soft ear mold placed inside the concha and ear canal. This provides increased safety and allows for the ear mold to be remade as the child grows. For newborns, it may be necessary to remake ear molds every month or so because of the amount of growth during this time period. ITE hearing aids may be considered for an older child who has stopped growing if the degree and configuration of the hearing loss permit. Some children cannot use traditional amplification systems because of auditory or physical limitations. Bone conduction hearing aids are recommended for children whose ears cannot accommodate air conduction systems, such as with binaural atresia. For a child who has usable hearing in only one ear, a contralateral routing of signal (CROS) hearing aid may be recommended, although studies have shown mixed results with this type of system.[44] When fitting a child with bilateral hearing loss, two hearing aids individualized to each ear are always fitted, unless otherwise contraindicated, because of the known benefits of binaural hearing, which include sound localization and hearing speech in noise. Even children with asymmetrical hearing loss should be fitted binaurally until such time that this is shown to be detrimental to performance.[44]

Technology. Another consideration when choosing hearing aids is technology. Advances in technology have provided the clinician with a wealth of options from which to choose. Hearing aids work by amplifying specific frequency regions according to the degree and configuration of the hearing loss. Advances in digital multichannel devices now allow for greater electroacoustic flexibility in shaping the desired response to address the specific hearing loss configuration, which makes them more effective than older, conventional hearing aids. Modern hearing aids are programmed using a computer as opposed to trimpots on the device, allowing for more possible adjustments. This technology can be useful when fitting young children, from whom limited auditory information is available. Hearing aids can be reprogrammed as additional information is obtained. This technology is also beneficial for children with progressive or fluctuating hearing loss. Additionally, it is important to fit hearing aids that have a wide bandwidth to provide audibility for high-frequency consonant sounds. Most children will benefit from choosing amplification with wide dynamic range compression (WDRC), which is designed to provide maximum audibility for soft sounds and simulate normal loudness growth.

Many hearing aids are available with a number of memories, allowing the parent or older child to switch programs for different listening situations. This may be especially useful for a listener with fluctuating hearing loss, because the gain and frequency response of the device can be different in each program. Another available option is a directional microphone, designed to favor signals in front of the listener rather than those from behind. However, there is little evidence documenting benefit from this technology in children. Therefore, one should proceed cautiously in recommending directional microphones for children. Children do not always face the person speaking and may benefit more from an omnidirectional microphone, which picks up sound equally from all sides. Many hearing aids with a directional microphone option allow for deactivation until the child is old enough to use it effectively.

Many hearing aids also offer automatic feedback reduction, which can be particularly useful for children who are likely to have objects close to their ears and when ear molds start to loosen and need to be replaced. It is important to choose a system that does not reduce gain, and thus reduce audibility, to avoid feedback. Hearing aids should also be equipped with a telecoil to allow for telephone conversation and coupling to certain assistive devices. Direct audio input and a microphone-telecoil (MT) switch should also be included.

Earmolds. A BTE hearing aid is coupled to an ear mold that retains the device on the ear and brings the sound into the listener's ear canal. The ear mold can also serve to modify the signal acoustically. Ear molds are available in a wide range of colors and materials to suit the child's preferences and degree and configuration of the hearing loss.

Other Features. Other features necessary for young children include tamper-proof battery doors, pediatric-sized ear hooks, and the ability to disable the volume control wheel, so that a young child cannot accidentally change the hearing aid volume. Many hearing aid manufacturers offer hearing aids in various colors. Children may accept their hearing aids more readily if they can participate in choosing the color themselves. Other accessories are available for holding hearing aids onto the ears.

Hearing Aids: Fitting Considerations

Amplification Targets. Hearing aids should be fitted to targets for gain and output based on a prescriptive method that is evidence-based and specifically developed for use with children.[44] Targets should be based on ensuring audibility for speech across a wide range of input levels, including audibility for the child's own voice.[44] The child's own ear canal size should be used in determining target sound pressure levels because the measured sound pressure may exceed that of an adult. When it is not possible during an office visit to obtain custom measures, age-appropriate normative data can be used.[44]

Verification. When fitting hearing aids for amplification, it is necessary to verify that specified targets are being met. Real ear measures of the sound pressure level in the individual ear should be done with the child's ear mold in place to ensure that the gain and output of the device are appropriate. It is necessary to verify gain for soft and moderate speech levels. Additionally, maximum output should be measured to ensure that the aid cannot produce sounds that would be uncomfortable for the listener or damaging to the ear. Aided testing in the sound booth, especially speech testing, is appropriate when used in conjunction with real ear measures. Other measures, such as outcome questionnaires and parent or teacher reports, also provide important information regarding the child's auditory abilities.[44]

Orientation. A new hearing aid fitting should include an orientation for the family accompanied by written material to take home. This orientation should include the following[44]:

- Wearing schedule and suggestions for keeping the child's hearing aid in place
- Insertion and removal
- Retention of the aids (including possible accessories such as Huggie Aids, Critter Clips toupee tape, and pediatric-sized ear hooks, all of which are designed to secure the aid to the ear)
- Care and cleaning of the aids
- Battery insertion and removal
- Battery life and safety (with provision of battery ingestion hotline)
- Moisture protection
- Turning aids on and off
- Provision of tools (e.g., listening stethoscope for parents, battery tester)
- Troubleshooting (e.g., feedback, dead battery, sound channel plugged with wax)
- Information regarding warranty and repair issues
- Follow-up schedule
- Telephone and assistive device coupling

Follow-up. At the time of fitting, a follow-up appointment schedule should be reviewed. Children with newly identified hearing loss should be seen at least every 3 months initially for audiologic monitoring and hearing aid checks.[44] Ear mold fit should be monitored, with replacement as necessary. Real ear measures should be performed periodically, especially on receipt of new ear molds. If hearing should change, hearing aids can be reprogrammed to match targets for the new hearing loss. Otologic management may be more important for a child with hearing loss as well. Otitis media needs to be managed promptly, especially if it creates a further reduction in hearing. Cerumen management is also important, because excess cerumen can block the ear mold sound bore, decreasing the amount of amplification the child receives. Academic and communicative progress of a hearing impaired child are best monitored using a team approach; this can include audiologists, speech-language pathologists, early intervention specialists, teachers of the deaf, classroom teachers, otolaryngologists, pediatricians, and parents.[44]

Assistive Listening Devices

In addition to hearing aids, other assistive listening devices might also be recommended. Most children with hearing aids will also use an FM system, especially in school. An FM system works by bringing the voice of a particular speaker directly to the listener via a wireless FM connection. This improves the signal-to-noise ratio and makes it easier for the child to hear in more competitive listening environments. There are various styles of FM devices, including those that are ear level, body worn, desktop, or classroom sound field. Other types of devices may be recommended as well, especially for a child with profound hearing loss, and include alerting devices (e.g., phone, doorbell) and devices with vibrating or high-volume signals, such as alarm clocks and smoke detectors. In addition, it is necessary to ensure that the child can use the telephone. Recommended hearing aids should be equipped with a telecoil to allow for telephone use and for coupling with certain assistive devices. For children who do not receive sufficient benefit from a telecoil, a teletypewriter may be recommended. It is important for the audiologist to spend time demonstrating telephone use to parents of even very young children so that no child is excluded from using the telephone.

Pediatric Cochlear Implantation

In a normally functioning organ of Corti, inner hair cells transduce mechanical energy initiated by an acoustic signal into electrochemical energy that is passed to the peripheral and central auditory systems to be perceived as sound. In the case of significant sensory hearing loss, the inner hair cells are reduced in number or function insufficiently so that an individual cannot understand speech effectively. A cochlear implant is a neural prosthetic device designed to replace the transduction function of inner hair cells in the organ of Corti. The cochlear implant system has two components. The externally worn component supplies the power to both components and is usually worn behind the user's ear. The external component picks up sound with a microphone, transforms the signal into a code suited for neural detection, and transmits this signal to the internal component. The internal component has an antenna and stimulator placed under the skin behind the ear and an electrode array implanted into the scala tympani through a mastoidectomy and cochleostomy. The internal component receives the signal from the external component and stimulates individual electrodes with the neural code. The internal device may return monitoring telemetry information to the external device. The external antenna is aligned and held in place with the internal antenna by magnets in the center of each. The standard of care is implantation into one ear; however, a number of patients have received bilateral cochlear implants seeking better sound quality, speech perception skills, and sound localization abilities.

Cochlear implant technology has progressed over the past few decades from single-channel devices, in which the electrode is placed outside the cochlea, to multiple-channel devices, in which the array of electrodes is implanted within the cochlea. Signal-processing capabilities have progressed as well. As a result of improved signal transduction capabilities, combined with improving educational, therapeutic, medical, and audiologic management, many adults can now be restored their functional auditory abilities[45-47] and many children can develop auditory function to the point where they use spoken language and are educated with their hearing peers.[48-52]

Despite the remarkable accomplishments of many people who are deaf and use a cochlear implant, the cochlear implant is not a cure for deafness. Although many adults and children are able to use sound for spoken communication, many cannot. These cochlear implant users may use sound as a support to a visual form of communication (e.g., speech reading or various forms of sign language) or may only use the cochlear implant to provide sound awareness. Children require special education and therapy to acquire the ability to learn in a mainstream setting.

Pediatric Cochlear Implant Team

Because outcomes vary widely with pediatric cochlear implantation, and success factors include those related to the child's hearing, education, speech and language abilities, development, health, and family, a pediatric cochlear implant team must represent diverse specialties. The role of the cochlear implant team is to determine whether the child is a candidate, perform clinical procedures relating to the function of the device, and provide or support therapeutic and educational services. Team members include the following:

- Surgical and medical support staff specifically trained to work with the very young child.
- Audiologic staff proficient in objective and behavioral hearing assessment methods to diagnose hearing loss and determine benefit from amplification in very young children before implantation is done. Once the device is implanted, the audiologist must understand the perceptual consequences of signal processing and electrical stimulation of the auditory nerve.
- Therapeutic staff who can assess a wide range of speech and language abilities, regardless of the communication modality and independent of hearing ability. The speech-language pathologist and/or therapist must be able to establish appropriate goals and design intervention strategies to increase the child's access to spoken and heard language.
- Staff who can address the psychosocial aspects of the family's involvement in the child's outcome and the family's expectations.
- Educational staff who address the child's environment for learning spoken language and work with the child's early intervention or educational program to ensure coordinated medical and educational collaboration.
- Developmental staff who can determine factors external to the child's hearing that may be related to the ability to develop spoken language.

Cochlear Implant Candidacy

The current U.S. Food and Drug Administration (FDA) guidelines for cochlear implant candidacy include children older than 12 months with severe to profound bilateral deafness (more than 70-dB HL pure-tone average) who receive little or no benefit from appropriate hearing aids. In older children, this may be quantified as less than a 30% score on the Multisyllabic Lexical Neighborhood Test (MLNT) or the Lexical Neighborhood Test (LNT).[53] In young children, this is quantified as a failure to progress on the Infant Toddler Meaningful Auditory Integration Scale (IT-MAIS) or the Meaningful Auditory Integration Scale (MAIS), which have a rated parent-guided interview format.[54,55]

Because of age and language ability differences, there is a battery of speech perception measures that are used in a pediatric cochlear implant program. In general, these tests are used to assign scores to the child's progress at increasingly difficult task levels. Levels progress from no sound awareness, to consistent sound awareness, to consistent pattern perception, to closed-set word identification abilities, to open-set word identification abilities, to key word identification in phrases and/or sentences and, finally, to open-set sentence identification.

In an attempt to organize and assess cochlear implant candidacy and to develop outcome expectations, Hellman and colleagues[56] devised the Children's Implant Profile (ChIP). The ChIP rates concern on a three-level scale of no concern, mild to moderate concern, and great concern in the following areas: chronologic age, duration of deafness, medical and radiologic, multiple handicap, functional hearing, speech and language abilities, family structure and support, expectations, educational environment, and availability of support services. To account for changes as to what constitutes levels of concern in each category, The Children's Hospital of Philadelphia Cochlear Implant Team modified the ChIP to include our experience and those of other centers working with children, as described in the following sections.

Chronologic Age. Currently, FDA guidelines suggest that children older than 12 months can be considered for implantation. Exceptions to FDA guidelines can be indicated to include children younger than 12 months. In the case of congenital or early-onset hearing loss, early implantation ensures that the child will have access to the sound provided by the electrical stimulation during as much of the critical period of language development as possible. For this reason, children younger than 2 years are categorized as no concern. As the age of implantation increases, the child's reliance on auditory information typically diminishes, whereas reliance on other visual forms of communication grows. The chronologic age of the cochlear implant candidate raises mild to moderate concern between approximately 2 and 6 years of age, and great concern when the child is older than 6 years.

Duration of Deafness. The duration of deafness is defined as the amount of time between the onset of severe to profound bilateral hearing loss and the cochlear implant evaluation. It is equal to the chronologic age in congenitally deaf children. It reflects auditory plasticity and neural degeneration in the absence of stimulation. The extent to which the deprived auditory periphery and cortex degenerates may increase with the amount of time that auditory input is deprived.[57,58] Also, there exists a critical period of language development—during the first 6 years of life—in which the brain demonstrates high neural auditory plasticity.[59] Duration of deafness also addresses the extent to which the child may have adapted using other forms of communication. The longer a child has adapted without auditory input, the longer it may take to learn to use sound effectively. Children for whom the duration of deafness is less than 2 years are included in the no concern category. Mild to moderate concern is assigned to children whose duration of deafness is between 2 and 6 years, and great concern for duration more than 6 years.

Otolaryngology. The otolaryngologist determines the medical aspects for cochlear implant candidacy. No concern for medical candidacy includes children in good health. Mild to moderate concern describes children with seizure or reactive airway disorders that can be monitored and controlled throughout the implantation process. Children with major airway disorders or severe cardiac issues may be classified in the great concern category. For all children being evaluated for a cochlear implant, radiography is performed to assess the status of the cochlea. Some causes of deafness include Mondini's malformation or dysplasia, in which there is deviation from the normal shape of the cochlea. As noted earlier, the cochlea may become partially or completely filled with bone after meningitis. Radiologically, the no concern category is used for cochleas that are normal and patent. Partially ossified or not completely formed cochleas constitute mild to moderate concern, and great concern is warranted when the cochleas are completely ossified or severely malformed. The otolaryngologist confirms that the child has received meningitis vaccine.

Multiple Handicaps. It is the philosophy of the CHOP cochlear implant program that if a child would benefit from more access to auditory stimulation in the context of developing spoken language skills, a cochlear implant is indicated, no matter how much the child is subject to handicapping condition(s). For the purposes of evaluating candidacy, no concern is the lack of any handicaps other than deafness. Mild to moderate concern is blindness, oral motor disorder, sensory integration issues, learning issues, or attention-deficit disorder or attention-deficit/hyperactivity disorder. Major concern is warranted for global developmental delay or two or more mild to moderate handicapping conditions. Because children are being implanted as young as 1 year of age, some multiple handicapping conditions, such as autism or mental retardation, may not be detected by the time of cochlear implantation.

Audiology. In addition to audiometric hearing levels described earlier, other aspects of the audiometric evaluation are relevant to assessing candidacy. Audiometric test reliability is graded into no concern, mild to moderate concern, or great concern if reliability is good, fair, or poor, respectively. Although hearing aid benefit is assessed through speech perception and audiometric measures, consistency of hearing aid use is also used to determine candidacy. If the hearing aid has been used inconsistently, speech perception scores may not reflect the child's true aided potential. Therefore, no concern is given for a history of consistent hearing aid use, mild to moderate concern for limited hearing aid use (worn more than 50% of the time), and great concern for no history of consistent use (worn less than 50% of the time). Finally, if hearing aids amplify sound to the point at which speech information is available to the child, and the child is able to use this information to develop speech and language skills, a cochlear implant may not be indicated. A child showing no hearing aid benefit is graded in the no concern category by the cochlear implant team. Depending on the amount of functional hearing aid benefit, there may be mild to moderate concern if the child demonstrates some functional hearing aid benefit or great concern for excellent functional hearing aid benefit.

Speech-Language Pathology. Acquisition of spoken language through the implant requires auditory skills. If a child demonstrates consistent auditory training and conditioned responses, there is no concern. There may be mild to moderate concern in children with limited auditory training or great concern in children with no auditory training. When there is some concern regarding a child's auditory training abilities, therapy may be suggested. A child's speech and language abilities are assessed whether the child has written, oral, or manual language. When a child has comprehension and expression of spoken language, emerging or present, the implant team will have no concern. When a child communicates using visual language only or when there is no formal language system in place, a child would be graded in the category of mild to moderate concern or great concern, respectively. Finally, if the child uses age-appropriate attempts to communicate, the desire to communicate will give a rating of no concern. If the child required intervention while taking turns to become engaged in age-appropriate communication, there is mild to moderate concern. A child requiring maximum intervention to elicit communication would be rated with great concern.

Social Work. Family structure and support are crucial to a successful outcome, no matter the form of intervention or communication. A social worker is able to assess the extent to which the family is actively involved with their child and can determine whether there are life stressors external to communication issues that could affect outcome. There is no concern when the family communicates with a child effectively, is actively involved in the child's therapeutic and educational program, and effectively copes with parental stress. Mild to moderate concern is warranted when some family members communicate with the child effectively, the family is not intact but still communicates and supports the child's needs, there is moderate parental stress, and appointments are occasionally canceled or broken during the evaluation process or by history. If a family does not communicate with the child effectively and is not intact, with issues that override the child's needs, and there is severe parental stress and a past history of noncompliance with medical regimens, the social worker may have great concern. There is no concern when a child's behavior is typical for age and there is effective parental control of behavior. In the event of sporadic parental control of a child's behavior or inconsistent engagement in therapy sessions, mild to moderate concern is warranted. Severely hyperactive, aggressive, or defiant behavior, poor parental control of the child's behavior, or consistent disengagement in therapy sessions constitutes major concern.

Parental expectations of the child's outcome with the implant are an important factor to consider in cochlear implant candidacy. Parents must realize that the cochlear implant will not fix the child's hearing and that the implanted child will remain deaf. The parents must realize that progress with the cochlear implant is not sudden and that extensive therapy is required. Parents must realize that their deaf children may always need support from assistive communication services and other deaf individuals. However, parents should expect that with consistent use, follow-up, and therapy, the child will have more access to sound and spoken language. With parents who realize that a cochlear implant will not restore normal hearing and have a rehabilitation or habilitation plan, the rating is no concern. Mild to moderate concern is justified when the parents believe that their child will move to a mainstream setting, with no support services, whose expectations are inflexible, and have no plan for rehabilitation. A cochlear implant team will have great concern if parents inflexibly believe that the cochlear implant will restore normal hearing. If the child is old enough to be able to understand that he or she is being evaluated for cochlear implantation, the child's expectations must also be similarly considered.

Education. The cochlear implant team should help parents make sure that their child's educational placement will maximize success. In so doing, the team has no concern when the child's current educational environment includes an auditory oral class or oral mainstream program. True total communication programs, in which spoken information is provided along with manual communication methods, is also an appropriate educational environment. If auditory-oral communication methods are inconsistently used, auditory therapy is limited, and the child is taught in the context of special education, the team may have mild to moderate concern. In an environment in which the educational philosophy is exclusively manual (American Sign Language only) and there is no auditory therapy, the team would have great concern about the child's candidacy. Similarly, the appropriateness of the child's future transitional educational placement is considered. Within the educational system, the level of availability of support services is evaluated. If staff are trained to work with cochlear implants, understand how to troubleshoot the device, and are equipped to handle minor problems, such as broken cords and drained batteries, the cochlear implant team will have no concern. When cochlear implant experience is limited, there may be mild to moderate concern. When teachers and therapists have no training or are not supportive of cochlear implant use, the team will have great concern. Finally, the ability of the parents to participate in their child's educational program is rated, given the parents' understanding of the educational system and their rights and provisions under the IDEA.

When completed, the ChIP is reviewed with the Cochlear Implant Team. If there are no concerns, appointments are made for final preoperative evaluations and the cochlear implant operation. If issues are identified with concern, some will warrant only more cautious expectations, whereas others may require that further evaluation or therapy occur before implantation is recommended. A number of categories indicating great concern may result in the decision not to perform implantation.

Postoperative Management

If a child receives a cochlear implant, follow-up care retains the multidisciplinary nature of the candidacy assessment.

Audiology. A child will have regularly scheduled programming appointments during which the parameters of the electrical stimulation are adjusted to suit the individual needs of the child. Initially, frequent appointments are scheduled, every 2 weeks, and are then spread out by the end of the first year of device use, every 3 to 6 months. After 1 year of use, the parameters are generally adjusted once or twice annually or as needed. At programming appointments, the signal-processing characteristics of the processor are manipulated and the amount of current delivered to each electrode is adjusted. Adjustment is required as a child's experience with stimulation progresses, as the ability to communicate the audibility of signals matures, and as the ability to demonstrate objective and qualitative preference develops. Signal-processing parameters are determined not only from a child's behavioral responses to sound but also from objective measures, such as the electrically evoked compound action potential and the electrically evoked stapedius reflex. The child's speech perception skills are assessed annually to determine cochlear implant efficacy compared with preimplantation abilities.

Speech-Language Pathology and Therapy. A child uses his or her cochlear implant to develop auditory, speech, and language skills. Therapy to acquire these skills is a crucial component of postoperative care. The duration of therapy recommended for each child will depend on the child's skills, availability of services, and consistency within educational and home environments. Therapy is often recommended on a twice-weekly basis until skills have progressed enough that therapeutic services are no longer necessary. It is important that auditory, speech, and language skills all be developed together. Periodic evaluation marks a child's progress and influences the focus of therapy. Not all children will progress to the level of spoken language relying only on audition. It is crucial that each child be considered individually and appropriate language provided. At the annual evaluation, formal speech and language assessments indicate progress.

Educational Consultation. The ongoing educational environment of a child with a cochlear implant must support oral communication methods. This does not necessarily exclude the use of manual forms of communication, but it may. Furthermore, the quality of the acoustic environment must be optimized to reduce background noise. The role of the educational consultant is to provide information to the parents of a child with a cochlear implant about the best educational options for that particular child. Once the family has chosen an educational route that is most compatible with such factors as for example, their educational philosophy and geographic proximity, the educational consultant can work with the educational agency and family to develop the Individualized Family Service Plan (IFSP) or Individualized Educational Program (IEP). The IFSP and IEP are formal outlines of educational goals and objectives that are required by law for any child with special needs. The IFSP is used for children 0 to 3 years old and the IEP for school-age children.

Otolaryngology. The surgeon annually checks the health status of the patient with the cochlear implant. A routine otologic examination is performed. Particular attention is devoted to examining the health of the skin flap in between the transmitting and receiving antennae. The placement and stability of the internal receiver are also checked. The child is assessed for tinnitus, vestibular problems, any pain associated with the device, and facial nerve involvement. In children with a cochlear implant, ear infections are treated more aggressively because of the possibility of infection spreading into the cochlea and potentially causing meningitis.

CHILDHOOD SPEECH AND LANGUAGE DISORDERS

In the first few years of life, children acquire skills at a tremendous pace. Critical to their ability to learn and interact with others is the development of a conventional communication system. The key components of such a system are language and speech. Language involves comprehension and expression in oral, written, graphic, and manual modalities.[60] Speech is the physical production of oral language.

Many children encounter difficulties acquiring language and/or speech skills. In addition, children may acquire these skills, but then experience a loss of one or more skills as a result of disease or injury. Because of the great variability in types of speech and language disorders, it is difficult to ascertain prevalence among children. Tomblin and colleagues[61] have found the prevalence of specific language impairment (SLI) to be 7.4% in monolingual English-speaking kindergarten children. This did not include children with language disorders related to developmental disabilities. A subsequent study on the same population of children found the prevalence of speech delay to be 3.8%.[62]

A speech-language pathologist is a licensed professional trained in the identification and treatment of those with speech and language disorders. The speech-language pathologist must determine the type and severity of the disorder and implement an appropriate plan of treatment. Ongoing evaluation of treatment efficacy as the child progresses is an essential component of the treatment plan.

Language Disorders

Any impairment in the understanding or use of language constitutes a language disorder. Speech-language pathologists refer to receptive language delays or impairments when children do not understand language at an age-appropriate level. Expressive language delay or impairment reflects difficulties using language appropriately. Receptive and expressive language deficits can be in the form (phonology, morphology, syntax), content (semantics), or function (pragmatics) of language.[63] Language disorders can be developmental (i.e., present at birth or at an early stage of language development) or acquired (i.e., occurring after a significant period of language development).

Specific Language Impairment

SLI reflects difficulties in acquiring age-appropriate language skills in the absence of any related mental deficiency, sensory and physical deficit, severe emotional disturbance, environmental factor, or brain damage.[64] Children can demonstrate an expressive language disorder in the presence of age-appropriate receptive language skills or a disorder of both receptive and expressive language skills. In theory, children's receptive language skills cannot be less developed than their expressive skills. That is, they need the language comprehension to support their development of expression. However, some children will perform more poorly on receptive language tasks because of other factors (e.g., attentional difficulties or auditory processing problems).

Developmental Language Disorders

Delayed or atypical development of language skills is a component of certain disabilities diagnosed in childhood. These include but are not limited to global developmental delay, mental retardation, pervasive developmental disorder–autism spectrum disorder (PDD-ASD), and language learning disability. In addition, language disorders are commonly seen in many genetic syndromes. In general, developmental language disorders differ from SLI in that the rate and extent of progress in gaining skills may be limited by the child's overall cognitive development. Language skills will be acquired at a much slower pace and many children will not reach age appropriate levels. In addition, the language characteristics in some developmental disabilities (e.g., PDD-ASD) are atypical, not following a usual sequence of acquisition. Many children with autism acquire some linguistic skills but struggle with using these skills for successful communication.[65] For example, a young child with autism may see a ball in a picture and label it "ball," but not ask for a ball that he wants to play with that is up on a shelf, out of his reach.

Other diagnoses that may affect language development include sensory impairments (hearing loss, visual impairment), maternal substance abuse, psychiatric disorders, and attention deficit hyperactivity disorder (ADHD). Selective mutism is a disorder in which children may have age- level language skills but do not communicate in particular environments. The speech-language pathologist plays a key role in determining if there is a language component to the problem and collaborating with a psychologist to facilitate communication in the environments in which the child is not communicating.

Acquired Language Disorder

An acquired language disorder occurs as a direct result of injury or disease. This may be a result of a focal lesion or diffuse injury. Causes include cerebrovascular accident, seizure disorder, tumor(s), infection, radiation, and traumatic brain injury (TBI). Common causes of TBI in young children are falls, car accidents, and abuse. Outcomes can be grossly predicted by the degree of coma, length of time in coma, and duration of post-traumatic amnesia.[66] Acquired language disorder differs from developmental language disorder in that children do not have the same communication skills that they once had. The challenge to speech-language pathologists and educators is that the injury occurs during the development of language skills. Therefore, children will be relearning skills and developing new language skills with a system that is not functioning normally. Language characteristics seen in acquired language disorder include language comprehension deficits (including verbal abstraction and drawing inferences), difficulty learning new linguistic material, problems expressing complex ideas, and poor organization of verbal and written information.[66] In addition, these children may exhibit word-finding problems and paraphasic errors (i.e., the substitution of inappropriate sounds, words, or phrases). Spoken or written language may sound inappropriate, irrelevant, fragmented, illogical, tangential, concrete, and confused. There are typically concomitant cognitive deficits related to attention, concentration, short-term memory, long-term memory, information-processing speed, and reasoning.

Assessment and Interventions

An assessment of a child's language skills requires a thorough history, including information regarding communication, medical, family, social, and educational backgrounds. Results of previous testing are important to obtain, including hearing and visual assessments and developmental and cognitive testing. For school-age children, it is critical to know about their academic performance. The evaluation incorporates standardized measures, therapeutic observations during unstructured and structured tasks, language analysis, and parent report. The child's language skills are compared with developmental norms and expectations of skills for children of the same chronologic age. The pattern of language skills indicates a general delay in skill acquisition, atypical or impaired characteristics, or skills that are within the range of acceptability for the child's age.

For children with delayed language skills, the speech-language pathologist identifies where along the developmental sequence the child's language skills fall and develops a plan to progress the child along the sequence. For children with impaired or atypical language skills, such as is seen in PDD-ASD, intervention focuses on developing functional communication skills within the environments in which that the child needs to communicate on a regular basis. These children will likely demonstrate splinter skills—that is, will have some skills that are at or close to age level and lack skills that emerge earlier in the typically developing child. For example, a child with PDD-ASD may be able to label a large number of pictures of common objects, but not be able to point to the same pictures when they are named by another individual. The development of functional communication skills may take the form of verbal communication or involve the use of augmentative and alternative forms of communication. Because social interaction skills can be so difficult for children with PDD-ASD, augmentative communication strategies focus on teaching the child that communication involves the exchange of information between two people. A popular method used for this training is the Picture Exchange Communication System.[67]

Assessment of children with acquired language disorders begins with identifying the level of coma that the child is in, or their general orientation to person, time, and place. The Rancho Los Amigos Coma Scale[68] offers an eight-step scale for use with children to describe the child's level of alertness, responsiveness, and general orientation. The language assessment identifies the areas and extent of deficit that the child is experiencing. Goals of treatment focus on improving residual functioning, structured tasks to develop functional and adaptive behaviors (language comprehension, simple verbal problem solving, and use of self-monitoring to detect and self-correct errors), and integrating communication skills within the classroom and educational program.

Outcomes of intervention vary significantly, depending on the severity and type of disorder. With appropriate intervention, many young children with SLI are able to gain age-level language skills. Other children will continue to struggle to acquire more advanced language skills over the years and will likely develop language-based learning difficulties. Children with cognitive impairments are likely to have lifelong language deficits. Speech-language therapy is provided to ensure that children meet their maximum potential for communicative success.

Speech Disorders

Developmental Articulation Disorders

Articulation errors are common in children. When errors are inappropriate for age or when they affect a child's intelligibility to others, they become clinically significant. Speech production requires integrity of the structures of speech, neuromotor skills, cognitive skills, and hearing. A speech disorder may result from difficulties in any of these areas. Errors in articulation are characterized by substitutions, omissions, or distortions of the sounds of speech. The speech characteristics of children with articulation disorders are variable.

Developmental phonologic disorder is a term often used to describe systematic speech sound errors in a child's language that are of unknown cause. Children with developmental phonologic disorders have difficulty perceiving and producing the features of speech sounds, such as place, manner, or voicing. Articulation describes the placement of the oral structures during speech production. For example, /g/ and /k/ are described as velar sounds, while /m/ and /b/ are described as labial sounds. These sounds are further categorized by the manner of production or how the oral air stream is managed. For example, /p/ is a stop plosive in which the air stream is obstructed and released. An /s/ is a fricative in which a continuous friction of air is maintained throughout the production of the individual sound. Voicing refers to the presence or absence of vibration of the vocal cords. Voicing is present for /b/ but absent for /p/, whereas both of these sounds are produced with the same place and manner of production.

Developmental phonologic disorders are the most common form of speech disorders. Because of differences in methodology and age and criteria used to define speech disorder, prevalence estimates vary from 2% to 13%.[62] Males are at increased risk for developmental speech disorders, with ratios varying from 1.5:1 to 3:1. The role of fluctuating or conductive hearing loss on speech development is controversial. Studies are also ongoing evaluating the possible role of genetics in this disorder. Children with phonologic disorders often have coexisting developmental language disorders. Early speech delay is also associated with reading and spelling disorders that occur later.

Motor Speech Disorders

Dysarthria

Dysarthria refers to motor speech disorders that result from deficits in motor control secondary to central or peripheral nervous system damage. Children with this diagnosis may exhibit weakness, paralysis, or incoordination of the musculature responsible for respiration, phonation, articulation, and resonation. Disorders of muscle tone and reflexes may also be present. Dysarthria is associated with unilateral and bilateral lesions of the upper or lower motor neurons, basal ganglia, cerebellum, and cranial and/or spinal nerves.[69] Dysarthria can also result from inflammatory processes, toxicity, metabolic disorders, or tumors. Different types of dysarthria can often be distinguished by clinical symptoms, such as rate, vocal quality, resonance, stress, and slurred articulation. Types of dysarthria include flaccid, spastic, ataxic, hypokinetic, hyperkinetic, and mixed types. Dysarthria can be congenital; it can appear in children with cerebral palsy, in syndromic conditions, or in isolation. It can also be acquired, such as in patients with brain injury or degenerative neurologic disorders.

Apraxia

Apraxia of speech is another type of motor speech disorder but one that is not well defined and whose features are somewhat controversial. Descriptions of apraxia often cite difficulties in motor planning and executing oral speech movements. Usually, there is no abnormality of tone, reflexes, or automatic acts. Nonspeech oral motor movements are typically not affected. Although there is wide disparity in the description of apraxia, most characterizations of the disorder include some of the following features: groping, searching, or effortful volitional oral movements, difficulty sequencing or transitioning from one sound to another, difficulty imitating speech, inconsistency in articulation with repeated productions of the same utterance, errors in vowels as well as consonants, and abnormalities of prosody, including rate, rhythm, and stress patterns. Although dysarthria is a more static condition, apraxia may have a developmental or maturational component. The site of lesion is not clear in apraxia, but is more commonly associated with cortical and white matter lesions.[70]

Structural Disorders

Speech errors may also result from abnormalities in the structures of the speech mechanism, such as the size and relative positions of the dental arches, cleft palate (overt or submucosal), craniofacial anomalies, and size and position of the tongue.

Ankyloglossia (tongue tie), or tethering of the anterior tip of the tongue, is rarely associated with speech problems. In those cases, children may be unable to mobilize the tongue to produce tongue tip sounds, such as /d/, /s/, and /l/.

Fluency Disorders

Fluency disorders are characterized by disruptions in the rate, rhythm, effort, and/or continuity of speech.[71] Typically, these disruptions result in a reduced ability to initiate, coordinate or maintain the proper movements required for speech production. In addition, fluency disorders frequently include affective, psychosocial, cognitive, and/or physiologic variables, which further complicate the problem.

The most common fluency disorder is stuttering, which is characterized by an abnormally high frequency and/or duration of stoppages in the forward flow of speech.[72] These disruptions usually present as the following:

- Repetitions of sound (m-m-m-mommy)
- Prolongations of sound (baaaaaall)
- Blocks of the airflow to support speech

Children who stutter frequently present with secondary behaviors that result when the individual attempts to hide from, avoid, or mask the basic stuttering behaviors. These may include head twitching, facial grimacing, moving the arms or legs, tapping the hands or feet, switching words, increasing tension, changing pitch or loudness, and avoiding talking secondary to fears of stuttering. Although it is typical for stuttering to develop slowly in a systematic fashion, children can present with severe behaviors close to onset.[73]

During language acquisition or periods of increased pressure, many children struggle with language formulation and organization. This is especially true between the ages of 2½ and 5 years, when language skills are emerging. These periods of uncertainty are frequently marked by dysfluencies in the child's speech. The most common types of normal dysfluency include hesitations, interjections (uhm, well, like), phrase revisions (I want, I need cake), and whole-word repetitions (my, my sister is nice). Guitar has proposed that normal dysfluencies should occur in less than 10% of a child's words.[72]

Treatment of fluency disorders is most successful when initiated before the development of any negative speech-related attitudes. As a result, early identification and intervention are imperative for successful treatment. Physicians should refer families to specialized programs or to speech-language pathologists who specialize in this type of disorder.

Voice Disorders

A voice disorder is an abnormality in vocal quality, pitch, or loudness; this may be congenital or acquired. Hoarseness and breathiness are common voice quality disturbances. Pitch deviations may be present, such as a pitch that is too high or too low for the child's age and gender. Vocal volume may be too low or too high for comfortable listening. There may be voice breaks or aphonia. The incidence of voice disorders in school-age children ranges from 6% to 23%.[74]

A voice disorder may result from anatomic, physiologic, or functional causes. Anatomic causes of voice disorders include structural anomalies such as webs or stenosis, growths in and around the larynx (e.g., papilloma, cysts or tumor), or local inflammation (viral infection or allergy). Physiologic causes include paralysis of the nerves supplying the larynx, either as an isolated occurrence or as a part of a more complex neurologic problem. Trauma to the larynx from a foreign body or prolonged intubation may cause structural and/or physiologic alterations in the voice.

On the other hand, functional voice disorders occur in the absence of a physiologic cause and are typically related to environmental or psychogenic factors. Causes of functional voice disorders can be characterized by imitation, faulty learning, psychological causes, or disturbed maturation during the period of voice change in children, which may cause strain in the vocal apparatus.[75] Functional voice disturbances are much less common than those secondary to physiologic or structural causes.

Often, both physiologic and functional components are present in the development of voice changes. For example, vocal nodules, the most common form of voice disorder in children, are structural changes of the vocal cords that occur as a result of misuse or overuse of the voice, such as excessive talking, emphatic talking, or screaming. Studies have shown that approximately 50% of children with voice disorders have vocal nodules.[76]

Resonance Disorders

Resonance refers to the amount of air in the oral and nasal cavities during speech. Hypernasality occurs when too much air escapes into the nose and may result from an overt or submucous cleft palate or dysfunction of the velopharyngeal mechanism. Velopharyngeal inadequacy (VPI) has various structural and physiologic causes, such as palatopharyngeal disproportion or neuromuscular disorder. Hyponasality refers to the condition in which too little air is present in the nose during speech. This is often seen with nasal airway obstruction, which can be caused by enlarged adenoids, swollen nasal turbinates, or nasal polyps.

Augmentative and Alternative Communication

For children who have insufficient speech skills to be functional communicators, augmentative or alternative forms of communication need to be investigated. There is a wide variety of types of augmentative communication options available, including manual signs, picture communication boards (in which the child points to a picture to convey a message), basic electronic communication devices with a limited number of recorded messages, and sophisticated computerized devices with language-based software that allow the child to compose novel, grammatically intact messages. Assessment focuses on identifying the appropriate techniques and equipment that the child can use to communicate at a level consistent with his or her cognitive and linguistic skills.

SWALLOWING AND FEEDING DISORDERS

Swallowing and feeding disorders comprise another area of assessment and intervention for speech-language pathologists. *Swallowing* is a complex task that requires the coordination of both neuromuscular and respiratory systems.[77] *Feeding disorders* is a more global term that includes swallowing difficulties, failure to thrive, failure to achieve developmental milestones related to feeding skills, and behavioral challenges related to food refusal and food selectivity. The ability to swallow safely (i.e., without aspiration) and feed effectively and efficiently can be directly related to various congenital and acquired medical issues (e.g., neurologic, gastrointestinal, cardiac, respiratory, genetic, anatomic).

General Considerations

Swallowing

The swallow is composed of four phases: (1) oral preparatory, (2) oral, (3) pharyngeal, and, (4) esophageal.[77] During the oral preparatory phase, a voluntary phase, the bolus of food is prepared (e.g., mastication, bolus formation) and transferred toward the base of the tongue. The lips remain closed, the soft palate is relaxed, and the airway is open. The oral phase involves the elevation of the tongue to move the bolus posteriorly into the pharynx. The pharyngeal phase is an involuntary stage that begins as the base of the tongue propels the bolus into the pharynx. During this phase, the soft palate is elevated and retracted to protect the nasopharyngeal region, the larynx is elevated, and the lowering of the epiglottis aids in directing food into the pyriform sinuses through the cricopharyngeal region and into the esophagus. In addition, the true and false vocal folds adduct to provide added protection against aspiration. The esophageal phase involves peristaltic action, which moves the bolus down the esophagus and through the esophageal sphincter into the stomach. Impairment in any of these phases is diagnosed as dysphagia.[78]

Children must adjust their swallowing skills to adapt to a changing anatomy and the introduction of various food textures over the first few years of life. In an infant, the coordination of sucking, swallowing, and breathing is extremely important. Over time, a child's ability to advance to thicker, higher textures is dependent on his or her oral-motor, gross and fine motor, and cognitive development, as well as maturation of the gastrointestinal tract.

Feeding

Disordered feeding behaviors most often stem from underlying medical issues that need to be addressed prior to focusing on the residual behaviors that have developed.[77] For both the child and parents, maintaining a pleasant and social mealtime environment can be extremely challenging as the focus turns to dealing with less desirable behaviors and monitoring the quantity of oral intake. Speech-language pathologists assist parents in determining the most appropriate textures and oral feeding strategies to provide increased acceptance and intake.

Assessment and Interventions

Swallowing and feeding assessments are completed by a speech-language pathologist as a member of a team of professionals (e.g., developmental pediatrician, gastroenterologist, nutritionist, psychologist, physical therapist, occupational therapist) who consider multiple factors that may be affecting a child's ability to feed orally. For the speech-language pathologist, a swallowing and feeding assessment involves obtaining a complete medical and feeding history, as well as completing an oral-motor examination and feeding observation. The child's positioning, respiratory status, behaviors, and level of alertness are carefully considered. If an aspiration risk is identified and clinical adjustments (e.g., different equipment, position changes) are unsuccessful, instrumental evaluations may be completed. Swallow function may be directly observed by speech-language pathologists via a video fluoroscopic swallow study (VFSS), also known as a modified barium swallow study (MBSS), which is a video x-ray taken from the lateral and/or anteroposterior view that allows for observation of the swallow phases. A second option for evaluating swallow safety is fiberoptic endoscopic evaluation of swallowing (FEES), which may be completed jointly with an otolaryngologist. This is a more invasive means by which to evaluate swallowing but allows for visualization of the pharyngeal area from above just prior to and immediately following the pharyngeal phase of the swallow.

The speech-language pathologist's role in the management of swallowing and feeding disorders includes optimizing oral-motor skills for bolus management and preparation, providing appropriate equipment (e.g., nipple, spoon, seating) and swallow strategies to elicit safe swallows, and varying size, taste, texture, and temperature of food. Most important, frequent contact with other team members and consideration of all the medical and psychological factors that may contribute to swallowing and feeding disorders are vital to maintain a consistent approach to feeding advancement.

SUMMARY

In summary, early identification, comprehensive assessment, and appropriate intervention are critical to optimizing the communication abilities of the pediatric population across childhood. Audiologists and speech-language pathologists are the professionals singularly qualified by their training and experience to provide comprehensive early detection, assessment, and intervention programs. These professionals work in collaboration with educators, social workers, family wellness counselors, psychologists, physical and occupational therapists, and otolaryngologists and other medical specialists to diagnose and evaluate each child with a communication disorder.

Critical to the success of children who have communication disorders and their families is the ongoing care and surveillance provided by the pediatrician. Moreover, the pediatrician plays a critical role in the identification of children with possible communication disorders, the medical diagnosis or etiology and other co-existing conditions, and the long-term follow-up care and support of the child and family. Box 3-3 provides ways to improve the follow-up of children who fail newborn hearing screening.

Today, early detection methods and the availability of early intervention programs provide an unprecedented opportunity for children who are born with or acquire

Box 3-3 Ways to Improve Follow-up of Children Who Fail Newborn Hearing Screening

Take responsibility.
Develop a protocol.
Obtain the family's contact information.
Connect the child with a "medical home."
Give office staff a lead role.
Offer broad-based institutional support.
Cross-train staff.
Communicate accurately and carefully.
Be sensitive to cultural and other differences.
Explain how hearing loss can hamper a child's speech and language development.
Use incentives, when appropriate, such as travel vouchers.
Perform the follow-up test while the parents are still in the hospital.
Combine the follow-up test with well-baby checkups.
Involve the entire family in the screening.
Equip parents with information for decision making.
Use a family-centered approach.

Adapted from National Institute on Deafness and other Communication Disorders (NIDCD): How Medical and Other Health Professionals Can Help Increase the Number of Infants with Return for Follow-up. Available at http://www.nidcd.nih.gov/health/hearing/professionals.asp

Table 3-2 Developmental Milestones for Communication Development

Age	Hearing	Receptive Language	Expressive Language (Speech)
Birth-3 mo	Reacts, startles, and awakens to loud sounds, including voices Increases or decreases sucking behavior response to sound Turns head toward speaker's voice	Seems to recognize caregivers voice, is soothed, and quiets to it Quiets or smiles when spoken to	Makes pleasurable sounds (cooing, gooing) Cries differently for different needs Smiles when sees caregiver
4-6 mo	Looks upward and turns toward the direction of a new sound Notices and enjoys toys that make sounds Pays attention to music Becomes scared by loud voice	Responds to "no-no" and changes in tone of voice	Babbles speechlike sounds Produces many different sounds, including *p, b, m* Vocalizes excitement and displeasure Makes gurgling sounds when left alone, playing with his or her own voice Makes sounds when playing with caregiver (reciprocal vocalizations) Begins to repeat sounds
7 mo- 1 yr	Turns and looks in the direction of the source of sounds, such as telephone ringing Exhibits listening behaviors when music present or to toys that make noise Responds to soft sounds as well as moderate and loud sounds	Listens when spoken to Recognizes words for common objects ("cup," "shoe," "milk") Begins responding to verbal requests ("come here"; "want more?") Responds to his or her own name Looks at objects or pictures when caregiver talks about them Enjoys games like peek-a-boo and pat-a-cake	Tries to communicate by action or gesture Babbles long and short groups of sounds (reduplicative, canonical babbling—tatata, bababa) Makes babbling sounds even when alone Shows enjoyment in the sound and feel of his or her own voice: plays with his or her voice Uses speech or noncrying sounds to get and keep caregiver's attention Imitates different speech sounds in response to caregiver Begins to try and imitate words Has one or two words (bye-bye; dada), although utterances may not be clear
1-2 yr	More attentive to video or books when there is a sound accompanying the activity	Points to simple body parts when requested ("nose," "mouth") Follows simple directions ("kiss the baby," "wave bye-bye," "give me the ball") Listens to simple stories, songs, and rhymes Understands simple "yes-no" questions ("Do you want more?") Understands simple phrases ("in the cup," "on the table") Enjoys being read to; attends to book or toy for about 2 minutes Points to familiar pictures in book when asked ("where's the doggie?") Knows 10-20 words	Number of words spoken (vocabulary) grows every month Asks for common foods by name Makes animal sounds, such as "moo" Starts putting two words together ("more cookie," "no more") Uses some two-word questions: ("Where mommy?" or "What's that?") Correctly pronounces most vowels and *n, m, p, h* at the beginning of words Begins to use other consonant sounds at the beginning of words Says 8-10 words Begins to use pronouns such as "mine"

Continued

Table 3-2 Developmental Milestones for Communication Development—cont'd

Age	Hearing	Receptive Language	Expressive Language (Speech)
2-3 yr		Knows about 50 words at 24 mo Knows meaning of or differences between (or both) descriptive words (go-stop, big-little, up-down) Knows spatial concepts ("in," "on") Knows pronouns (e.g., you, me, her) Understands "not now" and "no more" Follows simple directions ("put on your shoes"; "drink your milk" Follows two requests ("go get the book and put it on the table") Understands many action words (run, jump)	Says around 40 words at 24 mo Often asks for or directs attention to objects by naming them Speaks in two- or three-word "sentences" Answers simple questions Uses question inflection to ask for something ("my ball"?) Speech is understood by familiar listeners most of the time; strangers may not understand what is said Speech is becoming more clear; ends of words (final sounds) may still be left off Begins using more pronouns ("you," "I") Begins to use plurals ("shoes") and past tense of verbs ("jumped")
3-4 yr	Responds when called from another room Hears TV, CD, or radio at same level as other family members	Groups objects such as food, clothes Can identify colors Understands simple, "who," "what," "where," and "why" questions Has fun with language; enjoys poems; recognizes language absurdities, such as "Is that a dog on your head?"	Uses most speech sounds, but may distort some (e.g., *l, r, s, sh, ch, y, v, z, th)* (NOTE: these sounds may not be spoken correctly until 7-8 yr) Uses consonants in the beginning, middle, and end of words (although more difficult words may be distorted, as noted earlier) Talks about activities at school or at friends' homes Talks about feelings and ideas, not just describing the world around her or him Strangers usually understand much of the child's speech Uses a lot of sentences that have four or more words Can describe the use of objects such as "fork" and "car" Uses verbs that end in "-ing" (e.g., running, jumping) Answers simple questions "What do you do when you get hungry?" Can repeat full sentences Usually talks easily without hesitating or repeating syllables or words
4-5 yr		Understands spatial concepts such as "behind" and "next to" Understands complex questions Pays attention to short story and answers simple questions about it Shows understanding of most of what is said at home and in school *By 5 yr,* understands more than 2000 words; understands time sequences; carries out three-step directions; understands rhyming	Says about 200-300 different words Voice sounds clear, like other children's Use sentences that include details; can describe how to do things Can define words Tells stories and sticks to topic Communicates easily with other children and adults Speech is clear except for long, difficult, or complex words Uses the same grammar as his or her family Uses some irregular past tense verbs, such as "ran" and "fell" Can list items that are within a category such as animals or food Answers "why" questions *By 5 yr,* engages in conversation; speaks in sentences up to eight words and longer; uses compound and complex sentences; describes objects; uses imagination to create and tell stories

Adapted from the American Speech-Language-Hearing Association (ASHA): How Does Your Child Hear and Talk? 2006 (http://www.asha.org/public/speech/development/child_hear_talk.htm); National Institute on Deafness and Other Communication Disorders (NIDCD): Silence Isn't Always Golden, 2006 (http://www.nidcd.nih.gov/health/hearing/silence.asp); American Academy of Pediatrics: Childhood Hearing: A Sound Foundation in the Medical Home, 2005 (http://www.medicalhomeinfo.org/screening/ Screen Materials/PediaLink Launch Article.doc); Education Resources Information Center: (http://www.eric.ed.gov/); Coplan J: Normal speech and language development: an overview. Pediatr Rev 1995;16:91-100; and Better Hearing Institute: 2005 (http://www.betterhearing.org).

disorders in their abilities to communicate that may involve disorders of hearing, speech, and language. In addition, disorders of feeding and swallowing are included in those conditions that are within the scope of practice of professionals who specialize in childhood communication disorders. Because the pediatrician is critical to the early identification of all forms of communication disorders, we conclude this chapter with a checklist compiled from various sources to assist the physician in the detection of communication disorders in their patients throughout childhood. Table 3-2 provides developmental milestones for communication compiled from numerous sources. These are intended to assist the pediatrician in the identification of infants and children who are at risk for communication disorders at various ages. Collaboration among the pediatrician, audiologist, speech-language pathologist, and family provides the optimal model for the follow-up of at-risk children, as well as those diagnosed with various communication disorders.

ACKNOWLEDGMENTS

We wish to acknowledge our colleagues in the Center for Childhood Communication at the Children's Hospital of Philadelphia whose daily work has made lives better for children with communication disorders. This chapter is a reflection of the excellent services and compassionate care provided to families daily by those in audiology, speech-language pathology, social work, counseling, and education. We are proud to represent their efforts in this chapter. In particular we thank Joy Peterson and Roger Marsh for their assistance in the development of this chapter.

MAJOR POINTS

Newborn hearing screening using physiologic tests (OAE and ABR) can identify infants with permanent congenital hearing loss.

Comprehensive audiologic assessment requires both behavioral and electrophysiologic tests to delineate hearing sensitivity.

Functional auditory abilities are important to monitor over time.

Hearing aids are fitted as soon as audiologic and medical evaluations have confirmed the presence of hearing loss.

Other assistive listening devices such as FM systems are useful for children with various forms of hearing loss who listen to speech in background noise.

When traditional hearing aids are insufficient to provide speech audibility, the child is evaluated for cochlear implantation.

A multidisciplinary team, along with input from the family, is critical for optimal follow-up of children with hearing loss.

Language and speech disorders can be identified at early ages.

Feeding and swallowing disorders are within the scope of practice of speech-language pathologists.

The differential diagnosis of language impairments is critical in the assessment of children suspected of having other developmental disabilities.

REFERENCES

1. Kuhl PK, Williams KA, Lacerda F, et al: Linguistic experience alters phonetic perception in infants by 6 months of age. Science 1992;31;255:606-608.
2. Oller DK, Eilers RE, Urbano R, Cobo-Lewis AB: Development of precursors to speech in infants exposed to two languages. J Child Lang 1997;24:407-425.
3. Eilers RE, Oller DK: Infant vocalizations and the early diagnosis of severe hearing impairment. J Pediatr 1994;124:199-203.
4. Oller DK, Eilers RE, Neal AR, Schwartz HK: Precursors to speech in infancy: The prediction of speech and language disorders. J Commun Disord 1999;32:223-245.
5. Rescorla L, Mirak J: Normal language acquisition. Semin Pediatr Neurol 1997;4:70-76.
6. Rescorla L, Alley A: Validation of the language development survey (LDS): A parent report tool for identifying language delay in toddlers. J Speech Lang Hear Res 2001;44: 434-445.
7. Rescorla L: Language and reading outcomes to age 9 in late-talking toddlers. J Speech Lang Hear Res 2002;45: 360-371.
8. Rescorla L: Age 13 language and reading outcomes in late-talking toddlers. J Speech Lang Hear Res 2005;48:459-472.
9. Early identification of hearing impairment in infants and young children. NIH Consensus Statement 1993;11: 1-24.
10. Johnson JL, White KR, Widen JE, et al: A multicenter evaluation of how many infants with permanent hearing loss pass a two-stage otoacoustic emissions/automated auditory brainstem response newborn hearing screening protocol. Pediatrics 2005;116:663-672.
11. Prieve B, Dalzell L, Berg A, et al: The New York State Universal Newborn Hearing Screening Demonstration Project: outpatient outcome measures. Ear Hear 2000;21: 104-117.
12. American Academy of Pediatrics Joint Committee on Infant Hearing: Joint Committee on Infant Hearing 1994 position statement. Pediatrics 1995;95:152-156.
13. Fortnum HM, Summerfield AQ, Marshall DH, et al: Prevalence of permanent childhood hearing impairment in the United Kingdom and implications for universal neonatal hearing screening: Questionnaire based ascertainment study. BMJ 2001;323:536-540.

14. Centers for Disease Control and Prevention (CDC): Serious hearing impairment among children aged 3-10 years—Atlanta, Georgia, 1991-1993. MMWR Morb Mortal Wkly Rep 1997;46:1073-1076.

15. Holmes AE, Niskar AS, Kieszak SM, et al: Mean and median hearing thresholds among children 6 to 19 years of age: The Third National Health and Nutrition Examination Survey, 1988 to 1994, United States. Ear Hear 2004;25: 397-402.

16. Bess FH, Dodd-Murphy J, Parker RA: Children with minimal sensorineural hearing loss: Prevalence, educational performance, and functional status. Ear Hear 1998;19339-554.

17. Niskar AS, Kieszak SM, Holmes AE, et al: Estimated prevalence of noise-induced hearing threshold shifts among children 6 to 19 years of age: The Third National Health and Nutrition Examination Survey, 1988-1994, United States. Pediatrics 2002;109:987-988.

18. Carney AE, Moeller MP: Treatment efficacy: Hearing loss in children. J Speech Lang Hear Res 1998;41:S61-S84.

19. Bess FH, Tharpe AM: Unilateral hearing impairment in children. Pediatrics 1984;74:206-216.

20. Joint Committee on Infant Hearing: Year 2000 position statement: Principles and guidelines for early hearing detection and intervention programs. Pediatrics 2000; 106:798-817.

21. Northern J, Downs M: Hearing in Children, 5th ed. Baltimore, Williams & Wilkins, 2002.

22. Rapin I, Gravel J; "Auditory neuropathy": Physiologic and pathologic evidence calls for more diagnostic specificity. Int J Pediatr Otorhinolaryngol 2003;67:707-728.

23. American Academy of Pediatrics Periodicity Schedule: Recommendations for Preventive Pediatric Health Care. Elk Grove Village, Ill, American Academy of Pediatrics, 2000.

24. American Speech-Language-Hearing Association: Guidelines for Audiologic Screening, 1996. Available at http://www.asha.org/NR/rdonlyres/A13D0ECC-684B-4E33-BA0E-CAF6681CEDEB/0/v4GLAudScreening.pdf.

25. White KR: The current status of EHDI programs in the United States. Ment Retard Dev Disabil Res Rev 2003; 9:79-88.

26. National Center for Hearing Assessment and Management. Available at www.infanthearing.org.

27. White KR, Maxon AB: Universal screening for infant hearing impairment: Simple, beneficial, and presently justified. Int J Pediatr Otorhinolaryngol 1995;32:201-211.

28. Harrison M, Roush J, Wallace J: Trends in age of identification and intervention in infants with hearing loss. Ear Hear 2003;24:89-95.

29. Norton SJ, Gorga MP, Widen JE, et al: Identification of neonatal hearing impairment: Evaluation of transient evoked otoacoustic emission, distortion product otoacoustic emission, and auditory brain stem response test performance. Ear Hear 2000;21:508-528.

30. Gravel J, Berg A, Bradley M, et al: New York State Universal Newborn Hearing Screening Demonstration Project: Effects of screening protocol on inpatient outcome measures. Ear Hear 2000;21:131-140.

31. Office of Disease Prevention and Health Promotion, U.S. Department of Health and Human Services: Healthy People 2010. Available at www.healthypeople.gov.

32. Widen JE, Johnson JL, White KR, et al: A multisite study to examine the efficacy of the otoacoustic emission/automated auditory brainstem response newborn hearing screening protocol: Results of visual reinforcement audiometry. Am J Audiol 2005;14:S200-S216.

33. Cone-Wesson B, Vohr BR, Sininger YS, et al: Identification of neonatal hearing impairment: infants with hearing loss. Ear Hear 2000;21:488-507.

34. Rosenfeld RM, Culpepper L, Doyle KJ, et al; American Academy of Pediatrics Subcommittee on Otitis Media with Effusion; American Academy of Family Physicians; American Academy of Otolaryngology—Head and Neck Surgery: Clinical practice guideline: Otitis media with effusion. Otolaryngol Head Neck Surg 2004;130(5 Suppl): S95-S118.

35. American Speech-Language-Hearing-Association: Guidelines for the Audiological Assessment of Children from Birth to Five Years of Age, 2004. Available at http:www.asha.org/members/deskref-journals/deskref/default.

36. Gravel JS, Hood LJ: Pediatric audiologic assessment. In FE Musiek, WF Rintelmann (eds): Contemporary Perspective: Hearing Assessment. Boston, Allyn and Bacon, 1999, pp 305-326.

37. Jerger J: Suggested nomenclature for impedance audiometry. Arch Otolaryngol 1972;96:1-3.

38. Roush J, Bryant K, Mundy M, et al: Developmental changes in static admittance and tympanometric width in infants and toddlers. J Am Acad Audiol 1995;6:334-338.

39. Koebsell KA, Margolis RH: Tympanometric gradient measured from normal preschool children. Audiology 1986;25: 149-157.

40. Margolis RH, Bass-Ringdahl S, Hanks WD, et al: Tympanometry in newborn infants—1 kHz norms. J Am Acad Audiol 2003;14:383-392.

41. Widen JE, O'Grady GM: Otoacoustic emissions in the evaluation of children. In Glattke T, Robinette M (eds): Otoacoustic Emissions: Clinical Applications. New York, Thieme, 2002, pp 375-415.

42. Gorga MP, Neely ST, Ohlrich B,et al: From laboratory to clinic: A large-scale study of distortion product otoacoustic emissions in ears with normal hearing and ears with hearing loss. Ear Hear 1997;18:440-455.

43. Schmida MJ, Peterson HJ, Tharpe AM: Visual reinforcement audiometry using digital video disc and conventional reinforcers. Am J Audiol 2003;12:35-40.

44. American Academy of Audiology: Pediatric Amplification Protocol 2003. Available at http://www.audiology.org/NR/rdonlyres/53D26792-E321-41AF-850F-CC253310F9DB/0/pedamp.pdf

45. Waltzman SB, Cohen NL, Shapiro WH: Sensory aids in conjunction with cochlear implants. Am J Otol 1992 Jul;13:308-312.

46. Waltzman SB, Cohen NL, Roland JT Jr: A comparison of the growth of open-set speech perception between the

nucleus 22 and nucleus 24 cochlear implant systems. Am J Otol 1999;20:435-441.

47. Zwolan TA, Kileny PR, Ashbaugh C, Telian SA: Patient performance with the Cochlear Corporation "20 + 2" implant: Bipolar versus monopolar activation. Am J Otol 1996;17:717-723.

48. Bollard PM, Chute PM, Popp A, Parisier SC: Specific language growth in young children using the CLARION cochlear implant. Ann Otol Rhinol Laryngol Suppl 1999;177:119-123.

49. Cheng AK, Grant GD, Niparko JK: Meta-analysis of pediatric cochlear implant literature. Ann Otol Rhinol Laryngol Suppl 1999;177:124-128.

50. Meyer TA, Svirsky MA, Kirk KI, Miyamoto RT: Improvements in speech perception by children with profound prelingual hearing loss: Effects of device, communication mode, and chronologic age. J Speech Lang Hear Res 1998;41:846-858.

51. Osberger MJ, Fisher L, Zimmerman-Phillips S, et al: Speech recognition performance of older children with cochlear implants. Am J Otol 1998;19:152-157.

52. Cohen NL, Waltzman SB, Roland JT Jr, et al: Early results using the nucleus CI24M in children. Am J Otol 1999;20:198-204.

53. Kirk KI, Pisoni DB, Osberger MJ: Lexical effects on spoken word recognition by pediatric cochlear implant users. Ear Hear 1995;16:470-481.

54. Osberger MJ, Geier L, Zimmerman-Phillips S, Barker MJ: Use of a parent-report scale to assess benefit in children given the Clarion cochlear implant. Am J Otol 1997;18(Suppl):S79-S80.

55. Robbins AM, Renshaw JJ, Berry SW: Evaluating meaningful auditory integration in profoundly hearing-impaired children. Am J Otol 1991;12(Suppl):144-150.

56. Hellman SA, Chute PM, Kretschmer RE: The development of a Children's Implant Profile. Am Ann Deaf 1991;136:77-81.

57. Palmer CV, Nelson CT, Lindley GA 4th: The functionally and physiologically plastic adult auditory system. J Acoust Soc Am 1998;103:1705-1721.

58. Tyler RS, Summerfield AQ: Cochlear implantation: Relationships with research on auditory deprivation and acclimatization. Ear Hear 1996;17(Suppl 3):S38-50S.

59. Manrique M, Cervera-Paz FJ, Huarte A, et al: Cerebral auditory plasticity and cochlear implants. Int J Pediatr Otorhinolaryngol 1999;5(Suppl 1):S193-S197.

60. American Speech-Language-Hearing Association: Scope of Practice in Speech-Language Pathology. Rockville, Md, American Speech-Language-Hearing Association, 2001.

61. Tomblin B, Records N, Bukwalter P, et al: Prevalence of specific language impairment in kindergarten children. J Speech Lang Hear Res 1997;40:1245-1260.

62. Shriberg LD, Tomblin JB, McSweeny JL: Prevalence of speech delay in 6-year-old children and comorbidity with language impairment. J Speech Lang Hear Res 1999;42:1461-1481.

63. Lahey M: Language Disorders and Language Development. New York, Macmillan, 1988.

64. Kamhi A: Trying to make sense of developmental language disorders. Lang Speech Hear Serv Sch 1998;29:35-44.

65. Prizant B: Language acquisition and communicative behavior in autism: Toward an understanding of the "whole" of it. J Speech Hear Dis 1983;48:296-307.

66. Russell N: Educational considerations in traumatic brain injury: The role of the speech-language pathologist. Lang Speech Hear Serv Sch 1993;24:67-75.

67. Frost L, Bondy A: The Picture Exchange Communication System Training Manual, 2nd ed. Newark, Del, Pyramid Educational Consultants, 2002.

68. Malkmus D, Stenderup K: Rancho Los Amigos Coma Scale Revised. Communication Disorders Service. Rancho Los Amigos Hospital, Calif, Communication Disorders Service, 1974.

69. Darley FL, Aronson AE, Brown JR: Motor Speech Disorders. Philadelphia, WB Saunders, 1975.

70. Croot K: Diagnosis of apraxia of speech: Definition and criteria. Semin Speech Lang 2002;23:267-280.

71. Starkweather CW: Fluency and Stuttering. Englewood Cliffs, NJ, Prentice Hall, 1987.

72. Guitar: Stuttering: An Integrated Approach to Its Nature and Treatment, 2nd ed. Baltimore, Williams & Wilkins, 1998.

73. Yairi E: The formative years of stuttering: A changing portrait. Contemp Issues Commun Sci Disord 2004;31:92-104.

74. Campbell TF, Dollaghan C, Felsenfeld S: Disorders of language, phonology, fluency, and voice: Indicators for referral. In Bluestone C, Stool S, Kenna M (eds): Handbook of Pediatric Otolaryngology, 3rd ed. Philadelphia, WB Saunders, 1996, pp 1595-1606.

75. Wilson DK: Voice Problems in Children, 3rd ed. Baltimore, Williams & Wilkins, 1987.

76. Miller SA, Madison CL. Public school voice clinics. Part II: Diagnosis and recommendations—a 10-year review. Lang Speech Hear Serv Sch 1984;15:58.

77. Arvedson J, Brodsky L: Pediatric Swallowing and Feeding: Assessment and Management, 2nd ed. Albany, NY, Singular Publishing, 2002.

78. Rosenthal SR, Sheppard JJ, Lotze M: Dysphagia in the Child with Developmental Disabilities: Medical and Clinical and Family Interventions. San Diego, Calif, Singular Publishing, 1995.

CHAPTER 4

Hearing Loss in Children

JOHN A. GERMILLER, MD, PhD

Intact hearing during childhood is vital for proper development of communication, cognitive skills, and social and family interaction and for normal emotional development. Early recognition and prompt management of hearing loss are therefore critical. This chapter provides an overview of the causes, diagnosis, and management of hearing loss in children. More details on the evaluation and management of certain disorders causing hearing loss—for example, otitis media and cholesteatoma—can be found elsewhere in this text (see Chapters 3 and 5 through 7).

GENERAL CONSIDERATIONS

Hearing sensitivity is defined by a threshold level, which is the lowest intensity at which the child is able to detect a given sound, and is expressed relative to standards established for the population. Normal hearing is defined as the ability to detect sounds presented at 0 to 15 decibels (dB) in quiet conditions (Table 4-1). Mild hearing loss exists when thresholds are measured between 16 and 30 dB, moderate loss between 31 and 60 dB, severe loss between 61 and 90 dB, and profound loss above 90 dB. Hearing loss can be caused by a wide variety of conditions and may be reversible (e.g., hearing loss from otitis media with effusion) or permanent (e.g., most forms of sensorineural hearing loss).

Types of Hearing Loss

Hearing loss can be broadly divided into three categories. *Conductive hearing loss* occurs when there is any disruption of efficient sound conduction via the micromechanical apparatus that makes up the external and middle ears. These include disorders affecting the patency of the ear canal, vibration of the tympanic membrane, ensuing vibration of the ossicles, or mechanical fluid wave established in the cochlea. The prototypical condition causing conductive hearing loss is otitis media, in which middle ear effusion dampens the vibration

Table 4-1 Categories of Hearing Loss Severity

Category	Hearing Level (dB)
Normal hearing	0-15
Hearing loss	
Mild	16-30
Moderate	31-60
Severe	61-90
Profound	>90

of the tympanic membrane and ossicles, leaving the sensory apparatus of the inner ear unaffected. *Sensorineural hearing loss* (SNHL) occurs from any disruption of the transduction of sound into electrical potentials in the inner ear, or of the efficient transmission of those signals to the brainstem or higher order centers in the cortex. *Mixed hearing loss* is defined as hearing loss with conductive and sensorineural components.

Determining the degree to which a hearing loss is conductive or sensorineural is critical in the early evaluation, because each suggests different sites of lesion, which differ greatly in their cause, workup, and management. Fortunately, even basic audiometric testing usually can easily distinguish among the three broad categories of hearing loss, because inner ear sensitivity can be tested separately from the rest of the auditory system.

Hearing Assessment

All hearing assessment begins by presenting sound to the patient at a controlled intensity and then using various techniques to determine whether sound is detected. Sound is presented as speech, pure tones, or clicks, first through the air via loudspeakers, headphones, or ear canal inserts and then via bone conduction directly to the bone of the skull. Bone conduction directly vibrates the fluids of the cochlea, bypassing the sound-conducting apparatus of the external and middle ears. This directly tests cochlear sensitivity, and is the first critical step toward categorizing a given hearing loss as conductive, sensorineural, or mixed. Detection of sound is then determined by either a behavioral response or by various physiologic measurements (Box 4-1). Behavioral assessments are preferred, because they verify the integrity of the entire hearing response from the ear to the highest centers of the cortex. Physiologic assessments (e.g., the auditory brainstem response) are used when patients are unable to engage in adequate behavioral testing or when specific information is needed about distinct elements of the auditory system.

The gold standard for determining hearing levels in children and adults is the familiar audiogram, a behavioral test that reports the child's sensitivity for hearing speech as well as pure tones of distinct frequencies.

Box 4-1 Common Audiometric Assessments of Hearing

BEHAVIORAL TESTS (AUDIOGRAM)

Behavioral observation audiometry
Visual reinforcement audiometry
Play audiometry
Standard audiometry

PHYSIOLOGIC TESTING

Auditory brainstem response (ABR); also called brainstem auditory evoked response (BAER)
Otoacoustic emissions (OAEs)
- Spontaneous OAEs
- Evoked OAEs
  - Transient evoked OAEs (TEOAEs)
  - Distortion product OAEs (DPOAEs)

Audiograms can be obtained as early as 6 months of age by well-trained pediatric audiologists using various behavioral conditioning and observational techniques. In infants and young children, testing is most commonly done in a sound field, in which sound is presented by loudspeakers several feet away from the child. Although behavioral responses can be elicited in cooperative children, a sound field does not permit accurate distinction between hearing in the left and right ears separately. Older toddlers and children, on the other hand, can undergo ear-specific audiometry.

The most common physiologic tests are the auditory brainstem response (ABR) and otoacoustic emissions (OAEs). These can be performed at any age, do not require cooperation with behavioral tasks, and can be done with the child sedated or even under general anesthesia. ABR testing measures action potentials generated in the auditory nerve, auditory nuclei, and ascending pathways in the brainstem in response to sounds, generally clicks or pure tones, presented by either air or bone conduction. By varying the intensity of the sounds, a rough estimate of sound detection thresholds can be determined.

Otoacoustic emissions are minute sounds actually produced by the inner ear, specifically the outer hair cells, and can be detected using a sensitive microphone placed in the ear canal. A useful subset is evoked OAEs, which are emitted several milliseconds after the inner ear receives a test sound. OAEs are generally recorded as present or absent at each frequency, and provide information on the integrity of the cochlea. Thus, they are particularly useful for further localizing the site of lesion in children found to have a SNHL on prior testing. For example, absence of OAEs in an otherwise normal ear, with SNHL, generally suggests that the defect resides in the cochlea. These are often referred to as cochlear or sensory hearing losses and are the most common findings in SNHL. Less commonly, OAE signals are detectable in ears known to have SNHL. Because it suggests that hearing loss exists in the presence of intact cochlear hair cells, this combination (intact OAE combined with SNHL and/or absent ABR) suggests a site of lesion beyond the cochlea in the neural pathways, termed *retrocochlear pathology*.

Over the last 15 years, there has been a national movement to screen newborns for hearing loss, to facilitate the early detection of hearing impairment and thus carry out earlier interventions, such as hearing aids, before the onset of language development. The Year 2000 Joint Committee on Infant Hearing has published guidelines[1] for federally mandated universal newborn hearing screening programs. Screening of neonates is aimed at detecting unilateral or bilateral losses of 30 to 40 dB or more in the frequencies most important for speech (500 to 4000 Hz). Simplified forms of the physiologic tests, the ABR or OAEs, are used to identify those with possible hearing loss. Those who fail the screening are then referred to audiologists for more thorough follow-up diagnostic ABR and/or OAE testing.

Evaluation of Possible Hearing Loss

The evaluation of a child with hearing concerns begins with the history and physical examination, which help direct further workup (Box 4-2).

History

Important elements of the history are past episodes of otitis media, including episodes severe enough to

Box 4-2 Evaluation of Childhood Hearing Loss

HISTORY

Hearing History

- Onset and duration of hearing loss
  - Sudden, gradual, unknown
  - Results of prior screening tests, if known
  - Inciting factors (e.g., preceding severe infection)
- Stability or progression of hearing loss
- Associated symptoms—tinnitus, vertigo, otorrhea, otalgia
- Use of hearing aids

Risk Factors for Hearing Loss

- Otitis media history, including any complications
- Prior ear surgery
- Significant noise exposure
- Trauma (particularly skull fracture)
- History of severe infection
  - Bacterial meningitis
  - Other severe infections (viral, or requiring IV antibiotics)
- Ototoxic medication exposures—aminoglycoside antibiotics; chemotherapy agents (e.g., cisplatin)

Neonatal History

- Prolonged neonatal ICU stay
- Mechanical ventilation, ECMO
- Prematurity, especially if gestation less than 32 wk
- Hyperbilirubinemia, especially if required exchange transfusion
- Hypoxia
- Congenital infection (TORCH)
- Postnatal sepsis, IV antibiotics, and/or diuretics
- Results of newborn hearing screening

Family History of Hearing Loss

Other Medical History

- Known syndromes
- Systemic disorders, malignancy
- Blood dyscrasias

PHYSICAL EXAMINATION

- Pathology of the external and middle ear
  - Ear canal stenosis, microtia
  - Middle ear pathology
    - Tympanic membrane status and mobility (pneumatic otoscopy)
    - Middle ear effusions, mass lesions
- Syndromic features

AUDIOMETRIC EVALUATION (see Box 4-1)

IMAGING STUDIES

- Conductive or mixed hearing loss—high-resolution temporal bone CT
- Sensorineural hearing loss—high-resolution temporal bone CT and/or inner ear, brainstem MRI

ADDITIONAL EVALUATION FOR SENSORINEURAL HEARING LOSS

- Genetics evaluation
- Ophthalmology evaluation

Ancillary Laboratory Testing (as appropriate)

- Electrocardiography for prolonged QT (Jervell and Lange-Nielsen syndrome)
- Urinalysis for proteinuria, hematuria (Alport's syndrome)
- Thyroid function testing
- Titers for past infection (FTA-ABS, TORCH)
- Inflammatory indicators for autoimmune hearing loss (e.g., sedimentation rate)

cause tympanic membrane perforation, labyrinthitis, or meningitis. Any history of otologic surgery, including tympanostomy tubes, should be recorded. The nature of the hearing loss should be explored, particularly to determine whether it was of sudden or gradual onset, and whether it is stable, fluctuating, or worsening in severity. One of the most critical questions is the time of onset. Although this may not be known, parents usually know whether the patient passed newborn hearing screening, which is vital information. In older infants and children, the parents should be asked about when they first noticed abnormal responses to their voice or environmental sounds, and information on speech milestones should be sought. For example, did the parents notice a startle reflex in infancy, and what was the age at which the child spoke his or her first words? Were there any previously normal hearing tests, including newborn hearing screenings?

An important associated otologic symptom is otorrhea, because this may accompany tympanic membrane perforations and cholesteatoma. Foul-smelling otorrhea often accompanies acquired cholesteatoma. The existence of tinnitus and vertigo should be determined, but these are uncommon in children. The family history is especially important in the setting of suspected SNHL because it may suggest a genetic cause, which is often the case. An efficient technique is to inquire if any family members required a hearing aid during childhood or before the age of 40. A careful antenatal and perinatal history is important to identify risk factors for acquired SNHL. These include the presence of any prenatal maternal infections (especially rubella, cytomegalovirus [CMV], and toxoplasmosis), history of prematurity, severe neonatal infection requiring intravenous antibiotics, severe neonatal hyperbilirubinemia, neonatal hypoxia, and prolonged neonatal intensive care unit (ICU) stays, including any that required mechanical ventilation.

Physical Examination

Physical examination is mainly focused on identifying external or middle ear pathology, as well as identifying any features that accompany hearing loss syndromes. Abnormalities of the auricles should be noted, because they often accompany middle and occasionally inner ear malformations. In particular, congenitally hypoplastic and deformed auricles (microtia) frequently accompany ear canal stenosis or atresia. These malformations can occur in isolation or can accompany craniofacial malformation syndromes, such as the Treacher Collins syndrome and hemifacial microsomia. The ear canal and tympanic membrane are evaluated by otoscopy to determine the presence of middle ear effusion or perforation. Pneumatic otoscopy is helpful in confirming effusions and in assessing tympanic membrane compliance. The remainder of the examination should note any anomalies associated with hearing loss syndromes. Common examples include mandibular deficiency and microtia (Treacher Collins syndrome), preauricular tags (Goldenhar syndrome), preauricular pits and branchial cleft anomalies (branchio-oto-renal syndrome), pigment anomalies and dystopia canthorum (Waardenburg syndrome), and goiter (Pendred syndrome).

Audiometric Evaluation

A careful audiometric evaluation is critical for determining the quantity and character of hearing loss. Depending on age and neurologic status, this may involve behavioral testing, otoacoustic emissions, and sedated or nonsedated ABR testing, as described earlier. A practical approach is to coordinate these evaluations to follow soon after the otologic history and physical examination, later the same day if possible, to ensure that testing is not performed in the presence of middle ear effusions or obstructing cerumen. Such conditions should be managed first, before proceeding with further testing.

Imaging Studies

Temporal bone and/or brainstem imaging generally are not needed for hearing loss associated with uncomplicated otitis media, but are extremely valuable in evaluating other types of conductive hearing loss and SNHL. The most widely available study is high-resolution temporal bone computed tomography (CT), which evaluates the bony anatomy of the inner ear, status of the facial nerve and ossicles, and general status of the middle ear and mastoid. With modern techniques, image resolution is as fine as 0.5 mm. Magnetic resonance imaging (MRI) evaluates soft tissues better than CT, and in the past was used mainly to rule out mass lesions affecting the auditory nerves or brainstem. However, in recent years, new techniques have been developed (e.g., volumetric T2-weighted three-dimensional [3D] constructive interference in steady state [CISS] imaging) that can be performed rapidly, without contrast, and yield outstanding resolution of inner ear labyrinth structure, status of the internal auditory canal (seventh and eighth nerves), and brainstem, in one setting. Specific uses for different imaging modalities are discussed later in this chapter in the sections on individual types of hearing loss.

Ancillary Testing

Ancillary testing and subspecialist referrals are often required for further evaluation of some forms of hearing loss. For example, genetic testing and referral to a medical geneticist are often performed for SNHL. These are described later in the relevant sections.

CONDUCTIVE HEARING LOSS

Causative Factors

A wide variety of conditions cause conductive hearing loss (CHL) (Box 4-3). Because of its high prevalence, *otitis media* is the most common cause of hearing loss in children, primarily the conductive type. The most common pathophysiology is reduced sound transmission because of the presence of middle ear effusion, which is generally reversible once the effusions have been cleared through medical or surgical management. Hearing loss varies from mild to moderate levels. Less commonly, severe and/or repeated infection can result in permanent stiffening of the tympanic membrane and ossicular chain (*tympanosclerosis*), which is detected as a residual conductive loss after the resolution of middle ear fluid. A number of other conditions can cause CHL in the absence of effusion. Cerumen impaction, if severe, uncommonly causes a mild hearing loss. Severe *eustachian tube dysfunction*, even without effusion, can cause significant retraction or atrophy of the tympanic membrane (e.g., atelectasis, adhesive otitis media) severe enough to reduce sound conduction through the middle ear. Although hearing loss is often mild in the absence of middle ear fluid, these patients need referral to an otolaryngologist to be considered for tympanostomy tube placement and close monitoring to detect progression of their retraction pockets into cholesteatoma. *Tympanic membrane perforation* can cause CHL by a number of mechanisms. A perforation reduces the effective vibratory surface of the tympanic membrane, and chronic perforations are often associated with tympanosclerosis, which can contribute to hearing loss. These patients also require evaluation by an otolaryngologist to be considered for surgical repair. Surgical repair (tympanoplasty) is generally recommended, because closing the defect may improve hearing and will prevent the ingrowth of epidermis into the middle ear, which can result in cholesteatoma.

Cholesteatomas are cystic masses of normal skin that expand within the middle ear. They cause conductive hearing loss by direct mass effect or by erosion of the ossicular chain. Rarely, they can erode into the inner ear, resulting in sensorineural hearing loss—even profound unilateral deafness. Cholesteatomas are either acquired (most common) or congenital. Acquired cholesteatomas most commonly form from a retraction pocket of the tympanic membrane. In the setting of chronic eustachian tube dysfunction and negative middle ear pressure, a retraction pocket can progressively deepen until skin debris can no longer be shed out of the ear canal, resulting in expansion of the cyst into the middle ear and/or mastoid cavity. Acquired cholesteatomas less commonly arise from direct epidermal ingrowth through a perforation or surgical defect (tympanostomy). Congenital cholesteatomas form behind an intact tympanic membrane, and are thought to originate from trapped epithelial rests left in the middle ear during development. All cholesteatomas require surgical excision to prevent further expansion and erosion into the inner ear and nearby para-auditory structures, such as the facial nerve. *Otosclerosis* can cause CHL, but is rare in children. This is a disease of abnormal ossification and fixation of the stapes footplate, resulting in progressive hearing loss. Although frequently hereditary, it rarely is manifested during childhood. Finally, *ossicular and middle ear malformations* are an uncommon cause of CHL that is present at birth, often unilaterally. Various malformations are familiar to the pediatric otolaryngologist; these range from isolated ossicular malformations, such as congenital stapes fixation or absent ossicles, to aural atresia (congenital atresia of the ear canal, typically accompanied by ossicular anomalies).

Box 4-3 Causes of Conductive Hearing Loss

EAR CANAL ABNORMALITIES

Cerumen impaction
Foreign body
Ear canal malformation (aural atresia, stenosis)

TYMPANIC MEMBRANE ABNORMALITIES

Tympanosclerosis
Perforation
Eustachian tube dysfunction (severe)

MIDDLE EAR ABNORMALITIES

Middle ear effusion
- Acute otitis media
- Otitis media with effusion

Cholesteatoma
Neoplasm
Vascular anomalies (e.g., aberrant carotid artery)

OSSICULAR CHAIN ABNORMALITIES

Tympanosclerosis
Ossicular malformation
Congenital ossicular chain fixation
Otosclerosis

Evaluation

The two most critical components of the CHL evaluation are the physical examination and tympanogram.

The examination will detect common causes of CHL such as middle ear effusion, acute otitis media, and tympanic membrane (TM) perforation. Cholesteatoma can be suspected if the examination shows a white mass behind the TM or a deep retraction pocket, especially if associated with debris or otorrhea. Prompt referral to an otolaryngologist is essential. Tympanosclerosis may be suspected if the examination shows white calcific plaques within the TM (myringosclerosis). In some cases, the white plaques of myringosclerosis may not be distinguishable from cholesteatoma to the general practitioner, and referral to an otolaryngologist is warranted. Tympanometry helps evaluate CHL by assessing tympanic membrane stiffness, compliance, and mobility, and thereby can confirm the presence of effusion and severe eustachian tube dysfunction. Tympanometers are also very sensitive for TM perforations, even small ones, because a perforation of any size will transmit air pressure from the ear canal to the middle ear, causing the device to measure an abnormally large volume of air.

If the diagnosis is unclear after initial examination and tympanometry, referral to an otolaryngologist is warranted. A more detailed 3D examination can be performed in the office using the binocular microscope, if needed. Often, the diagnosis is then confirmed with temporal bone imaging. CT is preferred to MRI for evaluating CHL, because usually it provides better bony detail and fully evaluates the ossicles. CT can generally detect expansile middle ear masses, such as cholesteatomas, as well as many of the rarer middle ear malformations, such as congenitally absent ossicles or vascular anomalies.

Management

Management of CHL varies greatly depending on the associated cause. Recommendations for management of several common conditions causing CHL can be found elsewhere in the text (see Chapter 3). Although hearing can be improved in many types of CHL by medical or surgical management, hearing rehabilitation (amplification or bone conduction devices) may still be needed in some cases. Mild to moderate CHL not amenable to medical or surgical correction can be treated with standard hearing aids, assuming that the ear canals are normal. Hearing aids may also be beneficial for ears affected by severe tympanosclerosis or congenital stapes fixation. Although such patients may be candidates for surgical exploration to attempt to free the ossicular chain, the procedure fails in many patients and others do not elect surgery. In many of these patients, the amplification provided by standard hearing aids can overcome the ossicular stiffness and provide adequate sound to the inner ear.

On the other hand, for patients with moderate to severe CHL of various causes, standard hearing aids may not be adequate. For example, patients with ear canal atresia typically have severe losses (more than 50 dB) and lack an ear canal to deliver sound from a standard hearing aid. Other examples are patients with ossicular discontinuity resulting from congenital anomaly or surgery. Because their hearing losses are typically purely conductive, and the inner ears are normal, devices that can deliver sound via bone conduction can be extremely useful in such patients. Various bone vibration devices are available, worn externally or implanted in the skull near the inner ear. External bone conduction devices are worn with a headband to press them tightly against the mastoid bone; bone conduction hearing is thus achieved through transcutaneous vibration. These devices are effective, but can be cumbersome and uncomfortable and can result in skin complications from the pressure required to maintain good contact with the mastoid bone.

More recently, osseointegrated bone conduction implants have been developed and are gaining widespread acceptance. The familiar name for these devices is the bone-anchored hearing aid (BAHA). This term is a misnomer in that the devices are not actually hearing aids—that is, they are designed not necessarily to amplify sound, but rather to convert it into bone vibrations detectable by a normal cochlea. Osseointegrated bone conduction implants use a percutaneous titanium screw that becomes firmly integrated into the skull. Once osseointegration occurs, a small external processor or vibrator is snapped onto the osseointegrated screw abutment to provide direct bone conduction. These devices provide remarkably good hearing sensitivity, even in children with severe CHL. Often, they can provide hearing sensitivity in the normal range (less than 15 dB), because they bypass the sound conduction pathologic mechanism entirely to stimulate a normal cochlea.

SENSORINEURAL HEARING LOSS

Categories and Definitions

In discussing the causes of permanent sensorineural hearing loss (SNHL), disease entities are often placed into one of several broad categories, based on time of onset, heritability, or site of lesion. There can be confusion because each disorder, and certainly each individual patient, may fit into more than one category. The first distinction is *congenital versus acquired SNHL*. Congenital SNHL is present at birth and its detection is the target of newborn hearing screening programs. Acquired SNHL implies normal hearing at birth, with onset of hearing loss at some time later. Classic examples include SNHL after noise trauma, labyrinthitis, and skull fracture. These terms must be used with care to avoid confusion. For example, "acquired" hearing loss also includes certain hereditary hearing losses whose mutations are present at birth, but whose phenotype is not manifested until later in childhood or even adulthood. Several autosomal dominant hereditary hearing losses fall into this category. Furthermore, some congenital infections (e.g., cytomegalovirus) can result in hearing loss that has a delayed onset and/or progresses later in life.

The second major distinction is *genetic versus environmental SNHL*. In the United States, it is estimated that of all cases of congenital SNHL, approximately 50% are genetic and 50% are environmental. Environmental (epigenetic) causes of SNHL include ototoxic drugs, noise, infection, and trauma. Of importance, although the distinction of genetic or environmental is generally straightforward when discussing disease entities, it can be unclear in an individual child with hearing loss. For example, a child may be suspected of having a genetic hearing impairment because a few family members have hearing loss and the patient lacks risk factors for an acquired disorder. However, that child's SNHL cannot be conclusively categorized as hereditary unless genetic testing reveals a mutation, or unless clear evidence exists from inheritance patterns in the family pedigree. There are two more obstacles for categorizing individual patients as having genetic hearing loss: (1) at present, clinical genetic testing is available for only a small number of disease genes (albeit this is expected to expand rapidly in the coming decades); and (2) as with many genetic disorders, sporadic new mutations can occur in an individual and cause disease in the absence of any family history.

The last major distinction is *cochlear versus retrocochlear SNHL*. These two categories are sometimes called sensory and neural hearing loss, respectively. The terms indicate that the presumed site of the lesion is either in the cochlea, typically, the sensory auditory hair cells, or somewhere in the neural signaling pathways, anywhere from the afferents of the auditory nerve through the brainstem and higher centers. These are not true diagnoses, nor are they generally used to classify disease entities. Rather, they are descriptive audiologic categories useful for classifying hearing loss in individual patients. Although not all cases of SNHL fall neatly into one or the other, the distinction nevertheless can be useful for individual patients, because it can help direct further workup and rehabilitation efforts.

In the following discussions, the pathophysiology of SNHL is organized into genetic, environmental, and other causes that are not necessarily genetic or environmental (Box 4-4).

Box 4-4 Causes of Pediatric Sensorineural Hearing Loss (SNHL)

GENETIC DISORDERS

Genetic syndrome
Nonsyndromic SNHL

ENVIRONMENTAL CAUSES

- Labyrinthitis
  - Infectious—bacterial, viral
  - Meningitis
  - Inflammatory
- Ototoxicity
  - Medications
  - Hypoxic injury
  - Hyperbilirubinemia
- Trauma
  - Temporal bone fracture
  - Barotrauma
  - Noise

OTHER CAUSES

Inner ear malformation
Mass lesions
Central nervous system disorders
Idiopathic

Genetic Hearing Loss

As noted, approximately 50% of infants with SNHL are believed to have a genetic cause. Such figures are merely estimates, because many deafness genes remain unknown and, even for those that are known, we presently lack clinical tests for many of the associated mutations. Genetic hearing loss is either syndromic, occurring as part of a recognizable syndrome, or nonsyndromic. For example, in Usher syndrome, SNHL occurs together with retinitis pigmentosa. Among patients with genetic hearing loss, approximately one third of the cases are syndromic and two thirds are nonsyndromic. The final genetic distinction concerns inheritance patterns—autosomal dominant, autosomal recessive, X-linked recessive, and mitochondrial. The autosomal disorders predominate. The most common inheritance pattern for nonsyndromic hearing loss is autosomal recessive.

Syndromic Sensorineural Hearing Loss

Sensorineural hearing loss is a common feature of a large number of syndromes (Box 4-5). Syndromic hearing loss can be variable with regard to severity, age of onset, and progression. In many syndromes, hearing loss is often the first feature recognized, especially in the current era of universal newborn hearing screening. The following discussion highlights some of the hearing loss syndromes that are more commonly encountered in general otolaryngology practice, as well as a few less common syndromes toward which many otolaryngologists and geneticists direct certain special tests.

Box 4-5 Syndromes Associated with Sensorineural Hearing Loss

Pendred
Usher
Branchio-oto-renal
CHARGE
Waardenburg
Jervell and Lange-Nielsen
Alport

Pendred Syndrome. Pendred syndrome is an autosomal recessive syndrome of SNHL and thyroid abnormalities. Clinically, severe to profound SNHL is typically present at birth, and is frequently associated with malformations of the inner ear, including cochlear partitioning defects and enlarged vestibular aqueducts (see later discussion of inner ear malformations). Thyroid abnormalities can take the form of hypothyroidism, with or without goiter. However, it is uncommon for these abnormalities to present in the first decade of life, and many patients remain euthyroid throughout life. Pendred syndrome is caused by mutations in pendrin, a molecule believed to be involved in iodine transport. Historically, the syndrome has been diagnosed by an abnormal perchlorate discharge test, but today genetic testing for pendrin mutations (*SLC26A4*) is available.

Usher Syndrome. Usher syndrome is an autosomal recessive disorder characterized by retinitis pigmentosa, SNHL, and variable vestibular system pathology. Various types exist. Usher syndrome type I is the most severe type, with profound deafness at birth and severe vestibular dysfunction. It is caused by mutations in the *MYO7A* gene, which encodes a protein involved in proper functioning of the stereociliary bundle on sensory hair cells. Patients with type II Usher syndrome have less severe hearing impairment than in type I disease. Type III Usher's syndrome is characterized by intact hearing at birth that progressively deteriorates throughout life, without balance disturbance. In all forms of Usher syndrome, early referral to an ophthalmologist is important to monitor for retinitis pigmentosa and its associated vision loss. Hearing loss must be monitored especially carefully and managed aggressively in this syndrome because of the additional disability possible from multiple sensory impairments.

Branchio-oto-renal Syndrome. Branchio-oto-renal (BOR) syndrome is characterized by branchial apparatus anomalies—preauricular pits or cysts, branchial cleft cysts and sinus tracts, abnormal auricles—along with hearing loss and renal anomalies. It is an autosomal dominant disorder caused by mutations in the *EYA1* gene, which encodes a nuclear transcription factor. Malformations are commonly found in the external, middle, and/or inner ear. Accordingly, the resulting hearing loss is most often mixed (50%) and, less commonly, purely sensorineural (25%). Severity is variable, ranging from mild to profound.

CHARGE Syndrome. The CHARGE syndrome[2] (***c***oloboma, ***h***eart defect, ***a***tresia choanae, ***r***etarded growth and development, ***g***enital hypoplasia, ***e***ar anomalies/deafness) can include abnormalities of the external, middle, or inner ear, or any combination thereof. Sensorineural hearing loss is present to some degree in 75% of patients with the CHARGE syndrome, with about 35% having severe to profound loss. Mixed hearing loss is common because of the coexistence of inner and middle ear malformations. Malformations of the inner ear can be severe, including aplasia of the semicircular canals, severely malformed cochleas, and dilated, patent vestibular aqueducts. The severity of SNHL generally corresponds with the severity of the inner ear malformation. Cochlear implantation can be difficult in these patients as a result of the severity of inner ear malformation, high percentage of aberrant facial nerves, and difficulties with speech rehabilitation because of the frequency of cognitive delays in this population.

Waardenburg Syndrome. Waardenburg syndrome involves pigmentary anomalies, facial dysmorphic features, and variable hearing loss. The familiar facial and pigment anomalies include dystopia canthorum, heterochromic (multicolored) or hypochromic (brilliant blue) iris, synophrys, broad nasal root, and depigmentation of hair (white forelock) or skin (or both). It is inherited in autosomal dominant fashion, with high penetrance but variable expressivity. Hearing loss in Waardenburg syndrome can be unilateral or bilateral, progressive or stable, and of variable severity. There can exist various inner ear malformations as well as microscopic abnormalities, including abnormal organ of Corti and cochlear spiral ganglion.

Jervell and Lange-Nielsen Syndrome (Prolonged QT Syndrome). This is a rare autosomal recessive disorder of SNHL, with abnormal prolongation of the QT interval on electrocardiography. It is caused by defects in a potassium transporter and, accordingly, has manifestations in the heart and inner ear, organs dependent on large potassium gradients for their electrical activity. Hearing loss is generally severe to profound bilateral SNHL present at birth. Although rare, long QT syndrome must be considered in all cases of congenital bilateral severe hearing loss, given the fact that the hearing impairment is manifest well before the initial cardiac symptoms, which can be as severe as arrhythmia or even sudden death.

Alport Syndrome. Alport syndrome is characterized by hearing loss and nephritis, and is most commonly inherited as an X-linked recessive disorder. Progressive renal failure can occur. The diagnosis can be suggested by hearing loss associated with proteinuria and/or hematuria.

Nonsyndromic Genetic Hearing Loss

Nonsyndromic SNHL is defined as isolated sensorineural hearing loss from a genetic abnormality, with no other recognizable features of a known syndrome. Nonsyndromic genetic hearing loss is approximately twice as common as syndromic hearing loss. A large number of genes have been associated with nonsyndromic SNHL, although many remain poorly characterized. All inheritance patterns have been described. Over 40 genes have been linked to autosomal dominant nonsyndromic hearing loss; each is designated as *DFNAn*, where *n* is a number unique to each gene. Over 30 genes have been found for autosomal recessive SNHL, and carry the designation *DFNBn*. Finally, a smaller number of genes have been identified in association with X-linked hearing loss (*DFNn*), with mitochondrial inheritance.

Mutations in one gene product, *GJB2* (connexin 26), account for up to 40% to 50% of cases of nonsyndromic SNHL in the United States. This protein is a constituent of connexons, which make up the complex of intercellular gap junctions. In this autosomal recessive disorder, hearing loss is of variable severity; can be symmetrical, asymmetrical, or even unilateral; and can be stable or progressive. This variability is thought to result from the large number of different *GJB2* mutations that have been identified in the population. The most common mutation, *35delG*, has a carrier frequency of 2.5% in the European and European-American general population. Driven by this high prevalence, genetic testing for several common *GJB2* mutations has become available for clinical use.

In addition to *GJB2*, a wide variety of other genes that have various roles in inner ear structure and function, have been identified as causing nonsyndromic SNHL. Examples include genes for structural proteins, such as the unconventional myosins (myosins 7a and 15), tectorial membrane constituents (alpha- and beta-tectorin), several extracellular matrix molecules, transcription factors (e.g., *POU4F3*, *EYA4*), ion channels, and intercellular channels. Various cochlear functions can be affected, including auditory hair cell structure, cellular arrangement and function, maintenance of the endocochlear potential and fluid homeostasis, and proper structure of the vibratory and transduction apparatus. The common end result of many of these mutations is permanent loss of the fragile auditory hair cells.

Environmental Sensorineural Hearing Loss

This category includes all conditions causing SNHL not associated with gene defects. Environmental SNHL can be caused by a specific insult often a single event (e.g., labyrinthitis) or by cumulative damage to the inner ear over time (e.g., noise trauma) (see Box 4-4). Onset can be at any age, from the prenatal period through adulthood. Important causative categories are infectious, inflammatory, autoimmune, ototoxic, and traumatic factors.

Infectious and Inflammatory Causes (Labyrinthitis)

Labyrinthitis refers to inflammation of the inner ear, which can cause permanent hearing loss. Infectious labyrinthitis can be classified by the primary origin of the infection. *Tympanogenic labyrinthitis* originates from middle ear disease and thus is most commonly unilateral. It begins as acute or chronic otitis media, with inflammation entering the middle ear via the oval or round window or through an acquired defect (fistula). The latter can occur secondary to trauma (e.g., temporal bone fracture) or surgery, or from the bony erosion caused by cholesteatoma. Tympanogenic labyrinthitis can be serous or suppurative. Serous labyrinthitis is the more common type; this is a sterile inflammation of the labyrinth resulting from accumulation of bacterial toxins or inflammatory mediators in the inner ear. Suppurative labyrinthitis is a more acute and destructive form of tympanogenic labyrinthitis that results from direct bacterial invasion of the inner ear. It is characterized by severe, rapidly progressive SNHL and vertigo. Profound SNHL in the affected ear is not uncommon.

Meningitic labyrinthitis, a secondary complication of bacterial meningitis, results from spread of infection in the reverse direction, from the meninges or cerebrospinal fluid (CSF) directly into the inner ear. It is a suppurative labyrinthitis that is commonly bilateral. Sensorineural hearing loss occurs in 5% to 35% of patients and is often profound. Pathogens of note are *Haemophilus influenzae* and *Streptococcus pneumoniae*. Although immunization programs against these organisms have reduced the incidence of meningitis, it still remains the most common cause of acquired SNHL in childhood.

A third category, *hematogenic labyrinthitis*, is a heterogeneous group of conditions in which labyrinthitis is secondary to a systemic infectious or inflammatory disorder, such as viral and syphilitic infections or autoimmune diseases. Viral labyrinthitis can result from systemic mumps, measles, cytomegalovirus, influenza, parainfluenza, or herpes simplex virus infections. Congenital viral infections are important members of this category. Prenatal or perinatal infections with cytomegalovirus (CMV), rubella virus, or *Toxoplasma* are an important cause of congenital hearing loss. The incidence of SNHL is particularly high in congenital CMV infection (up to 30% to 60% in cytomegalic inclusion disease).

Hearing loss can also occur in asymptomatic congenital CMV infection, and is frequently fluctuating and progressive. New-onset viral labyrinthitis can also occur sporadically in later childhood and cause acquired SNHL, but this is uncommon. A typical presentation would be abrupt onset of hearing loss and vertigo in the setting of an otherwise unremarkable viral infection. Mumps is the most common cause of this type of acquired viral hearing loss, which is most often unilateral. Syphilitic labyrinthitis results most commonly from congenital infection, but can also result from acquired systemic disease in later childhood. The presentation and course of hearing loss and vestibular symptoms are variable. Autoimmune labyrinthitis is rare in children. It is often associated with systemic disease, such as rheumatoid arthritis, vasculitides, and Wegener's granulomatosis. Autoimmune labyrinthitis is the suspected mechanism in many cases of idiopathic sudden-onset SNHL, which is rare in children. Adults with this condition often improve with systemic steroids, consistent with the concept of an autoimmune cause in many cases.

Ototoxicity

Like the brain, the cochlea is among the most metabolically active organs in the body, and lacks the capacity for regeneration after injury. Consequently, its sensitive tissues are subject to injury from a wide variety of toxic insults. Sensorineural hearing loss occurs after such insults, mainly from the loss of auditory hair cells. Many of these can occur in the setting of severe perinatal illness (Box 4-6). Prolonged hypoxia or anoxia can result in SNHL of variable severity. Infants who survive prolonged mechanical ventilation and intensive care unit stays, as well as extracorporeal membrane oxygenation (ECMO) therapy, must be carefully tested for hearing loss. Such infants often have multiple ototoxic exposures beyond hypoxia, including exposures to aminoglycoside antibiotics and loop diuretics (see later). Hypoxia can affect many levels of the auditory system, from the cochlea to the central auditory pathways.

Ototoxic medications cause direct or indirect damage to auditory hair cells. The classic example is the aminoglycoside antibiotics, which cause dose-dependent hair cell loss by inducing apoptosis. Loop diuretics affect the stria vascularis, which resembles the kidney in its high metabolic rate and ion pumping activity required to maintain the endocochlear potential. Diuretics are not thought to injure the hair cells directly, but rather contribute to hair cell death by disrupting the homeostasis of the inner ear. They are also thought to potentiate the direct toxic effects of ototoxic antibiotics on the inner ear.

Hyperbilirubinemia can cause sensorineural hearing loss if bilirubin levels are extremely high. The site of injury in the auditory system appears to be retrocochlear—specifically, the neurons of the auditory ganglia and/or cochlear nuclei. Therefore, hyperbilirubinemia is the prototypical condition causing auditory neuropathy, a condition in which cochlear function is intact but neural transmission of sound information to the cortex is disorganized or absent. The expression of the disorganized auditory input can be variable; some children can even perceive distinct sounds at near-normal levels, but are unable to process speech because of the neural dyssynchrony. Unique among types of SNHL, bilirubin-associated auditory neuropathy can spontaneously improve in some patients during the first few years of life.

Box 4-6 Neonatal Risk Factors for Sensorineural Hearing Loss

- Positive family history
- Syndromic findings associated with SNHL (see Box 4-5)
- Severe perinatal disease
  - Prematurity: <32 wk gestation
  - Prolonged neonatal ICU stay
  - Hypoxia
  - Prolonged mechanical ventilation
  - Extracorporeal membrane oxygenation (ECMO)
- Severe infection
- Meningitis
- Hyperbilirubinemia, especially if requiring exchange transfusion
- Ototoxic medications
  - Aminoglycosides, loop diuretics
- Congenital infection
  - Cytomegalovirus
  - Rubella
  - Toxoplasmosis
  - Syphilis

Trauma

Trauma to the inner ear can cause SNHL. The most common occurrence is temporal bone fracture, particularly if the fracture involves the otic capsule, the extremely dense bone encasing the inner ear. This requires considerable energy, and therefore other neurologic deficits and complications frequently coexist with SNHL as a result of skull fracture. When SNHL occurs, it is typically immediate and profound. Acute vestibular dysfunction can also be present. Rarely, severe barotrauma, such as that associated with explosions, can cause shock waves in the fluids of the inner ear, which can rupture delicate cochlear membranes. Similarly, noise-induced SNHL can occur abruptly after intense noise exposure or can develop cumulatively over longer periods of exposure to less intense noise. Loss of hair cells, as well as disrupted stereociliary bundles, is observed histologically.

Other Disorders Causing Sensorineural Hearing Loss

Malformations of the Inner Ear

Inner ear malformations are a surprisingly common finding in the inner ears of children with SNHL. In fact, studies have indicated that about 20–30% of children with SNHL will have anatomic abnormalities detectable on temporal bone imaging.[3] Inner ear malformations can be associated with both hereditary and nonhereditary SNHL. Sporadic malformations may occur by presumed localized teratogenesis during the early development of the inner ear as a result of putative toxic insults during the first 8 weeks of gestation. The cause is rarely determined. Such malformations can be asymmetrical or even unilateral. Less commonly, certain heritable disorders are associated with macroscopic malformations visible on temporal bone imaging, often bilaterally. These include Pendred, branchio-oto-renal (BOR), and CHARGE syndromes.

Inner ear malformations cause SNHL with variable severity, symmetry, and degree of progression. As a general rule, the severity of hearing loss correlates with the severity of malformation. In severe malformations, there is typically profound hearing loss because of the absence of sensory epithelia. However, in even the most dysplastic cochleas, neural elements (rudimentary forms of the spiral ganglion) are often present, such that hearing rehabilitation is sometimes possible with electrical stimulation (e.g., with cochlear implantation).

Malformations can range from subtle defects in the partitions between cochlear chambers to complete absence of the inner ear (Box 4-7). The most common inner ear malformation is the enlarged vestibular aqueduct (EVA). This refers to dilation of the endolymphatic duct and sac, seen on CT scans as a dilation of their bony boundary, the vestibular aqueduct (Fig. 4-1). The remainder of the labyrinth is typically normal. Although EVA can accompany other malformations, it can cause SNHL even in isolation. The SNHL is of variable severity and, in a distinct subgroup of patients, progresses throughout childhood and young adulthood, often in stepwise decrements associated with minor head trauma. The mechanism of SNHL development is unknown, but one theory has postulated that the dilated vestibular aqueduct allows transmission of intracranial pressure to the inner ear, resulting in accumulated damage over time, and that head traumas cause spikes in pressure that further rupture delicate membranes in the inner ear.[4] Therefore, in patients with EVA, the importance of helmet use is emphasized for contact sports, and many otolaryngologists advise avoiding certain activities (e.g., boxing), in which head trauma is inevitable.

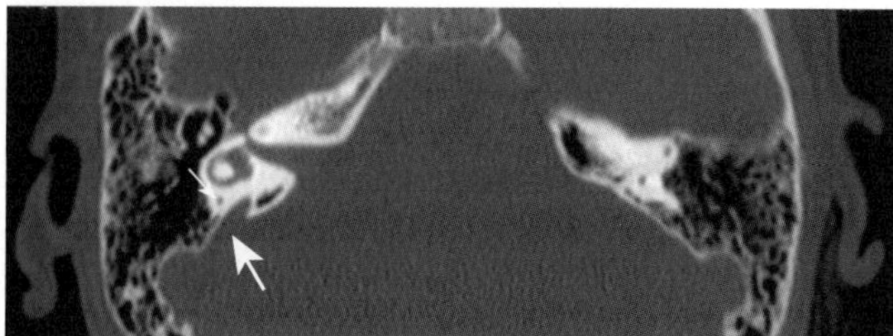

Figure 4-1. Enlarged vestibular aqueduct (EVA), right ear. This axial temporal bone CT scan reveals a dilated, cone-shaped bony vestibular aqueduct in the right temporal bone (*large arrow*), whose diameter should normally be less than that of the posterior semicircular canal (*small arrow*).

Box 4-7 Inner Ear Malformations

- Endolymphatic duct/sac malformations
  - Enlarged vestibular aqueduct (EVA)
  - Dilated endolymphatic sac (usually with EVA)
- Cochlear malformations
  - Incomplete cochlear partitioning (Mondini's dysplasia)
  - Cochlear hypoplasia
  - Cochlear aplasia
- Vestibular malformations
  - Semicircular canal dysplasias
- Combined cochleovestibular malformations
  - Common cavity dysplasia
  - Cochleovestibular aplasia (absent inner ear, Michel's aplasia)
- Cochlear nerve malformations
  - Cochlear nerve aplasia
  - Cochlear nerve hypoplasia

Cochlear partitioning defects refer to poorly developed bony walls and membranes between adjacent turns of the cochlear ducts. Incomplete partitioning is detectable on routine temporal bone CT and MRI scans and can vary in severity from subtle changes in the apical turn to a widened, almost cystic, cochlea in severe cases. These malformations are often referred to as Mondini dysplasia. Severe deformity typically results in profound SNHL, but milder deformities can cause milder loss that can progress over time, sometimes in stepwise fashion, as for EVA. The most severe types of inner ear malformation, almost always associated with profound SNHL, are the common cavity deformity (rudimentary inner ear, with the entire cochlea and vestibular labyrinth represented by a common cystic structure), cochlear hypoplasia, and cochlear aplasia (Michel's aplasia).

Inner ear malformations accompany several syndromes. In CHARGE syndrome, inner ear malformation occurs in almost all cases, with nearly universal aplasia of the semicircular canals, utricle, and saccule, and with most patients also having cochlear partitioning defects of variable severity. BOR syndrome frequently includes cochlear hypoplasia and EVA. Middle ear malformations, including abnormal ossicles, also are common in both CHARGE and BOR syndromes, resulting in mixed hearing loss. In Pendred syndrome, there is a high prevalence of EVA and incomplete partitioning cochlear malformations. In fact, now that genetic testing has become more widely available, many specialists routinely test for Pendred mutations when patients have these findings on initial imaging studies. Mondini-type malformations are also common in DiGeorge syndrome, Klippel-Feil syndrome, and Waardenburg's syndrome.

Of importance, all patients with inner ear malformations are believed to be at increased risk for bacterial meningitis compared with children with normal anatomy. Meningitis in these patients results from ascending (tympanogenic) infection and is more likely in dysplastic than in normal ears, because the former provides a more direct route for infection to ascend to the meninges. This concept of deficient barriers between the cochlea and CSF is supported by the frequent (20%) observation of CSF leaks when surgical cochleostomy is created in these patients during cochlear implantation. Although the relative risk of meningitis in children with SNHL and malformations is unknown, most experts recommend that children with inner ear malformations receive immunizations against the organisms causing bacterial meningitis, particularly *H. influenzae* and pneumococci.

Tumors and Related Mass Lesions

Although neoplasms and other space-occupying lesions are known causes of SNHL in adults, especially unilateral or asymmetrical SNHL, they are uncommon in children. Various pediatric malignancies, particularly brainstem tumors, can cause unilateral SNHL, with a retrocochlear pattern. Other lesions include endolymphatic sac tumors, which can erode the inner ear, and meningiomas, which can compress the cochlear nerve or auditory brainstem. Vestibular schwannomas (acoustic neuromas) can occur in children, but are exceedingly rare. They must certainly be considered in patients with familial neurofibromatosis type 2, because affected patients may manifest their first tumors in late childhood or adolescence. Although not a tumor, cholesteatoma, as described earlier, is a mass lesion that can erode into the inner ear and cause SNHL. Finally, brainstem compression associated with Chiari type I malformation can cause SNHL, however, hearing loss is rarely an isolated symptom. One important finding common to many of these disparate lesions is unilateral retrocochlear hearing loss (unilateral auditory neuropathy). This finding on audiometric testing, especially in the presence of other neurologic signs and symptoms such as cranial nerve deficits, should prompt consideration of mass lesions and evaluation with gadolinium-enhanced MRI.

Idiopathic Sensorineural Hearing Loss

When genetic causes, syndromes, environmental causes, malformations, and space-occupying lesions are ruled out, SNHL is considered to be idiopathic. In congenital idiopathic SNHL, one can speculate on roles for new mutations, mutations in presently unknown deafness genes, occult infections or toxic insults during gestation, or even developmental accidents, such as vascular disruption to the inner ear during development. In other cases, subtle malformations, too small to be detectable with modern imaging techniques, might be postulated to exist. Fortunately, regardless of whether a cause can ever be ascertained, most patients benefit from amplification (hearing aids), and most with severe to profound idiopathic SNHL can benefit from cochlear implantation. Future advances in hearing loss research and genetic studies may eventually allow understanding of the underlying cause in cases presently lumped together as idiopathic.

Associated Disorders in Other Organ Systems

A number of other organ systems can be abnormal in patients with SNHL. These disorders often prompt the use of certain screening tests, particularly because SNHL is frequently the first disorder to be detected in patients with multisystem disease. Renal disease can occur in BOR, Alport's, and DiGeorge syndromes, as well as after therapy with certain ototoxic medications, many of which can be nephrotoxic as well (e.g., aminoglycosides, chemotherapeutic agents). Therefore, if any of these are suspected, the initial workup of SNHL may include urinalysis and renal ultrasound examination to detect nephritis and renal anomalies. Ophthalmologic disorders include retinitis pigmentosa in Usher syndrome, colobomata in CHARGE syndrome, and retinopathy of prematurity, among others. Ophthalmologic referral is important to rule out these disorders, as well as to optimize vision, since patients already suffer sensory compromise from their hearing loss. Cardiac disease can include arrhythmias from prolonged QT syndrome, as well as congenital heart defects (e.g., CHARGE and DiGeorge syndromes). Electrocardiography easily detects QT abnormalities, and is frequently used as an inexpensive screening test when SNHL cannot be ascribed to other causes. Finally, cognitive impairment is not uncommon in the deaf population. Approximately 30% to 40% of children with SNHL have an additional disability, and 13% of hearing-impaired schoolchildren are also mentally retarded, visually impaired, or both. Conditions associated with both SNHL and cognitive impairment include congenital infections (CMV, rubella), neonatal insults (hypoxia, prematurity, kernicterus, ECMO), acquired infections (meningitis), and malformation syndromes (CHARGE).

Diagnosis and Evaluation

Traditionally, the workup for SNHL has involved a somewhat indiscriminate battery of tests and referrals ordered at the time of diagnosis, with the hope that an anomaly or syndrome associated with SNHL may be detected. As a result of advances in genetics and imaging, however, the SNHL workup is gradually becoming more focused and more likely to yield an underlying cause.

History and Physical Examination

The initial history and physical examination rarely determine the cause of the SNHL, but rather provide information to direct further workup. Often, the findings can place a patient into one of the broad categories of SNHL described earlier, such as hereditary, syndromic, or acquired hearing loss. Important elements of the otologic history and physical have been presented (see Box 4-2). Once hearing loss is known to be SNHL, the critical historical data include time of onset, stability and progression, family history of hearing loss, and perinatal and neonatal history in cases of suspected congenital hearing loss. Perinatal and neonatal history should include questions on prenatal infection, mechanical ventilation, prematurity, jaundice, and severe infection requiring intravenous antibiotics (see Box 4-6). Although physical examination in SNHL usually reveals unremarkable middle ears, it is critical because it may identify pathology, such as middle ear effusion, that could add a superimposed conductive hearing loss component that may be reversible. Physical examination may also identify physical features of certain syndromes.

Audiometric Evaluation

Audiometric evaluation of SNHL uses behavioral audiometry whenever possible, supplemented with physiologic tests in some cases. Young infants usually require ABR testing to confirm hearing loss, assess its severity, and determine whether it is sensorineural, conductive, or mixed. As described earlier, when SNHL is first identified, otoacoustic emission testing is often performed early in the workup to help direct attention to the site of a lesion in the cochlea or retrocochlear apparatus.

Imaging Studies

Imaging studies are performed to detect inner ear malformations, as well as less common lesions of the inner ear and brainstem. High-resolution temporal bone CT is excellent for detecting macroscopic inner ear malformations such as incomplete partition of the cochlea and enlarged vestibular aqueducts. Temporal bone CT, however, has several limitations. Because it cannot distinguish fluid from soft tissue, CT is unable to discern the eighth nerve; detect mass lesions of the brainstem, cerebellopontine angle, or internal auditory canal; or delineate nonossified scar tissue in the labyrinth (as can occur after labyrinthitis). If such conditions are suspected, MRI is indicated.

Historically, MRI has been inferior to CT at resolving the fine structure of the cochlea and labyrinth, thus presenting a dilemma in the evaluation of SNHL. Because malformations are far more common than mass lesions, most patients historically have undergone CT alone, with MRI reserved for special cases. Today, however, at some centers, new volumetric T2-weighted 3D scanning protocols for high-resolution MRI have become available that provide not only submillimeter resolution of the inner ear structure, but also allow its reconstruction in any arbitrary plane. Thus, they simultaneously can detect inner ear malformations and tumors, mass lesions, and other brainstem abnormalities. The technique takes advantage of the fact that cochlear fluids show up bright on T2-weighted images, whereas the dense surrounding bone of the otic capsule is dark. Temporal bone MRI therefore not only allows analysis of the gross structure of the cochlea and labyrinth, but also can reveal some of its fine membranous internal architecture (Fig. 4-2). For example, the integrity of the basilar membrane of the cochlea and even the neurosensory epithelium of the

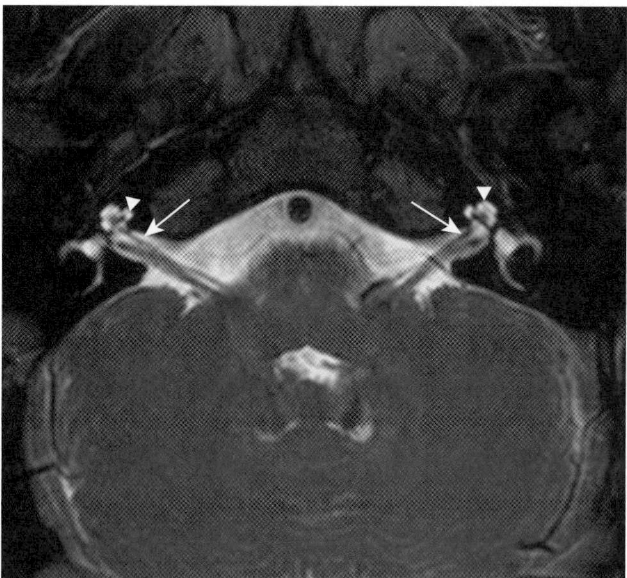

Figure 4-2. High-resolution inner ear magnetic resonance imaging (MRI). Volumetric T2-weighted 3D MRI allows detailed microanatomic resolution of inner ear architecture, as well as cranial nerves and brainstem. In this axial noncontrast section, the individual nerves of the internal auditory canals are well delineated, as are the fine structures of the semicircular canals, vestibule, and cochlea. Some of the membranous partitions of the inner ear, such as the basilar membrane of the cochlea (*arrowheads*), are discernible. *Arrows*, cochlear nerves.

vestibular system can often be resolved. It also allows detailed analysis of specific structures not aligned with the cardinal axes. For example, such protocols allow all four nerves of the internal auditory canal to be discerned as they exit the cranial cavity. The presence of a cochlear nerve is critical, particularly when cochlear implantation is being considered. Newer MRI protocols, such as the 3D CISS method, can be completed in less than 10 minutes, and without intravenous contrast. The main disadvantage of MRI is its poor discrimination of bone, so CT is still preferred if concerns exist about bony architecture, such as mastoid configuration, ossicular status, and facial nerve course.

Genetic Evaluation

A referral to a medical geneticist is recommended in most cases of bilateral SNHL unless there is clear evidence for a nonhereditary cause of the condition. Such specialists will determine inheritance patterns in families and can help integrate disparate physical and other features into patterns suggesting known syndromes. Genetic testing can be performed to detect mutations in several hearing loss genes. In 2006, clinical genetic testing was widely available for *GJB2* and *GJB6* (connexins 26 and 30, respectively), *SLC26A4* (Pendred syndrome), and the mitochondrial *A1555G* mutation. This list is growing each year, and high-throughput screening tools capable of querying multiple deafness genes are being developed. In addition to helping determine the cause, the geneticist also coordinates genetic counseling for the families to explain the implications of genetic findings for future offspring.

Other Diagnostic Studies

As noted earlier, SNHL can be accompanied by a number of defects in other organ systems detectable by certain routine tests, so the latter are commonly used in the workup for the cause of SNHL. Electrocardiography can detect the characteristic of long QT syndrome (Jervell-Lange-Nielsen syndrome), and urinalysis can detect the proteinuria and/or hematuria that can accompany Alport's syndrome. Renal ultrasound is sometimes used to detect renal malformations, such as those accompanying BOR syndrome. Serology is typically used in a targeted fashion if there are concerns about specific disorders. For example, TORCH (***T**oxoplasma*, ***o**ther* infections [e.g., syphilis], ***r**ubella*, ***c**ytomegalovirus*, and ***h**erpes simplex*) titers can be ordered if concerns exist for prenatal or perinatal infection, as can fluorescent treponemal antibody absorption (FTA-ABS) testing if risk factors for syphilis are suspected. Finally, thyroid function testing is sometimes used if Pendred syndrome is suspected, although it should be noted that thyroid function is most commonly normal during childhood, even in patients homozygous for pendrin mutations.

Other Specialists

As noted earlier, referral to an ophthalmologist should be considered after the diagnosis of SNHL. This provides diagnostic and therapeutic benefit. Retinal pathology, such as that found in Usher's syndrome, can be detected by examination or electroretinography. Other visual disturbances can be detected and corrected in other cases as well. It has been estimated that visual deficits, usually refractive errors, exist in over 50% of patients with severe SNHL, so it is critical that these be diagnosed and corrected early to minimize the disadvantage of a second sensory handicap. Referral to other specialists, including those in cardiology, nephrology, and endocrinology, is sometimes needed based on all the test results. Finally, referral to a developmental pediatrician is warranted in the setting of multisensory disorders, multiple disabilities, and cognitive delays.

Management

Because SNHL in children is generally not reversible, principles of management are focused mainly on auditory rehabilitation, detecting and minimizing additional reversible causes of hearing loss, and minimizing progression of existing hearing loss.

Auditory Rehabilitation

Amplification

Auditory rehabilitation should include early referral to an audiologist for a hearing aid evaluation. Children can be fitted and receive hearing aids even in early infancy. Early amplification is critical to maximize the development of central auditory and language centers during the rapid neurologic development that occurs during early childhood. Any auditory input, however weak, will help promote development of cortical centers for speech and language processing. This fact should be emphasized to parents because they will be responsible for ensuring the child's compliance with the hearing aid, which can be difficult. During school age, simple measures such as preferential seating in the classroom can make a large difference in improving the ratio of the signal (teacher's voice) to the classroom noise. Similarly, wireless microphone-loudspeaker combinations (often referred to as frequency modulation [FM] systems, although not all work by FM technology) also help in the classroom by improving the signal-to-noise ratio. Both classroom strategies can help patients with all degrees of hearing loss, even those with near-normal hearing, excel in a noisy classroom environment.

Cochlear Implantation

Cochlear implantation can provide dramatic benefits to patients with severe to profound SNHL who derive minimal or no benefit from hearing aids. The cochlear implant is a linear array of electrodes that is implanted in the first spiral turn of the cochlea, and stimulates the auditory nerve (cochlear spiral ganglion) electrically. It is surgically placed in a region of the cochlea that receives and processes sound frequencies most important for speech (500 to 4000 Hz). Current devices use an electronic receiver-stimulator unit implanted under the parietal scalp. An externally worn microphone and speech processor convert environmental sound into coded electromagnetic signals that are transmitted across the intact scalp to the internal device, which then electrically stimulates specific regions of the auditory nerve.

The cochlear implant has been approved for children since 1990 and, because of its remarkable success in treating deafness, its indications have broadened since then. At present, the devices are implanted in children as young as 12 months, with some receiving implants at even younger ages in special circumstances. Although performance varies from patient to patient because of many factors, many children develop excellent speech understanding and speech production, including open-set speech recognition, which means understanding speech sounds with no environmental context, visual input, or lip reading. Speaking on the telephone is a form of open-set speech recognition and is achieved by many cochlear implant recipients. Performance data in children have clearly shown a benefit for early implantation in language development. Children who undergo implantation before age 3, and especially before age 2, can catch up to their normal-hearing peers in language development in as few as 1 to 2 years, and many are able to attend mainstream schools at the beginning of kindergarten. Although such high levels of performance are not reached by some patients, the vast majority derive at least some benefit from electrical stimulation. Some patients plateau at closed-set or context-assisted speech understanding. Finally, certain others, particularly those with significant cognitive impairment or other disabilities, may gain only sound awareness or augmentation of lip-reading skills, which nevertheless still provide significant improvement in their quality of life.

Inner ear malformation does not preclude cochlear implantation. Patients with enlarged vestibular aqueducts and cochlear partitioning defects can receive implants, and most derive significant benefit. Cochlear implantation is also possible, albeit challenging, in more severe deformities, such as cochlear hypoplasia and common cavity deformity; however, the outcome is more variable, probably because of variation in the amount of neural elements that remain present in the walls of the dysplastic cavities. MRI is particularly useful in making the decision to attempt implantation because it can ascertain the presence and caliber of the cochlear nerve, the target of the electrical stimulation.

Preservation of Residual Hearing

When SNHL is diagnosed, the clinician must ensure that all reversible sources of hearing loss are treated, because these can be additive with the SNHL and increase disability. The most common is otitis media. Although the detection of otitis media is important in all patients, its diagnosis and aggressive management in the SNHL population are critical, because hearing thresholds can be reduced by an additional 30 or 40 dB by a chronic middle ear effusion. Close monitoring is critical during the otitis-prone years in early childhood. Similarly, parents should be counseled that extra diligence is needed, to protect the ears from excessive noise exposure throughout the child's lifetime.

Future Prospects in Therapy

Humans and other mammals lack any significant natural ability to regenerate the sensory tissues of the inner ear and, as a result, SNHL has historically been viewed as generally permanent and untreatable. However, great strides have been made in the last 2 decades in auditory neuroscience research, and in understanding the development and molecular physiology of the auditory sensory cells and the mechanisms of regeneration in other animal species (birds, in particular). Recently, several laboratories have demonstrated,[5] for the first time, the ability to induce regeneration of lost cochlear sensory hair cells in mammals as a result of experimental cell or gene therapy. Although similar human therapies are many years from clinical application, the future holds promise for possible biologic therapies for SNHL in at least some deaf children.

SPECIAL CONSIDERATIONS

Mixed Hearing Loss

In mixed hearing loss, there are components of both SNHL and CHL. Many of the causes of mixed hearing loss overlap with those causing SNHL (see earlier). For example, both BOR and CHARGE syndromes can cause mixed hearing loss, with the conductive component due to middle ear and ossicular malformations. The diagnostic workup and management of mixed hearing loss need to be individualized, but will include the elements described for both CHL and SNHL. For example, if a large conductive component is present, the clinician may combine CT scanning and MRI in the evaluation, because of the former's ability to evaluate the ossicular chain. Beyond imaging studies, however, the remainder of the evaluation is focused on identifying the underlying cause of the sensorineural component.

Unilateral Hearing Loss

Unilateral hearing loss (UHL) presents some unique considerations in evaluation and management. Many of the same conditions that cause bilateral SNHL can cause unilateral disease. Inner ear malformations are a surprisingly frequent cause (40%, even more prevalent than in bilateral SNHL). As described earlier, tumors and other space-occupying lesions are a known but uncommon cause of UHL, and therefore MRI is being used more often for the initial workup of UHL in children. Newer MRI protocols have the advantage of detecting both mass lesions and inner ear malformations in these patients. Although genetic disorders more commonly produce bilateral losses, they can cause asymmetrical or even purely unilateral hearing loss. As one example, unilateral involvement has been described in several cases of *GJB2* mutations. Overall, a genetic cause is suspected in 2% to 13% of those with unilateral hearing loss, so genetics referral should be considered in these patients if imaging does not reveal an anatomic cause.

The clinical presentation of UHL can be enigmatic because, before the advent of neonatal hearing screening, it often went unnoticed for years, often until the child's first elementary school screening tests. This made its time of onset and duration impossible to determine. Only recently has it become widely recognized that unilateral hearing loss can affect school performance significantly. Whereas patients were formerly told just to rely on the "good" ear, many centers are currently emphasizing hearing aid trials in unilateral hearing loss, unless the hearing loss is too severe to benefit from amplification. Restoration of bilateral hearing in these patients has been shown to improve speech understanding in noise, which is important in the classroom setting.

Hearing Loss in the Newborn

Failing a newborn hearing screening (NBHS) can be a worrisome event for new parents. It is important to realize that NBHS is only a screening evaluation, and can yield both false-positive and false-negative results. It is done on each ear individually, and so will typically detect congenital UHL as well as bilateral loss. It is important to note that screening programs are specifically designed to provide sound in the mild hearing loss range (approximately 30 to 40 dB), so NBHS programs can be expected to miss cases of mild hearing loss. Prompt referral to an audiologist for follow-up screening is vital, because infants with confirmed hearing loss should begin auditory rehabilitation as soon as possible, including being fitted for hearing aids or even being evaluated for cochlear implantation, to avoid missing auditory input during the critical early years of language development. Finally, neonates with a significant family history or perinatal risk factors (see Box 4-6) should be referred for follow-up audiologic evaluations, regardless of whether they pass NBHS. This recommendation is based on the fact that certain high-risk infants may have fluctuating losses or progressive SNHL that is not detectable until later in infancy. Some notable examples are children with severe hyperbilirubinemia, congenital CMV infection, and many types of autosomal dominant genetic hearing loss.

SUMMARY

Hearing loss in children is relatively common and its early detection is critical. Prompt referral for audiometric testing and/or otolaryngologic evaluation is indicated for parental hearing concerns, failed screenings, or a family history of hearing impairment. Beyond the initial detection of a hearing loss, the first consideration should be determination of its severity and categorization of the broad type of loss—conductive, sensorineural, or mixed. Once these are known, subsequent evaluation can focus on determining the diagnosis. Underlying conditions causing conductive hearing loss are distinct from those causing sensorineural hearing loss, and therefore their evaluation and management algorithms differ substantially. Many forms of hearing loss, particularly conductive losses, are potentially reversible, and many others are

MAJOR POINTS

Hearing loss in children is categorized as conductive or sensorineural. Conductive loss usually originates in the external or middle ear, and sensorineural loss originates in the inner ear, auditory nerve, or higher centers. Mixed hearing loss has components of both. The distinction is critical, because they differ greatly in cause, evaluation, and management.

Conductive hearing loss has various causes, the most common of which is middle ear effusion. Many forms are reversible by medical and/or surgical management.

Critical components of the evaluation of conductive hearing loss are the physical examination and the tympanogram. If the cause is not clear, noncontrast CT of the temporal bone can be valuable.

Sensorineural hearing loss (SNHL) can be congenital or acquired, genetic or environmental. The site of lesion can be sensory (cochlear) or neural (retrocochlear), a distinction that can often be made on audiometric testing.

Continued

MAJOR POINTS—cont'd

Approximately 50% of all cases of congenital SNHL are believed to have a genetic cause. Of these, most are not part of a syndrome.

Mutations in connexin 26 are the most common genetic cause of SNHL in the United States, accounting for up to 40% of nonsyndromic cases.

Syndromes commonly associated with SNHL include Pendred, Usher, branchio-oto-renal, Waardenburg, and CHARGE syndromes.

Acquired environmental causes of SNHL are varied and include labyrinthitis (viral and bacterial), ototoxic exposures including medications and hypoxic insults, and trauma.

Inner ear malformations are found in about one third of all children diagnosed with SNHL. The most common is the enlarged vestibular aqueduct (EVA). Many malformations are accompanied by progressive hearing loss.

Inner ear malformations carry an increased risk of bacterial meningitis. Appropriate immunizations and aggressive management of otitis media are critical.

Basic evaluation of hearing loss includes history and physical examination and the audiometric assessment. Risk factors for hearing loss, such as family history, history of otitis media and meningitis, trauma, and exposure to ototoxic medications, should be determined. The physical examination focuses on identifying middle ear pathology and any physical features of hearing loss syndromes.

The gold standard for hearing assessment is the familiar audiogram. More specialized physiologic testing is also available for children unable to be tested by behavioral audiograms and for testing specific parts of the auditory pathway.

Imaging is important in the evaluation of hearing loss. Temporal bone CT detects bony malformations and middle ear pathology. Newer MRI protocols detect inner ear malformations and intracranial pathology, and assess the status of the auditory nerves.

Genetics consultation is critical when the cause is unclear or when there is a positive family history of hearing loss.

Amplification (hearing aids) should be instituted as soon as possible after the diagnosis of permanent hearing loss. Cochlear implantation is an excellent option for children with bilateral severe to profound loss who fail to benefit from amplification.

amenable to rehabilitation with amplification or cochlear implantation.

REFERENCES

1. Joint Committee on Infant Hearing, American Academy of Audiology, American Academy of Pediatrics, American Speech-Language-Hearing Association, Directors of Speech and Hearing Programs in State Health and Welfare Agencies: Year 2000 position statement: Principles and guidelines for early hearing detection and intervention programs. Pediatrics 2000;106:798-817.
2. Blake KD, Prasad C: CHARGE syndrome. Orphanet J Rare Dis 2006;1:34.
3. Park AH, Kou B, Hotaling A, et al: Laryngoscope 2000;110:1715-1719.
4. Jackler RK, De La Cruz A: Laryngoscope 1989;99:1238-1242.
5. Izumikawa M, Minoda R, Kawamoto K, et al: Auditory hair cell replacement and hearing improvement by *Atoh1* gene therapy in deaf mammals. Nat Med 2005;11:271-276.

SUGGESTED READING

Germiller JA, Kazahaya K: Labyrinthitis. In Burg FD, Polin RA, Ingelfinger JR, Gershon AA (eds): Current Pediatric Therapy, 18th ed. Philadelphia, Elsevier, 2006.

Gurtler N, Lalwani AK: Etiology of syndromic and nonsyndromic sensorineural hearing loss. Otolaryngol Clin North Am 2002;35:891-908.

Hereditary hearing loss. Available at http://webhost.ua.ac.be/hhh.

Hone SW, Smith RJ: Medical evaluation of pediatric hearing loss. Laboratory, radiographic, and genetic testing. Otolaryngol Clin North Am 2002;35:751-64.

Li H, Roblin G, Liu H, Heller S: Generation of hair cells by stepwise differentiation of embryonic stem cells. Proc Natl Acad Sci U S A 2003;100:13495-13500.

Li XC, Friedman RA: Nonsyndromic hereditary hearing loss. Otolaryngol Clin North Am 2002;35:275-285.

Lieu JE: Speech-language and educational consequences of unilateral hearing loss in children. Arch Otolaryngol Head Neck Surg 2004;130:524-530.

Morton CC, Nance WE: Newborn hearing screening—a silent revolution. N Engl J Med 2006; 354:2151-2164.

Preciado DA, Lawson L, Madden C, et al: Improved diagnostic effectiveness with a sequential diagnostic paradigm in idiopathic pediatric sensorineural hearing loss. Otol Neurotol 2005;26:610-615.

Smith RJ, Bale JF Jr, White KR: Sensorineural hearing loss in children. Lancet 2005;365:879-890.

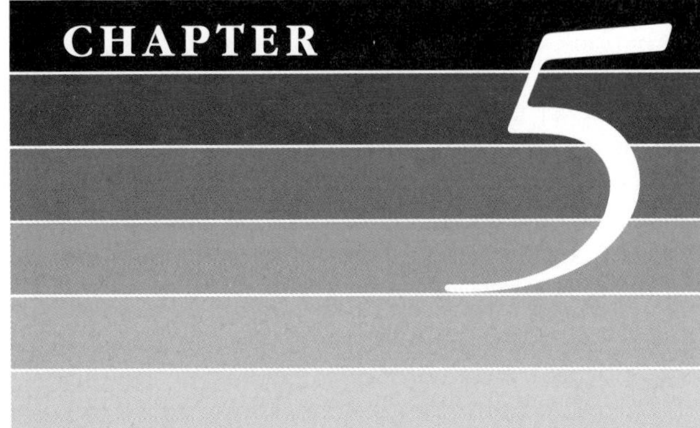

Otitis Media

LISA M. ELDEN, MD

Otitis media (OM) is one of the most common reasons that children visit their physicians, with an estimated 5.2 million acute otitis media (AOM) episodes occurring yearly.[1] From 1980 to 2006, the incidence of AOM increased, partly because more children attended daycare centers. The disease is expensive and the cost of treament of OM in the United States has been reported to be between $3 billion and $5 billion.[2] Treatment strategies are beginning to change because of concerns about the emergence of resistant bacteria caused by antibiotic overuse. In addition, studies have indicated that antibiotics have limited benefit in the treatment of AOM. Because acute infections have been shown to resolve spontaneously without significant sequelae when patients are carefully observed, guidelines have been devised that propose a period of observation before antibiotics are prescribed in otherwise healthy children as an option for management. Although the morbidity of untreated AOM is potentially severe, such a policy has proven to be successful in certain countries (Netherlands and Sweden), but remains controversial in the United States. It is clear that this strategy does not apply to all children and is highly dependent on age and the presence of coexisting illness. Controversy also exists regarding the timing and treatment of chronic otitis media with effusion (OME) because the effect of the associated mild, fluctuating hearing loss on speech and language development is not clear.

DEFINITIONS

Otitis media implies inflammation of the middle ear that usually spreads to contiguous structures, including the mastoid and surrounding air cells of the temporal bone. The associated middle ear effusion (MEE) may be serous, mucoid, purulent, or bloody in nature, but the type of effusion does not always provide information as to the cause or pathogenesis. AOM and OME should be considered as different stages of a continuum. Although in the early stages of AOM it is possible to have myringitis with a red, inflamed tympanic membrane (TM), the diagnosis cannot be confirmed without the finding of MEE. Erythema of the TM can also be found in crying or febrile children. To differentiate AOM from OME, there must also be a history of rapid onset within 24 to 48 hours and one or more signs or symptoms of inflammation, including otalgia, otorrhea, fever, and irritability.[3] OME is defined as MEE without signs of AOM. OME may occur with or without a preceding AOM. OME is considered chronic (COME) if it has been present for longer than 3 months. Recurrent AOM is defined as a new episode of AOM that occurs more than 4 weeks after a preceding infection. Chronic suppurative otitis media (CSOM) is further defined by the presence of otorrhea, which occurs when MEE drains through a pressure-equalizing tube (PET) or through a perforation of the TM.

Atelectasis refers to thinning and collapse of the TM, which may occur as a result of eustachian tube dysfunction that leads to negative pressure of the middle ear or from scarring of the weakened TM. Retraction pockets are isolated areas of atelectasis or thinning that may progress to cholesteatoma. *Adhesive otitis media* is the condition in which part of or the entire TM becomes adherent to the promontory (floor of the middle ear) or the structures within the middle ear, including the ossicles. It is considered a complication of otitis media; it may be progressive in nature, but can result in associated ossicular erosion, conductive hearing loss, and cholesteatoma development.

ANATOMY AND PATHOPHYSIOLOGY

The middle ear system includes the mastoid posteriorly and structures related to the eustachian tube (ET) anteriorly—the nose, nasopharynx (NP), and palate (Fig. 5-1). The ET normally maintains a healthy middle ear by (1) providing a means of ventilating the middle ear by allowing middle ear pressure to equilibrate with ambient pressure, (2) protecting against nasopharyngeal pressure variations and ascending pathogens, and (3) allowing for drainage of middle ear secretions into the nasopharynx. OM develops when ET dysfunction occurs with the development of negative pressure in the middle ear space. It is usually preceded by a viral upper respiratory tract infection that leads to edema and congestion of the respiratory mucosa, including that of the middle ear, mastoid, and ET. The ET is normally closed at rest, but periodically opens with movement of the palate to ventilate the middle ear. When the ET isthmus—that part of the ET that enters into the NP—becomes edematous, the ET cannot properly ventilate air into the middle ear system. Air eventually diffuses out of the middle ear space, causing retraction of the TM and the development of MEE. The MEE may persist as noninfected serous otitis media or become infected with viruses or bacteria. If the ET dysfunction is sustained, potential pathogens in the nasopharynx may be aspirated into the middle ear and mastoid cavities. Viruses are rarely the sole pathogen and account for only 20% of middle ear infections.

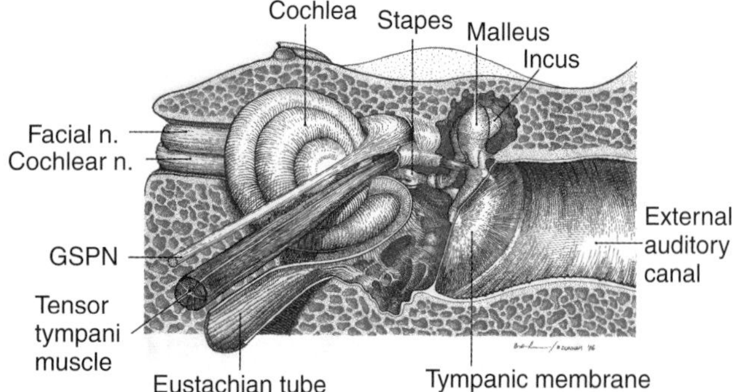

Figure 5-1. Anatomy of the middle ear and eustachian tube. GSPN, Greater sphenopalatine nerve.

Young children and infants are more prone to OM because they have ETs that are shorter, more horizontal, and functionally more immature than those in older children and adults. Most children have mature systems by 5 to 7 years of age. Children with chronic inflammation of the NP, as seen in those with allergic rhinitis or enlarged or chronically inflamed adenoids, are more likely to have persistent problems throughout their early childhood. Severe gastroesophageal reflux may also result in inflammation of the ET.

Children with craniofacial anomalies that affect palatal and nasopharyngeal function may have ET dysfunction that persists throughout their lifetime. Children more likely to be affected have craniofacial abnormalities such as unrepaired cleft palate or midface anomalies as seen in Apert's syndrome, Crouzon's syndrome, Treacher Collins syndrome, Down syndrome, or other skull base malformations.

Other children at higher risk include those born with immune disorders, including ciliary dyskinesia, immunoglobulin deficiencies (especially immunoglobulin A [IgA] deficiency and hypogammaglobulinemia), T-cell deficiencies (e.g., 22q deletion syndrome), combined T- and B-cell deficiencies, and phagocyte defects (e.g., telangiectasia or complement disorders). In addition, children on corticosteroid therapy or chemotherapy, and those with acquired immune disorders, including human immunodeficiency virus (HIV) infection or ET dysfunction secondary to radiotherapy, are more likely to develop OM.

NATURAL HISTORY

After every episode of AOM, fluid may persist in the middle ear for weeks to months that may be associated with hearing loss, discomfort, and less often imbalance (Fig. 5-2). If treated successfully with antibiotics, it may remain sterile. Alternatively, OME may develop de novo without bacterial infection and follow a similar pattern. Periodically, nasopharyngeal secretions may be aspirated

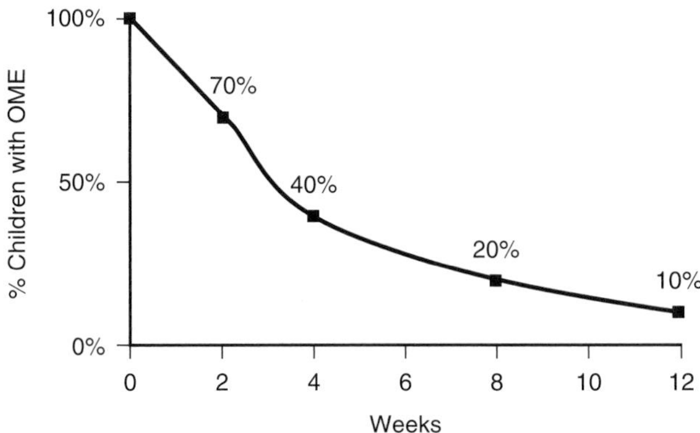

Figure 5-2. Duration of otitis media with effusion (OME) following an episode of acute otitis media.

into the middle ear because of negative pressure in the middle ear, which can lead to recurrent infection. In some cases, structural changes of the eardrum may develop, partly caused by high negative middle ear pressure. Despite the high prevalence of OME episodes, most last only 2 months and spontaneously resolve without treatment, usually in the spring and summer months.[4,5]

It is clear that the incidence of OM has been increasing. A Finnish study comparing AOM cases diagnosed in 1978 to 1979 with those diagnosed in 1994 to 1995 found that the rates of medical and surgical treatment for recurrent OM increased during those periods.[6]

EPIDEMIOLOGY AND RISK FACTORS

Nonmodifiable Risk Factors

Age. The peak age-specific attack rate occurs between the ages of 6 and 18 months and the overall prevalence of OM is highest in children who are 1 to 3 years of age.[7] This increased risk is thought to relate to the immature ET. Children who have AOM before 6 months of age or OME before 2 months of age are at increased risk for ongoing middle ear problems compared with those whose ear disease develops later. If a child has not had OM before the age of 3 years, he or she is unlikely to develop severe or recurrent middle ear disease. The prevalence of OM decreases after age 3 years until a second smaller peak occurs at 5 to 7 years. This second peak is thought to represent those children with ongoing ET dysfunction and/or those with developing adenoid pathology. The growth rate of lymphoid tissue, including adenoids and tonsils, is greatest as children approach 5 to 7 years old. The size of adenoid tissue may be less important than the effect of associated inflammation on the ET, because researchers have shown that OM occurs less frequently after removal of the adenoid in this age range, regardless of the size of the adenoid pad.[8]

Race. OM was originally thought to be less prevalent in African American children than in white children, but more recent cohort studies have shown that the incidence of OM is similar in black and white infants.[9] In contrast, Native American and Alaskan Native children who are younger than 1 year of age have been shown to have three times the number of OM-associated outpatient visits and hospitalization rates compared with other U.S. children.[10] This may be explained by the fact that these children are more likely to have patulous (chronically open) ET compared with the more commonly inflamed and closed ET seen in most cases of OM.[11] Similar findings have been noted with Down syndrome children, but this group also has dynamic problems that increase the tendency for nasopharyngeal contents to be aspirated into the middle ear space.[9]

Socioeconomic Status. The rates of OME are higher in infants who live in cities than in those who live in the suburbs and in lower income groups compared with those in higher socioeconomic groups, respectively. This increased risk in city children probably relates to their exposure to more crowded conditions, both in living situations and in daycare settings, where they may be exposed to more children.[12]

Genetic. Children whose parents and siblings have had significant OM have been shown to have an increase in the number and duration of infections. From a prospective study of 168 sets of twins and seven sets of triplets followed during their first 5 years of life, the estimate of heritability in regard to the duration of OME was .73 ($P < 0.001$), suggesting a strong genetic base to the disease.[13,14] The genes that may account for the genetic predilection for developing OM include those controlling cytokine production and function. Specifically, a Finnish study reported an association between interleukin-1 alpha 889 and recurrent OM.[15] Another study reported an association between surfactant protein A gene locus and susceptibility to severe respiratory syncytial virus (RSV) and AOM infections.[16]

Season. The incidence of OME is highest in the winter and lowest in the summer.[17] In children ages 2 months to 2 years studied in Finland, this seasonal variation correlated with the increased incidence of upper respiratory tract infection (URTI) that occurred in the winter. Rhinoviruses and RSV infections were the most common concurrent viral infections,[18] and are thought to cause the ET swelling that leads to middle ear involvement.

History of Premature Birth. In some studies, children born prematurely have been shown to be at increased risk of developing OM. This increased susceptibility may relate to the narrowed head shape that sometimes occurs because the neonates spend most of their time sleeping. Such anatomic changes or the use of previous long-term indwelling nasotracheal or nasopharyngeal tubes in these infants can lead to later ET dysfunction.

Presence of Other Siblings in the Home. Children with older siblings at home are at increased risk of OM, most likely because they are exposed to more upper respiratory infections, especially if the siblings are of school age.

Other nonmodifiable risk factors include craniofacial malformations and immune deficiencies (see earlier).

Modifiable Risk Factors

Second-hand Smoke. With respect to preventable risk factors, the risk of OME or AOM is higher in children exposed to second-hand smoke. In addition, recurrent OM has been found to occur more frequently in children who have been exposed to smoke prenatally (gestational) as well as passive smoke exposure after birth.[19]

Daycare Attendance. Most studies examining the impact of daycare (attendance as a risk factor for OM) suggest that the critical number that increases the risk of OM is six or more children, regardless of whether this exposure is in a daycare or a home center. This is especially true if entry occurs before the first year of life.[20] From large longitudinal studies at 10 U.S. centers, investigators found that the incidence of common childhood infections, including OM, is higher during the first 2 years of life for those in child care, but differences are not statistically significant by age 3 years.[21] Of these children, 10% had PETs placed by the age of 3 years. The effect of frequent exposure to an increased number of children appears be partly independent of age factors. These studies have demonstrated that the prevalence of URTI and OM is higher among 3- and 4-year-old children when they first enroll in daycare centers at this later age, compared with the prevalence in children who had already been exposed in daycare settings.[22]

Breast-feeding. Although most clinicians agree that children who have been exposed to a URTI have less risk of OM, the evidence from studies supporting this impression has been mixed. The discrepancy may stem from variability in reported duration of the URTI. More recent studies using multivariate models have suggested that the lower risk of OM in children who are breast-fed may be more significant if the duration of breast-feeding is longer than 6 months. This protective effect may last for months after breast-feeding has stopped.[9,23]

Pacifier Use. Pacifier use in young children has been associated with a twofold increased risk of OM in those attending daycare compared with those who did not attend daycare.[24]

Gastroesophageal Reflux. Some data from an uncontrolled study of gastroesophageal reflux disease (GERD) and OM in children undergoing myringotomy for MEE have shown that pepsin and/or pepsinogen protein levels are 1000 times higher than reference serum levels, suggesting a possible correlation between GERD and OM.[25] Gastric acid may reflux to the opening of the ET in the NP and possibly even enter the middle ear space, resulting in inflammation that then leads to infection.

MICROBIOLOGY

Viral Acute Otitis Media

Viruses account for only 20% of AOM cases and are more commonly found (65%) as part of a mixed viral and bacterial infection. RSV and rhinovirus are the most common viruses found in MEE infections, followed by parainfluenza, influenza, enteroviruses, and adenovirus.[26] Patients with MEEs infected with viral and bacterial pathogens have higher concentrations of inflammatory mediators than those with bacterial AOM alone, which may result in worse clinical outcomes.[27]

Bacterial Acute Otitis Media

The two more common bacterial pathogens are *Streptococcus pneumoniae* (25% to 40%) and nontypable *Haemophilus influenzae* (35% to 50%), followed by *Moraxella catarrhalis*, which is isolated in 3% to 20% of cases.[28,29] Group A streptococci and *Staphylococcus aureus* are isolated in 1% to 10% of cases.[29] The bacteria causing infections in infants and neonates are usually the same as those in older children, but gram-negative enteric bacteria, including *Escherichia coli*, *Klebsiella* species, and *Pseudomonas aeruginosa*, and less common pathogens, including *S. aureus* and group A streptococci, may be responsible for 20% of AOM cases in this age group[30,31] (Tables 5-1 and 5-2).

Table 5-1 Microbiology of Acute Otitis Media

Organism	Primary Organism Cultured (%)
Haemophilus influenzae	35-50
Streptococcus pneumoniae	25-40
Moraxella catarrhalis	3-20
Viruses	5-20
No growth	1-15
Other bacteria	1-10

Table 5-2 Microbiology of Otitis Media with Effusion

Organism	Primary Organism Cultured (%)
Other bacteria, including nonpathogenic	45
No growth	30
Haemophilus influenzae	15
Moraxella catarrhalis	10
Streptococcus pneumoniae	7

Other bacterial organisms that have been isolated from MEEs include *Mycoplasma pneumoniae*, *Chlamydia trachomatis*, and *Mycobacterium tuberculosis*. Anaerobic bacteria, including *Peptostreptococcus*, *Fusobacterium*, and *Bacteroides* species, are rarely isolated from MEEs from acutely infected ears, but are more common in those with CSOM and underlying cholesteatoma.[32]

Pathogens in Otitis Media with Effusion

Thirty percent of cultures from MEEs in patients with OME do not grow bacteria and are considered sterile. The more common pathogens account for only 32% of all positive cultures (*S. pneumoniae*, 7%; *H. influenzae*, 15%; *M. catarrhalis*, 10%), with the remaining considered to be nonpathogenic bacteria alone or in combination with viruses.[30-32]

Antibiotic Resistance

To treat OM effectively, the most important pathogen to address is *S. pneumoniae* because it is less likely to resolve spontaneously without treatment compared with *H. influenzae* and *M. catarrhalis*.[33,34] The rate of penicillin-resistant strains of *S. pneumoniae* varies greatly worldwide (from less than 1% in Netherlands to 10% to 40% in the United States and more than 80% in parts of the Far East).[35] In the United States, the rates of penicillin resistance have increased dramatically throughout the 1990s, especially in children attending daycare. A primary cause of this increased rate involves the indiscriminate use of amoxicillin and cephalosporins for the treatment of AOM and OME. The risk factors most often cited for the emergence of penicillin resistance are daycare attendance, treatment of nonresponsive and recurrent AOM, age younger than 2 years, and recent antibiotic therapy.[36]

The mechanism by which bacteria develop resistance to penicillin and cephalosporins relates to alteration of the penicillin-binding proteins in the bacterial cell wall. Overall, the rate of resistance is 40% in children attending daycare and 17% in all children with AOM.[37] In Israeli studies, *S. pneumoniae* strains were found that are also resistant to macrolides (10% to 30%), trimethoprim-sulfamethoxazole (TMP-SMX) (50%), and second- and third-generation cephalosporins, and 17% were multidrug resistant to three or more antibiotics.[38-40] The rates of resistance caused by β-lactamase-producing bacteria have been estimated to be as high as 20% to 50% for *H. influenzae* and almost 100% for *M. catarrhalis*.[41] Thoughtful reduction in antibiotic use may lead to a decrease in the number of resistant organisms.

PREVENTION

To reduce the need for antibiotics, various preventive strategies have been explored but generally have limited benefit. The more commonly studied interventions include the following.

Vaccines. Most studies have focused on preventing *S. pneumoniae*-related infections because it is the most common pathogen. Although the 23-valent polysaccharide vaccine covers 90% of all known pneumococcal infections in older children and adults, it is not efficacious in children most susceptible to OM (i.e., those younger than 2 years). Therefore, the vaccine only provides marginal benefit in preventing OM in older children who have not outgrown their disease.[42] In contrast, pneumococcal conjugate vaccines, in which the pneumococcal capsular saccharides are coupled to a carrier protein, are effective in children as young as 2 months, and they become even more effective in preventing invasive pneumococcal disease after they have been administered at 2, 4, and 6 months of age. Although they are powerful against invasive diseases, such as meningitis and pneumonia, they are less helpful in preventing mucosal infections, such as AOM. The clinical impact of pneumococcal vaccination in children followed for up to 3 to 5 years is limited in that it reduces the number of OM office visits by only 8%.[43]

Viral vaccines have also been shown to reduce the frequency of AOM. Specifically, influenza virus vaccine reduces the incidence of AOM during flu season, with a 30% to 36% relative reduction, but this protective effect disappears at 1-year follow-up and is more effective for children older than 2 years.[44]

Xylitol. Xylitol is a polyol that inhibits the growth of *S. pneumoniae* and its adherence to epithelial cells. The use of gum and syrup has been shown to reduce the risk of AOM in a randomized clinical trial (RCT) in a child care setting.[45] However other studies have suggested that it is less effective when the child has a concurrent URTI, so it may offer only limited benefit.[46]

Probiotic Bacteria. *Lactobacillus rhamnosus* has been studied for OM prevention in an RCT of daycare children to ascertain the effects of long-term consumption of milk containing probiotic bacteria. Although the effects were modest and not statistically significant, there were favorable trends of fewer days absent from daycare, fewer URTIs and AOM episodes diagnosed by physicians, and fewer prescribed antibiotics in the children taking *Lactobacillus* supplements. To date, the evidence is insufficient to recommend the use of *Lactobacillus* on a routine basis.[47]

Reduction of Pacifier Use. From studies of well-baby clinics, infants whose parents were randomized to limit the duration of time that the infants used pacifiers were compared with those whose parents allowed unlimited pacifier use. Those infants who had restricted use had one third fewer episodes of AOM.[48] However, some studies have shown that pacifiers are protective in reducing the risk of sudden infant death syndrome (SIDS), so it may be more appropriate to avoid counseling parents of OM-prone children to reduce pacifier use until their infants are older than 6 months.

Treatment of Allergy. Although it appears that children who have allergies that lead to nasal congestion are more likely to have ongoing OM, few studies have been done to examine the clinical impact of preventive treatment.

Antibiotics. Antibiotic prophylaxis has been shown to be successful in preventing AOM, but the impact is small and this practice is discouraged, because it promotes the development of emerging resistant organisms. From meta-analysis studies, it has been shown that it would be necessary to give 11 months of antibiotics to prevent one episode of AOM in 1 year.[49]

DIAGNOSIS

History and Physical Examination

To diagnose AOM more accurately, a new definition of AOM has been proposed by expert panels. This states that three components must be present to diagnose AOM: (1) a history of acute onset within 48 hours of presentation; (2) presence of MEE; and (3) signs or symptoms of middle ear inflammation.[23,50,51] The most common symptoms of AOM include ear pain or ear pulling, irritability, and low-grade fever. Less common symptoms are nausea and imbalance. Older children also usually complain of a blocked ear, with decreased hearing and a "popping" sensation.

OME is defined as fluid in the middle ear, without signs or symptoms of AOM.[52,53] Children with OME present in a more subtle manner, complaining of intermittent otalgia, imbalance, and hearing loss. Very young children may be more symptomatic at night, with frequent awakenings and, when mild hearing loss has been present, may have speech and language delays.

Otoscopy and Pneumatic Otoscopy

The physical examination of a normal TM reveals a pale gray and usually translucent eardrum. The middle ear landmarks include the short process and manubrium (or handle) of the malleus, which are in contact with the eardrum, and the chorda tympani nerve and incudostapedial joint posterosuperiorly, which are deep or medial to the TM but are usually visible through the eardrum (Fig. 5-3).

In AOM, the TM is thickened and edematous and sometimes pale yellow pus can be seen through the TM (Fig. 5-4). In the early phases of AOM (myringitis), the TM may be reddened, but diagnosis of ear disease cannot be confirmed unless a middle ear effusion is present. The strongest positive predictor of AOM is a bulging tympanic membrane that obliterates normal landmarks, followed by the finding of reduced mobility and then an opaque tympanic membrane.[50] Redness alone is the least predictive because of the potential for false-positive results that can occur when the child cries. Occasionally, there may be a red effusion when hemorrhage has occurred in an inflamed middle ear.

In OME, the TM is usually mildly inflamed, sometimes with overlying blood vessels spread out in a radial fashion throughout the eardrum. The middle ear effusion may be thin and clear, with or without air bubbles, especially

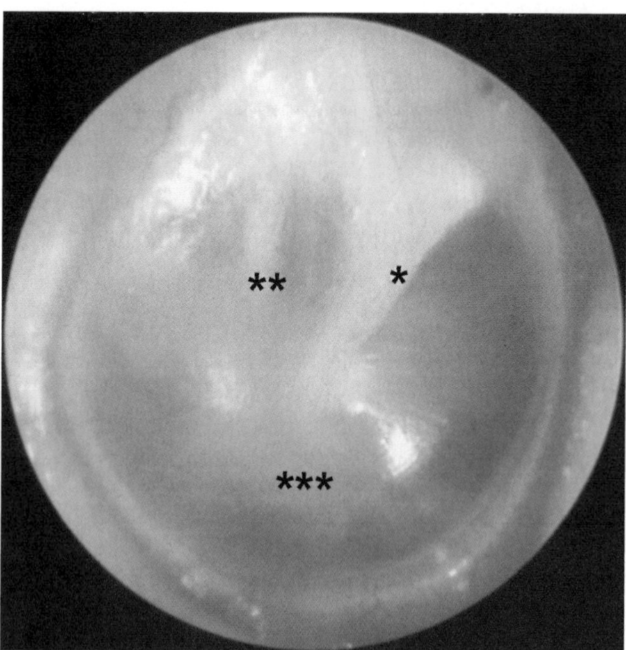

Figure 5-3. Normal tympanic membrane. The tympanic membrane is translucent, allowing visualization of the middle ear structures, including the short and long processes of the malleus (*), incudostapedial joint (**), promontory, and round window niche (***).

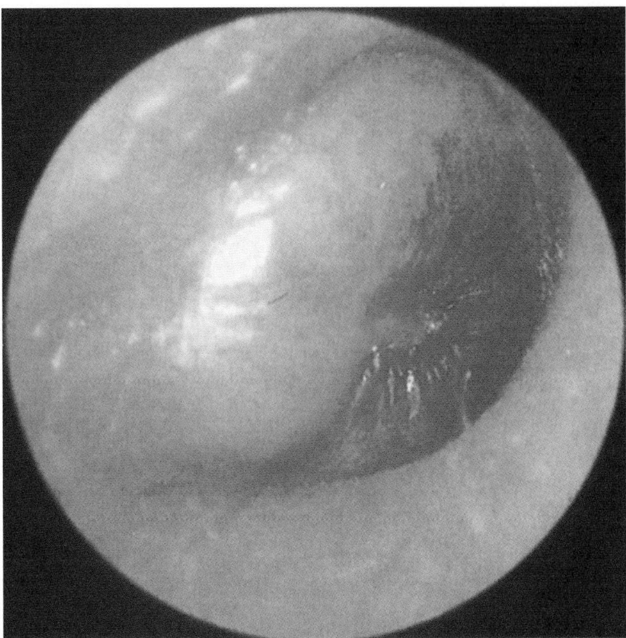

Figure 5-4. Acute otitis media. The tympanic membrane is inflamed and bulging.

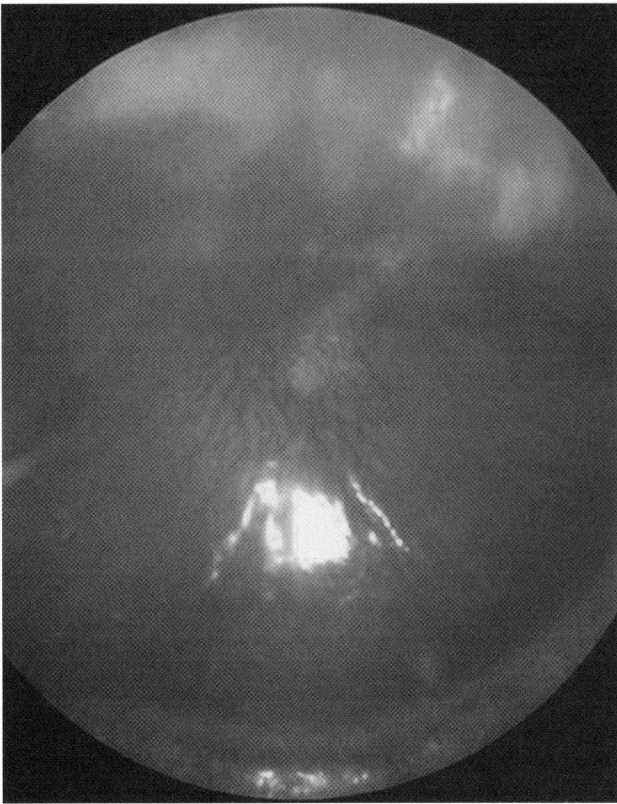

Figure 5-5. Otitis media with effusion. The tympanic membrane is amber pink and retracted, with a foreshortened malleus.

when serous effusion is present. It may be pale yellow or white if mucus is present. The TM is often diffusely retracted or concave (Fig. 5-5).

With CSOM, there is generally an associated perforation or draining tube present (Fig. 5-6). The otorrhea may be pale mucus or purulent in nature when a bacterial infection is present or pasty white with a fungal *Candida* infection. In some cases, pink granulation tissue may be seen and, if present in the inferior quadrants of the TM, a hidden and infected retained tube should be suspected (Fig. 5-7). Less often, the otorrhea relates to an underlying retraction pocket or cholesteatoma. It is important to ensure that the ear is reexamined once the exudate has been fully treated to exclude an underlying cholesteatoma. A cholesteatoma is more likely to be present if an attic or posterior superior retraction pocket is seen containing white keratin, granulation, or yellow wet debris (Fig. 5-8).

In addition to retraction pockets, long-standing changes that can occur related to middle ear disease include tympanosclerosis and atelectasis. Tympanosclerosis appears as white plaques containing calcium and phosphate in the middle fibrous layer of the three-layered TM; this tends to stiffen the TM. Tympanosclerosis or myringosclerosis is more commonly seen in the area of the pars tympani and often forms a horseshoe pattern in the lower half of the TM. It may change in pattern and distribution with time and is more commonly seen in children who have had tubes placed, but has also been reported in children who have had a history of OM without

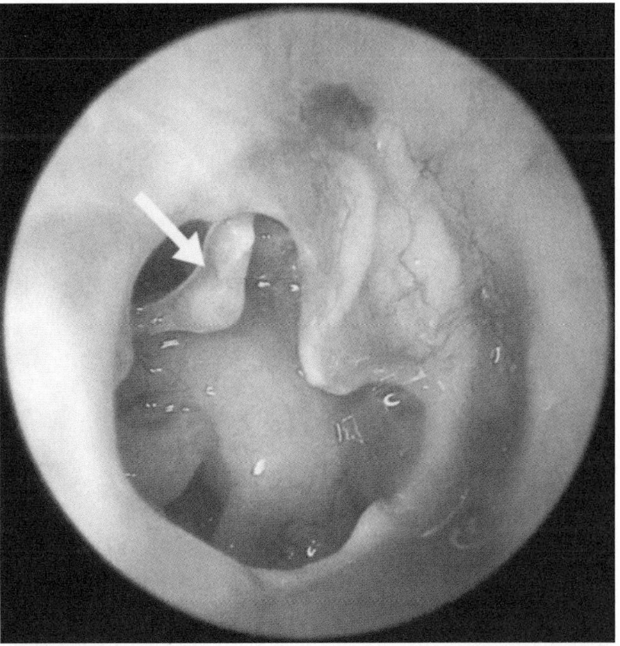

Figure 5-6. Perforation of posterior half of tympanic membrane. The partially eroded incudostapedial joint can be seen through the perforation *(arrow)*.

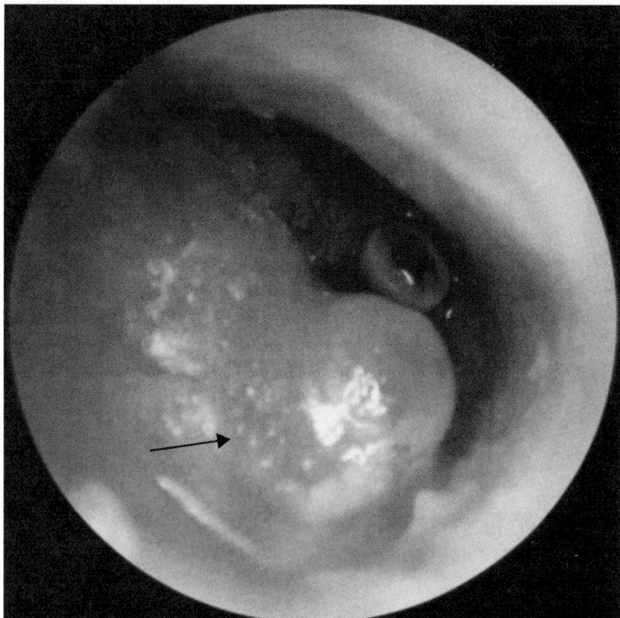

Figure 5-7. Ventilating tube in tympanic membrane, with associated infected granuloma *(arrow)*.

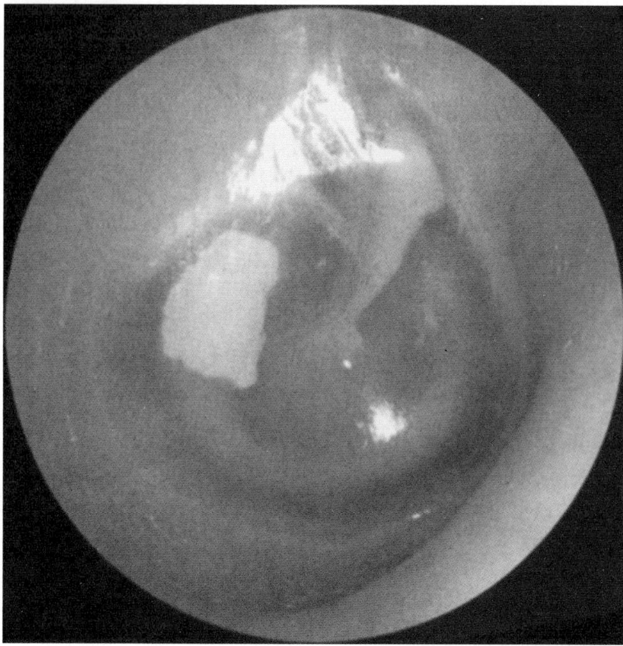

Figure 5-9. Myringosclerosis (tympanosclerosis) in the tympanic membrane, which resulted from calcium deposits in the middle fibrosis layer of the tympanic membrane.

tubes (Fig. 5-9). Tympanosclerosis is rarely associated with hearing loss. Atelectasis or thinning of the TM is a more ominous finding and may develop because of chronic negative pressure in the middle ear space. In more severe cases, there may be associated long-standing mild hearing loss that only improves if the ear is ventilated with a tube. The TM is usually thinned, drapes over the ossicles, and may lie on the floor of the middle ear or promontory. In some cases, adhesive otitis media develops, in which the TM may become adherent and fixed to the middle ear floor, covering the ossicles so they become "skeletonized." Hearing may or may not be affected (Fig. 5-10).

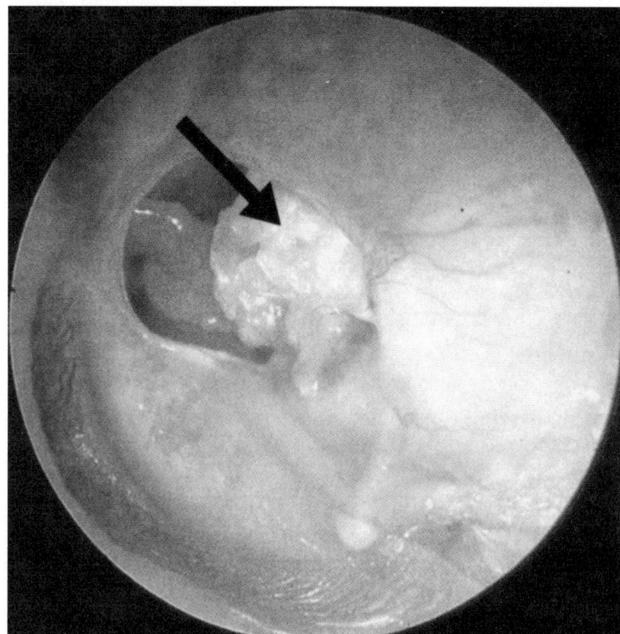

Figure 5-8. Cholesteatoma *(arrow)* seen through posterior superior tympanic membrane perforation.

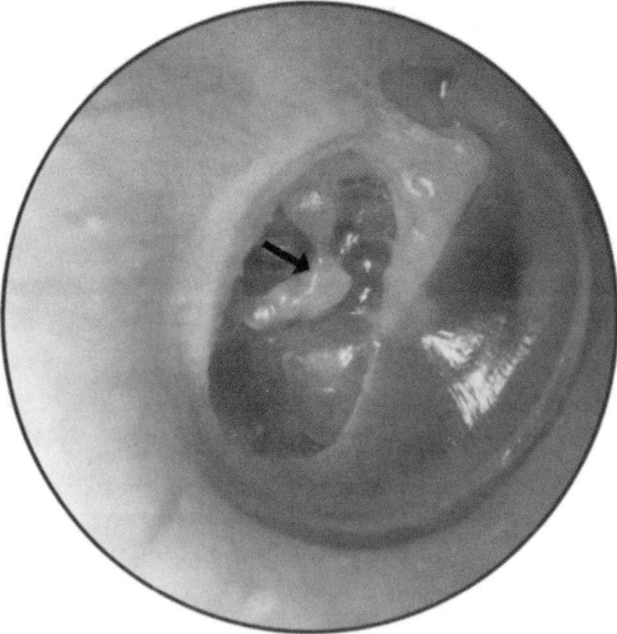

Figure 5-10. Severe atelectasis and retraction of the tympanic membrane with skeletonized ossicles. The distal tip of the incus is eroded and separated from the stapes *(arrow)*.

Accuracy of Diagnosis

Proper use of pneumatic otoscopy is critical in the diagnosis of AOM and OME to document the presence or absence of movement of the TM on insufflation. However, studies have shown that the learning curve to master this skill is steep.[54] When properly performed, pneumatic otoscopy is the most accurate test to diagnose AOM or OME when compared with the gold standard of incision and drainage by myringotomy. Meta-analysis studies have revealed a pooled sensitivity of 94% (95% confidence interval [CI], 91% to 96%) and specificity of 80% (95% CI, 75% to 86%) for a validated observer compared with myringotomy.[55]

Supplementary Tests

Because the diagnosis of OM is often made with some uncertainty, supplementary objective tests such as tympanography and acoustic reflectometry may be helpful to confirm the presence of MEE. Tympanograms are accurate in excluding disease because type A, or a normal pressure curve with normal compliance, is 90% to 95% sensitive and specific. A type B, or flat, tympanogram, which occurs when there is absence of TM movement, is less accurate, with a sensitivity of 81% and specificity of 74% in confirming the presence of MEE.[56] Instead, this pattern may represent a false-positive recording that occurs when an occlusive seal cannot be maintained between the probe and the ear canal or when the ear canals are excessively compliant, as in young infants. The presence of a type C tympanogram, or negative pressure with normal or reduced compliance, implies that ET dysfunction with a secondary vacuum effect exists in the middle ear. The sensitivity of a type C tympanogram (with pressure recordings of −200 to −400 mm H_2O) is 94%, but this test finding is less specific in ruling out the presence of MEE compared with tympanocentesis findings (62%) (Fig. 5-11).[56] Mobility of the TM may still be present on pneumatic otoscopy. However, if MEE is present, such mobility is usually minimal.

Acoustic reflectometry with spectral gradient analysis is also helpful in determining the probability of the presence of MEE, is inexpensive to use, and does not require that a seal be maintained between the ear canal and probe. However, it is not widely available in most physicians' offices.

Tympanocentesis is a needle aspiration of the eardrum that is usually performed using an 18-gauge spinal needle attached to a tuberculin syringe. Tympanocentesis (or myringotomy, when an incision is made) is considered the gold standard in confirming the presence of MEE and provides a means to obtain bacterial cultures in very sick children. However, even when topical anesthetic is used, tympanocentesis is difficult to perform and sometimes risky in sick and uncooperative children.

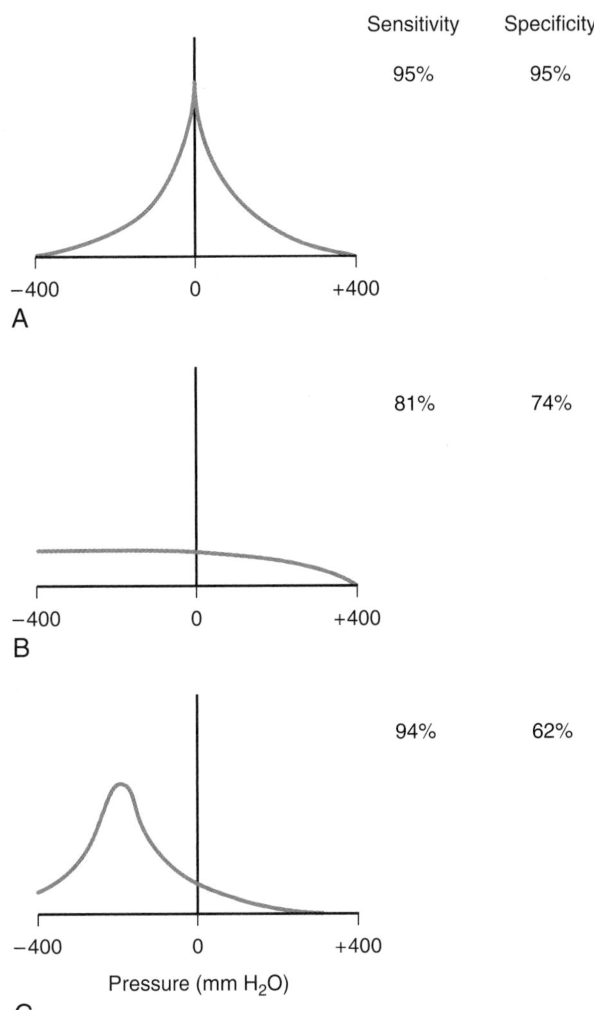

Figure 5-11. Sensitivity and specificity of type A, B, and C tympanograms relative to findings on tympanocentesis.

TREATMENT OF ACUTE OTITIS MEDIA

Development of a New Treatment Paradigm

The new paradigm that has been formulated for AOM treatment is observation versus antibiotic therapy. The rationale for its use is that antibiotics prescribed for AOM account for 25% to 50% of all outpatient antibiotics and are partly responsible for the global finding that bacteria, especially *S. pneumoniae*, *H. influenzae*, and *M. catarrhalis*, are becoming increasingly resistant to these medications.[57] Accordingly, expert panels and various medical societies have been forced to examine the benefits and choice of antibiotic used for AOM. Several expert groups, including the Therapeutic Working Group sponsored by the Centers for Disease Control and Prevention (CDC), along with the American Academy of Pediatrics (AAP), in 2000, and the Joint Committee of the American Academy of Pediatrics (AAP) and American

Academy of Family Practitioners (AAFP), in 2004, established separate guidelines based on reviews of scientific literature.[1,23]

Using the best available studies, including RCTs and cohort studies of patients with suspected AOM treated with antibiotics versus those treated with observation, the AAP-AAFP panel concluded that 80% of children not treated with antibiotics have spontaneous resolution of symptoms within 2 to 7 days of onset of symptoms. With this information, the AAP-AAFP panel has suggested that a period of observation may be appropriate for certain patients with AOM. Theories to explain this unexpectedly high spontaneous resolution rate include the possibility that the MEE eventually drains down the ET, despite the presence of an inflamed middle ear, that the infection is sometimes viral, or that the body's local or systemic immune system functions to cure the infection without the need for antibiotics. Other researchers, including some panel members of the CDC group, thought that this high resolution rate, derived from historical data, may reflect a falsely high estimate related to inaccuracy of diagnosis, in that some of the reviewed studies may have included children with OME, not AOM, in their treatment groups.[1,29] In some of these studies, the criteria for diagnosis of AOM were not made using more rigorous definitions currently recommended. Furthermore, it is highly likely that some of the children in these studies were inappropriately prescribed antibiotics, especially those who may have illnesses or conditions, such as teething, that can cause irritability and ear pain.

As a result, the guidelines differ as to whether observation should be an option in children with AOM. Although the AAP-AAFP panel included an option of observation in its guideline, the CDC group did not make any recommendations for observation.

In contrast, both groups agreed that antibiotics provide only minimal benefit in reducing the duration of symptoms compared with observation alone. Treatment with antibiotics has been shown to increase clinical resolution rates by 12% (95% CI, 3% to 22%) at 2 to 7 days; this implies that eight children must receive initial antibiotics to achieve one successful clinical outcome beyond clinical observation alone.[23,29,50,51] However, controversy exists as to how long it actually takes for symptoms to resolve with observation versus antibiotic treatment. The AAP-AAFP panel reviewed literature suggesting that most symptoms improve by day 2 of observation, but the CDC Advisory Group, which reviewed many overlapping papers, stated that symptoms (pain and fever) do not resolve until days 4 to 7.[1,23,29,57-60] With such inconsistency in time to resolution of symptoms, it is important to consider the quality of life of the child and parental concerns in determining who may be a candidate for observation.

Finally, both groups agreed that mastoiditis and suppurative complications associated with OM are rare and, when present, occur with similar incidence in those observed only and in those treated with antibiotics (0.59% versus 0.17%, respectively; $P = .212$).[23] Furthermore, the incidence of meningitis does not seem to be higher in observed groups, especially in fully immunized children who have been treated with pneumococcal vaccine.

Although they differ in regard to the option of observation, both sets of guidelines have stressed the need for improving accuracy in diagnosis to differentiate AOM from OME, and they both promote "judicious" use of antibiotics. Benefits of careful use of antibiotics are that there should be better control over emerging resistant bacteria and there will be fewer patients exposed to the side effects of antibiotics. These side effects have been reported to occur as often as 15% to 17% of the time and include rashes, diarrhea, and gastrointestinal upset. Both panels have recommended that physicians continue to be sensitive to patient pain, parental anxiety, and potential significant sequelae that may occur, especially in those patients whose parents may be less compliant in following recommendations. The strategy for withholding antibiotics has been shown to be successful in countries such as the Netherlands, where the health care system is designed to promote better follow-up care than is typically seen in the United States. To allow the model to succeed, it is essential that children who are observed be given appropriate analgesia for pain control, such as ibuprofen or acetaminophen.

The AAP-AAFP panel has specified that not all children with AOM are candidates for observation. Very young children or those with immune problems, genetic problems, craniofacial anomalies, known underlying OME, or recent AOM in the previous 30 days are more likely to suffer ill consequences from observation alone and should not be considered candidates for this option. The panel has also specified that the observation option must be used only if there is a high probability that the parent will be compliant in returning for evaluation if symptoms of AOM persist over the next 72 hours.

In summary, the AAP-AAFP guidelines have recommended an option of observation in cases of AOM that are uncomplicated, nonrecurrent, and nonpersistent and take into consideration three variables that should be considered before observation is chosen—patient age, certainty of diagnosis, and severity of illness.[61] Specifically, any patient younger than 6 months should be treated with an antibiotic, even when the diagnosis of AOM is uncertain. The observation option is recommended for children 6 months to 2 years of age whose baseline health is good. who are not seriously ill at presentation, and who have an uncertain diagnosis. The option of observation is available for children older than

Table 5-3 Options for Treatment of Acute Otitis Media (AAP-AAFP Guidelines)

Age of Child	Certain Diagnosis	Uncertain Diagnosis
Younger than 6 mo	Antibiotics	Antibiotics
6 mo-2 yr	Antibiotics	Antibiotics, if severe illness; observe if nonsevere illness*
2 yr or older	Antibiotics, if severe illness; observe if nonsevere illness*	Observe

*Nonsevere illness—fever < 39°C and/or mild otalgia; severe illness—fever >39°C and/or moderate to severe otalgia.

Guidelines from the Joint Committee of the American Academy of Pediatrics (AAP) and American Academy of Family Practitioners (AAFP); American Academy of Pediatrics Subcommittee on Management of Acute Otitis Media: Diagnosis and management of acute otitis media. Pediatrics 2004;113:1451-1465.

2 years, with nonsevere illness at presentation and uncertain diagnosis; it is also recommended when the diagnosis is certain (Table 5-3). In prospective studies, 25% of those children eventually required antibiotics on follow-up within 48 to 72 hours.

With regard to follow-up, the guidelines have suggested that the observed patient be contacted or seen within 72 hours so that he or she may be treated if symptoms persist. Other authors and practitioners have advocated a "safety net prescription" be given to children who are observed at initial assessment, with instructions to use it if symptoms persist.[51] Although not specified in the guidelines, many have advocated that the patient be reevaluated in 6 weeks to ensure that the MEE clears and within 2 weeks if the patient has other developmental delays or recurrent symptoms.

Medical Therapy

Choice of Antibiotics

Although controversy exists as to whether observation is an option, both expert panels have similar recommendations regarding choice of antibiotic. Table 5-4 summarizes antibiotics that may be given.

The antibiotic chosen initially to treat uncomplicated, nonrecurrent AOM has traditionally been geared to cover the more common pathogens, including *S. pneumoniae*, *H. influenzae*, and nontypable *M. catarrhalis*. Although a large number of species exist that are resistant to amoxicillin and cephalosporins, evidence has suggested that no antibiotic outperforms amoxicillin as the first-line drug to treat AOM in patients who are not allergic to penicillin (in either standard or high-dose forms). Higher-dose amoxicillin (80 mg/kg/day in two divided doses for 5 to 10 days) has been shown to be more effective than standard dosing (40/mg/kg/day) in that it increases the higher minimum inhibitory concentration (MIC) of penicillin to kill intermediate and some highly resistant strains of *S. pneumoniae*. In addition, although there is a relatively high prevalence of β-lactamase–producing *H. influenzae* and *M. catarrhalis*, AOM caused by these organisms is more likely to resolve spontaneously. Amoxicillin has a relatively low incidence of side effects, is cost-effective, and is palatable to children.

Children who have uncertain allergy to β-lactams or nonanaphylactic allergy are advised to take oral cephalosporins, such as cefdinir, cefuroxime, or cefpodoxime. Some advocate cefdinir because it is dosed once daily and tastes good.

Initial therapy in uncomplicated AOM in patients who have type 1 allergy (anaphylaxis or history of hives) to penicillin or cephalosporins should be treated with one of the following antibiotics: azithromycin, clarithromycin, or erythromycin. The newer macrolides, azithromycin and clarithromycin, act against AOM pathogens by a different mechanism than that for the antibiotics acting against bacteria that produce β-lactamase (including cephalosporins and preparations containing clavulanate). They are bacteriostatic and inhibit bacterial protein synthesis. Unfortunately, up to 30% of *S. pneumoniae* and *H. influenzae* strains have begun to display increasing resistance to the macrolides.[62] Even though the mechanism of action of trimethoprim-sulfamethoxazole differs from that of the more common antibiotics, it is rarely chosen because of the high resistance rate of *S. pneumoniae* to this antibiotic.

Table 5-4 Consistency of Guidelines for Antibiotic Treatment of Acute Otitis Media

Guideline	Recommended Dosage
All recommend as first-line	Amoxicillin, 80-90 mg/kg/day
All recommend as second-line	Amoxicillin-clavulanate; most recommend extra-strength (ES) form, 80-90 mg/kg/day
Recommend as second-line	Cefdinir, 14 mg/kg/day Cefpodoxime, 10 mg/kg/day Cefprozil, 30 mg/kg/day Ceftriaxone, 50 mg/kg/day Cefuroxime axetil, 30 mg/kg/day
Not recommended by any guideline unless pathogen known to be sensitive, history of severe allergic reaction to penicillin or amoxicillin, or combined with another antibiotic effective against additional organisms	Azithromycin Cefaclor Cefixime Ceftibuten Clarithromycin Clindamycin Erythromycin-sulfisoxazole Loracarbef Trimethoprim-sulfamethoxazole

Treatment Options When Initial Antibiotics Fail

In general, if symptoms persist after a child has taken the first-line antibiotic for 48 to 72 hours, the child should be reevaluated in the office or by phone. Antibiotics should then be prescribed to cover β-lactam–producing organisms. Specifically, amoxicillin-clavulanate, 90 mg/kg/day, should be given in two divided doses, up to 4 g, or the modified extra-strength (ES) version that lowers the dose of clavulanate in children with a history of intestinal upset should be prescribed. Other options include cefdinir, cefuroxime, cefpodoxime, and ceftriaxone, 50 mg/kg, IM or IV, in three daily doses for noncompliant children.

Quinolones have been evaluated in several trials because there is growing evidence that they are safe in pediatric patients despite early concerns about the effects of these antibiotics on bone growth. Gatifloxacin and levofloxacin are highly effective at eradicating *H. influenzae* and for the treatment of multidrug-resistant and highly penicillin-resistant stains of *S. pneumoniae* (90% to 94% clinical cure rate).[37] However, they have not yet been licensed for use in children.

For children who fail second-line antibiotics or those who have severe ongoing symptoms, cautious use of clindamycin is recommended. Clindamycin is 93% to 95% effective in treating infection due to highly resistant *S. pneumoniae*, which is the most likely organism to cause ongoing symptoms.[51]

Other Medical Therapies for Acute Otitis Media

Analgesia. Regardless of whether the child is treated by observation or with antibiotics, pain control is paramount in the management of AOM. For mild to moderately severe pain, ibuprofen or acetaminophen is usually effective. Codeine should be limited for use in those with severe pain, and other narcotics should be prescribed only when the child can be properly monitored for the side effect of respiratory depression. Topical benzocaine (Auralgan Otic, Americaine Otic) provides additional but brief (30 to 60 minutes) improvement in pain control compared with acetaminophen or ibuprofen and appears to be more effective in children older than 5 years.[63]

Corticosteroids. Most studies evaluating the effect of corticosteroids (oral and intranasal) in the treatment of AOM have shown only minimal and short-term benefit. As a result, steroids are not routinely recommended. However, there may be a role for them in the treatment of severely atopic children with severe nasal congestion and coexisting AOM.

Antihistamines and Decongestants. Antihistamines and decongestant are not recommended for AOM. In one study, combination therapy with antihistamines and decongestants did show a 24% reduction in treatment failures, but the number of patients needed to treat is 11; however, this may be of value in treating symptoms related to the associated nasal congestion.[58]

Complementary and Alternative Medicine. Complementary and alternative medicine (CAM) therapies that have been used for the treatment of AOM include homeopathy, acupuncture, chiropractic medicine, and nutritional and herbal supplements. It is difficult to measure the number of parents who have used these modalities. Their use remains controversial and evidence is limited as to their efficacy.[64]

Tympanocentesis. This may be considered an option for treatment of severe pain, but it provides only limited benefit because it does not routinely allow for drainage of the MEE.

Treatment of Recurrent Acute Otitis Media

Recurrent AOM in children is defined by the occurrence of three or more ear infections over a 1-year period. These patients are more likely to be young (6 to 18 months) and at higher risk if they attend daycare. Guidelines have recommended high-dose amoxicillin, amoxicillin-clavulanate, cefdinir, cefprozil, cefpodoxine, cefuroxime, or ceftriaxone for each individual episode, depending on the level of resistance in the community. Antibiotic prophylaxis reduces the incidence of AOM by 0.09 episode per patient month, which implies that 11 months of therapy are necessary to prevent one episode of AOM.[49] Although use of these agents is discouraged for routine therapy in healthy children, there may be greater clinical impact for children with immune disorders or craniofacial anomalies. Traditionally, amoxicillin or trimethoprim-sulfamethoxazole has been recommended for prophylaxis, rather than other antibiotics, to reduce the development of bacterial resistance.

Surgical intervention is considered using PETs for recurrent AOM when four to six infections occur within a 6- to 12-month period. However, children with fewer episodes of AOM, but who also have underlying medical problems or chronic or fluctuating OME, may benefit from tube placement sooner.

COMPLICATIONS

The complications of OM can be divided into those involving the temporal bone and those that are extratemporal, which mostly involve structures around or in the brain.

Intratemporal Complications

Mild hearing loss caused by persistent MEE is usually conductive and temporary in nature. The impact of this mild, fluctuating, and sometimes persistent hearing loss on speech and language is uncertain and is discussed in further detail later. Although rare, sensorineural hearing loss that occurs as a result of AOM is usually permanent. Infections of the middle ear can progress to other structures in the temporal bone, resulting in mastoiditis, petrositis, and labyrinthitis. Finally, facial nerve paralysis can occur as a complication of AOM because the facial nerve courses through the middle ear. Pressure from MEE and inflammation can cause neuritis when the bone overlying this nerve is dehiscent, which occurs in up to 55% of these cases. In more severe cases, the infection can lead to erosion of the bony canal, affecting neural function. More chronic complications occur when structural changes occur in the eardrum, including tympanosclerosis, which rarely is associated with hearing loss, perforation of the eardrum with or without otorrhea, hearing loss, atelectasis, adhesive OM, retraction pockets, and cholesteatoma. Less often, ossicular erosion is seen when the eardrum has had long-standing atelectasis accompanied by chronic middle ear dysfunction. This can lead to erosion of the long process of the incus, the portion of the ossicular chain with the most tenuous blood supply. The distal incus becomes fibrotic and eventually erodes. The hearing loss usually starts as mild but can progress to a maximal conductive 60-dB hearing loss when complete ossicular discontinuity occurs.

Extratemporal Complications

Extratemporal problems include meningitis, epidural abscess, sigmoid sinus thrombosis, and otic hydrocephalus when infection spreads to adjacent intracranial locations. These complications are discussed in depth in Chapter 7.

TREATMENT OF OTITIS MEDIA WITH EFFUSION

OME is a common occurrence following AOM, but can also occur without preceding AOM. Overall, the prognosis for spontaneous resolution of MEE is good, but it may be present for weeks to months throughout the cold and flu season. Often, there is associated hearing loss that may be unilateral or bilateral, persistent or fluctuant, and tested hearing levels may be borderline normal (less than 20 dB) or fall in the mild hearing loss (20 to 40 dB) to moderate hearing loss range (more than 40 dB). The impact of such hearing loss on speech and language is variable and the timing of treatment is controversial. Although many children remain asymptomatic, OME may affect their quality of life when pain and, less often, imbalance are present. In addition, there is a higher risk of developing recurrent AOM when MEE persists. With time, permanent structural changes of the TM can occur, including atelectasis, retraction pocket, and less frequently, cholesteatoma.

Guidelines for the treatment of OME were originally proposed by the Agency for Healthcare Policy and Research (now the AHRQ) in 1994, which made recommendations for otherwise healthy 1- to 3-year-olds.[55] A more recent update of this guideline (2004) has expanded its target population to include children 2 months to 12 years old, with or without developmental disabilities that can predispose to OME and its sequelae. These broader guidelines have reinforced the need for accurate diagnosis using pneumatic otoscopy to confirm the presence of MEE and to distinguish OME from AOM. Recommendations focus on the close monitoring of children; this includes periodic hearing assessment and consideration of level of speech and language development (see later). Studies remain inconclusive about the direct effects of prolonged OME and the effects of persistent unilateral or bilateral mild hearing loss (20 to 30 dB) that often accompany OME on speech and language. However, it is clear that children in unfavorable child care environments, including those in which the primary caregiver has a lower educational level or socioeconomic status (SES), are at higher risk for language delays. Compared with children in favorable child care environments, hearing loss related to OME affects school performance and language development more significantly.[65]

The guidelines for treatment of OME also include negative recommendations—asymptomatic children should not be screened for OME in population screening programs because it is highly prevalent and usually resolves spontaneously without significant sequelae. Unfortunately, studies have shown that parents and caregivers are unable to determine when mild hearing loss is present, so it is often difficult to estimate how long such a hearing loss may have been present. Furthermore, the longer that MEE has been present, the less likely that it will clear. As a result, the primary care physician and educators must monitor speech and language development in children with persistent middle ear fluid to ensure that they do not fall behind their peers. More studies need to be done that assess the effect of duration of mild hearing loss on speech and language development in very young children with OME.

Persistent moderate hearing loss (30 to 50 dB) that occur less frequently and in patients with underlying sensorineural hearing loss have definite negative consequences for speech and language development. Bilateral myringotomy and tube placement should be performed sooner in these children than in those with mild hearing loss.

Medical Therapy

With regard to treatment options, the guidelines have discouraged the use of antihistamines and decongestants because most evidence has shown that they are ineffective for the treatment of OME. Antimicrobials and corticosteroids have limited short-term efficacy and should not be used routinely to manage the patient with OME. Allergy management as a treatment for OME has not been recommended because of insufficient data about the effect on OME. However, some authors and clinicians have continued to advocate this treatment for subgroups of children.[66]

Finally, complementary and alternative medicine therapies are not recommended because of a lack of scientific evidence documenting their efficacy.

Surgical Therapy

Tympanocentesis. Tympanocentesis is an office-based procedure used to aspirate and culture MEE. It may relieve pain, but the symptoms may rapidly recur if ongoing inflammation from AOM or OME is present.

Myringotomy. Myringotomy in children is usually performed under general anesthesia because an incision is required to suction the MEE. Unlike tympanocentesis, myringotomy is more effective in draining effusion. In RCTs, myringotomy alone was not found to be as effective as antibiotics in treating uncomplicated AOM; the addition of myringotomy to antibiotic does not provide additional benefit.[67] Myringotomy alone (without adenoidectomy; see later) is not recommended to treat COME because the incision closes in a few days and does not provide long-term ventilation. Laser-assisted myringotomy has been described as an alternative to traditional myringotomy and can prolong the duration of patency of the incision to several weeks. Although promoted as an office procedure that can be performed with topical anesthetic in cooperative patients, it has not been widely used in pediatric practices. Furthermore, randomized trials comparing these patient outcomes with those of controls have not been conducted to establish efficacy.[55]

Bilateral myringotomy with the placement of a PET is the most commonly recommended therapy and is useful for recurrent AOM, AOM with acute complications related to the infection, and COME. General anesthetic is necessary for most children. The procedure is performed under microscopic guidance. A small incision in the eardrum is made to aspirate the MEE and to place the grommet-shaped tube, which remains suspended in the opening of the eardrum. Children are considered candidates if they have had four episodes of AOM in 6 months or six AOM episodes in 1 year. Given the seasonal variation in the risk of AOM, PETs are more likely to provide benefit when placed in the fall or winter. Placement of PETs should be considered sooner when recurrent AOM occurs with underlying OME that fails to clear, especially if the child is symptomatic with hearing loss, irritability, or poor sleep, if significant structural changes of the eardrum are seen, or if the child has coexistent developmental delays or immune disorders. Although PETs reduce future AOM episodes by 56% (95% CI, 17% to 77%), there may be ongoing episodes of recurrent otorrhea that are treatable with antibiotic drops.[68] PET placement with or without mastoidectomy is recommended when the following acute complications occur related to AOM—mastoiditis, acute facial nerve paralysis, or vertigo suggestive of labyrinthitis (not imbalance only).

Timing for placement of PET for OME is more controversial. The AAP-AAFP guidelines have stated that MEE can be monitored for a 3-month period unless the child is at increased risk for speech and language delays, learning problems, or more than mild hearing loss is suspected.[53,55] In some cases, duration of symptoms may be difficult to determine because the mild degree of hearing loss is hard to detect without formal testing. Parents of patients with mild hearing loss often are unaware of the presence of any hearing abnormalities. During this period of observation, the clinician should document the laterality, duration of effusion, and presence and severity of associated symptoms (e.g., subjective hearing loss, irritability, or pain) at each assessment of the child with OME. Hearing testing is recommended when the MEE has persisted for 3 months and at any time with high-risk children. The guidelines have recommended that children with persistent OME who are not at risk should be reexamined at 3- to 6-month intervals until the effusion resolves or until significant hearing loss (more than 20 dB) or structural abnormalities of the TM are identified. Finally, placement of PETs should be performed when structural changes have occurred and considered an option when the OME with hearing loss has been present in both ears for 3 months or in one ear for 6 months. It is the preferred initial procedure when a child becomes a surgical candidate.

PETs have been proven highly effective in reducing the incidence of AOM and in reducing the prevalence of MEE. Depending on the style and size of the tube used, most PETs remain in place for 12 to 14 months.[55] There is a 10% risk of the development of transient episodes of otorrhea, which may occur during a URTI or when the ear is exposed to water. Topical antibiotic drops, including ofloxacin (Floxin) and ciprofloxacin with dexamethasone (Ciprodex), which also contains steroids, have been approved by the U.S. Food and Drug Administration (FDA) for use in patients with tubes or for those who have perforated eardrums. Usually, a short 5- to 10-day course of drops is effective in treating otorrhea. Oral antibiotics do not routinely hasten the resolution of symptoms for uncomplicated episodes of otorrhea. In young children (younger than 3 years), otorrhea more often relates to the associated URTI and the usual bacteria are cultured (*S. pneumoniae*, *H. influenzae*, or *M. catarrhalis*). In older children, otorrhea occurs more often when a preexisting perforation or PET is present and the ear has been exposed to water, especially when it is not chlorinated. The most common bacterial pathogen is *P. aeruginosa* and, less often, *S. aureus*.[68] Persistent or recurrent otorrhea occurs less frequently. Cultures are often necessary to determine the organism involved. Although most chronic discharge is related to bacterial infection, fungal infections, including *Candida* and *Aspergillus* species should be considered if the patient has been on long-term antibiotic drops or if there has been a history of water exposure. Clotrimazole (Lotrimin) drops and frequent microscopic débridement are usually effective in treating fungal infections. Although unusual, methicillin-resistant *Staphylococcus aureus* (MRSA) has become more prevalent in this population. In addition to treating with topical antibiotics effective against MRSA, frequent débridement and sometimes trimethoprim-sulfamethoxazole given orally or, less often, intravenous antibiotics are necessary to eradicate the drainage.

Tube blockage occurs in 4% to 10% of cases, but tubes usually can be unblocked with suction or microscopic débridement in the office. Alternatively, the tubes can be unblocked with a course of otic drops that includes 3% hydrogen peroxide drops for several days, followed by antibiotic drops for 1 week to ensure that the middle ear remains clear when the tube is opened. Although structural changes are more common in TMs of children who have had tubes placed, these small areas of focal scarring, tympanosclerosis, and shallow retraction pockets are usually benign and are seen at the site where the tube had been located. Several studies have shown that these changes have no long-term effects on hearing in children who have had tubes.[55] Persistent TM perforations, which may require repair, have been reported in 2% of children after placement of short-term tube (grommet-shaped) tubes and in up to 17% of those with longer acting T-shaped tubes.[69]

Adenoidectomy. Approximately 20% to 25% of children who have had tubes have OM relapse once the tube extrudes.[8,55] When a child needs repeat surgery for OM, the guidelines suggest that adenoidectomy be considered, because it results in a 50% reduction in the need for future operations. The two separate groups of patients that may benefit most from adenoidectomy are children older than 4 years with COME (79% relative decrease in COME) and those older than 2 years with recurrent AOM who have had ongoing AOM after a first set of PETs has extruded (52% relative decrease in AOM).[70] Furthermore, the beneficial effect of adenoidectomy in the older age group appears to be independent of adenoid size. This therapy is not recommended in children with cleft palate or submucous palate because they are at significant risk of developing velopalatine insufficiency (VPI), resulting in hypernasal speech. Adenoidectomy with myringotomy (without tube insertion) has comparable efficacy as a PET alone in children 4 years or older but is more invasive than PET alone, and should not be considered before tubes are placed unless a distinct indication exists, such as coexisting adenoiditis, chronic sinusitis, or chronic nasal obstruction.[8,55] Complications associated with adenoidectomy include postoperative bleeding (less than 0.5%), short-term VPI (2.4%) (this is rarely permanent, even in a child with a normal-appearing palate), and infection-related complications. Tonsillectomy is not recommended for treatment of OME because there is limited evidence of benefit and higher risks are related to the procedure.

SUMMARY

Recent evidence-based reviews have provided guidelines for the diagnosis and management of AOM and OME. Areas of ongoing controversy mostly relate to whether a period of observation is reasonable instead of initial antibiotic therapy for AOM. However, expert panels have agreed about the choice of antibiotics and that quality of life should be considered in determining who may benefit from observation. Ongoing surveillance of these patients is necessary to ensure that complication rates remain low with this new treatment paradigm. Further studies are also

MAJOR POINTS

- Otitis media (OM) is common; antibiotics have been traditionally used for primary therapy to lower the risk of complications and alleviate symptoms.
- The diagnosis of OM is made with uncertainty in some cases because the tympanic membrane (TM) is difficult to visualize in young children.
- It is difficult to differentiate noninfected middle ear effusion (MEE) from acute disease and both can resolve spontaneously without antibiotic therapy.
- Overuse of antibiotics in the treatment of OM has led to the development of antibiotic-resistant bacteria, with worldwide implications.
- Guidelines have been developed to reduce the indiscriminate use of antibiotics. These guidelines stress the importance of improving diagnostic accuracy and make recommendations for observing some patients judiciously—patients who are less likely to suffer complications of the disease.
- Antibiotics should not be used to treat asymptomatic chronic otitis media with effusion (COME).
- The timing of surgical treatment of COME, which may be associated with hearing loss, remains controversial.
- Close monitoring is warranted to ensure that speech and language development are not hindered and that structural changes of the TM do not occur.

needed to determine the impact of OME on speech and language development in certain more vulnerable subgroups of children. In following these paradigms, physicians should be reminded that clinical judgment remains important. Specifically, it is important to consider variables that are not included in the guidelines, including quality of life and possibly evolving structural changes of the TM that may develop in the course of COME, because these may become permanent with time.

REFERENCES

1. Marcy M, Takata G, Shekelle P, et al: Management of Acute Otitis Media: Evidence Report/Technology Assessment No. 15 (AHRQ Publication No. 01-E010). Rockville, MD, U.S. Department of Health and Human Services, 2000.
2. Gates GA: Cost-effectiveness considerations in otitis media treatment. Otolaryngol Head Neck Surg 1996;114:525-530.
3. Gates GA, Klein JO, Lim DJ, et al: Recent advances in otitis media, 1: Definitions, terminology and classification of otitis media. Ann Otol Rhinol Laryngol 2002;111:8-18.
4. Castagno LA, Lavinsky L: Otitis media in children: Seasonal changes and socioeconomic level. Int J Pediatr Otorhinolaryngol 2002;62:129-134.
5. Casselbrant ML, Brostoff LM, Cantekin EI, et al: Otitis media with effusion in preschool children. Laryngoscope 1985;95:428-436.
6. Joki-Erkkila VP, Pukander J, Laippala P: Alteration of the clinical picture and treatment of pediatric acute otitis media over the past two decades. Int J Pediatr Otorhinolaryngol 2000;55:197-201.
7. Teele DW, Kelin JO, Rosner B: Epidemiology of otitis media during first seven years of life in children in greater Boston: A prospective, cohort study. J Infect Dis 1989;160: 83-94.
8. Gates GA, Avery CA, Prihoda TJ, et al: Effectiveness of adenoidectomy and tympanostomy tubes in the treatment of chronic otitis media with effusion. N Engl J Med 1987;317:1444-1451.
9. Bluestone CD:. Studies in otitis media: Children's Hospital of Pittsburgh-University of Pittsburgh Progress Report—2004. Laryngoscope 2004;114:1-25.
10. Curns AT, Holman RC, Shay DK, et al: Outpatient and hospital visits associated with otitis media among American Indian and Alaska Native children younger than 5 years. Pediatrics 2002;109:E41-1.
11. Bluestone CD, Klein JO (eds): Otitis Media in Infants and Children. Management Update. Philadelphia, WB Saunders, 2004.
12. Daly KA, Hoffman HJ, Casselbrant ML, et al: Panel report. I: Epidemiology, natural history and risk factors. Ann Otol Rhinol Laryngol 2005;194(Suppl):8-15.
13. Casselbrant ML, Mandel EM, Fall PA, et al: The heritability of otitis media: A twin/triplet study. JAMA 1999;282: 2125-2130.
14. Casselbrant ML, Mandel EM, Rockette HE, et al: The genetic component of middle ear disease in the first 5 years of life. Arch Otolaryngol Head Neck Surg 2004;130:273-278.
15. Joki-Erkkila VP, Puhakka H, Hurme M: Cytokine gene polymorphism in recurrent acute otitis media. Arch Otolaryngol Head Neck Surg 2002;128:17-20.
16. Löfgren J, Ramet M, Renko M, et al: Association between surfactant protein A gene locus and severe respiratory syncytial virus infection in infants. J Infect Dis 2002;185:283-289.
17. Rovers MM, Straatman H, Zielhuis GA, et al: Seasonal variation in the prevalence of persistent otitis media with effusion in one-year old infants. Paediatr Perinat Epidemiol 2000;14:268-274.
18. Vera S, Kleemola M, Blomqvist S, et al: Epidemiology of documented viral respiratory infections and acute otitis media in a cohort of children followed from two to twenty-four months of age. Pediatr Infect Dis J 2001;20:574-581.
19. Lieu JE, Feinstein AR: Effect of gestational and passive smoke exposure on ear infections in children. Arch Pediatr Adolesc Med 2002;156:147-154.
20. Dewey C, Midgeley E, Maw R: The relationship between otitis media with effusion and contact with other children in a British cohort studied from 8 months to $3^1/_2$ years. The ALSPAC Study Team. Avon Longitudinal Study of Pregnancy and Childhood. Int J Pediatr Otorhinolaryngol 2000;55:33-45.
21. National Institute of Child Health and Human Development Early Child Care Research Network: Child care and common communicable illnesses: Results from the National Institute of Child Health and Human Development Study of Early Child Care. Arch Pediatr Adolesc Med 2001;155:481-488.
22. Bradley RH; National Institute of Child Health and Human Development (NICHD) Early Child Care Research Network: Child care and common communicable illnesses in children aged 37 to 54 months. Arch Pediatr Adolesc Med 2003;157:196-200.
23. American Academy of Pediatrics Subcommittee on Management of Acute Otitis Media: Diagnosis and management of acute otitis media. Pediatrics 2004;113:1451-1465.
24. Jackson JM, Mourino AP: Pacifier use and otitis media in infants twelve months of age or younger. Pediatr Dent 1999;21:255-260.
25. Tasker A, Dettmar PW, Panetti M, et al: Is gastric reflux a cause of otitis media with effusion in children? Laryngoscope 2002;112:1930-1934.
26. Heikkinen T, Thint M, Chonmaitree T: Prevalence of various respiratory viruses in the middle ear during acute otitis media. N Engl J Med 1999;340:260-264.
27. Chonmaitree T, Owen MJ, Patel JA, et al: Effect of viral respiratory tract infection on outcome of acute otitis media. Pediatrics 1992;120:856-862.
28. Pelton SI: Otitis media. In Long SS, Pickering LK, Prober CG (eds): Principles and Practice of Pediatric Infectious Diseases, 2nd ed. Philadelphia, Churchill Livingstone, 2003, pp 190-198.

29. Pichichero ME, Casey JR: Acute otitis media: Making sense of recent guidelines on antimicrobial treatment. J Fam Pract 2005;54:313-322.

30. Turner D, Leibovitz E, Aran A, et al: Acute otitis media in infants younger than two months of age: Microbiology, clinical presentation and therapeutic approach. Pediatr Infect Dis J 2002;21:669-674.

31. Kenna M: Diagnosis and management of acute otitis media and otitis media with effusion. In Wetmore RF, Muntz HR, McGill TJ, et al (eds): Pediatric Otolaryngology: Principles and Practice Pathways. New York, Thieme, 2000, pp 263-279.

32. Bluestone CD, Stephenson JS, Martin LM: Ten-year review of otitis media pathogens. Pediatr Infect Dis J 1992;11:S7-S11.

33. Dowell SF, Butler JC, Giebink GS: Acute otitis media: Management and surveillance in an era of pneumococcal resistance. Nurse Pract 1999;24(Suppl 10):1-9.

34. Barnett ED, Klein JO: The problem of resistant bacteria for the management of acute otitis media. Pediatr Clin North Am 1995;42:509-517.

35. De Neeling AJ, Van Leeuwen WJ, Van Klingeren B, et al: Epidemiology of resistance of *Streptococcus pneumoniae* in the Netherlands. Presented at the 36th Interscience Conference on Antimicrobial Agents and Chemotherapy, New Orleans, September 1996 (abstract C57).

36. Marchant CD, Dagan R: Bacteriologic efficacy of antimicrobial agents. In Rosenfeld RM, Bluestone CD (eds): Evidence-Based Otitis Media, 2nd ed. Hamilton, Ontario, BC Decker, 2003, pp 256-267.

37. Segal, N, Leibovitz E, Dagan R, Leiberman A: Acute otitis media—diagnosis and treatment in the era of antibiotic resistant organisms: Updated clinical practice guidelines. Int J Pediatr Otorhinolaryngol 2005;69:1311-1319.

38. Leibovitz E, Dagan R: Antibiotic treatment for acute otitis media. Int J Antimicrob Agents 2000;15:169-177.

39. Leibovitz E, Dagan R: Otitis media therapy and drug resistance. Part I: Management principles. Infect Med 2001;18:212-216.

40. Leibovitz E, Dagan R: Otitis media therapy and drug resistance. Part II: Current concepts and new directions. Infect Med 2001;18:263-270.

41. Bluestone CD, Stephenson JS, Martin LM: Ten-year review of otitis media pathogens. Pediatr Infect Dis J 1992;11:75-115.

42. Rovers MM, Schilder AGM, Zielhuis GA, Rosenfeld RM: Otitis media. Lancet 2004;363:465-473.

43. Fireman B, Black SB, Shinefield HR, et al: Impact of the pneumococcal conjugate vaccine on otitis media. Pediatr Infec Dis J 2003;22:10-16.

44. Clements DA, Langdon L, Bland C, Walter E: Influenza A vaccine decreases the incidence of otitis media in 6- to 30-month-old children in daycare. Arch Pediatr Adolesc Med 1995;149:1113-1117.

45. Tapiainen T, Luotonen L, Kontiokari T, et al: Xylitol administered only during respiratory infections failed to prevent acute otitis media. Pediatrics 2002;109:E19.

46. Allenstein, Gondim LM, Suhonen J, et al: Xylitol release pacifier in the prevention of acute otitis media. In Lim DJ, Bluestone CD, Casselbrant ML (eds): Abstracts of the Eighth International Symposium on Recent Advances in Otitis Media. Fort Lauderdale, Fla, BC Decker, 2003, p 101.

47. Hatakka JK, Savilahti E, Pönkä A, et al: Effect of long term consumption of probiotic milk on infections in children attending daycare centres: Double-blind, randomised trial. BMJ 2001;322:1327.

48. Niemelä M, Pihakari Ok, Pokka T, Uhari M: Pacifier as a risk factor for acute otitis media: A randomized controlled trial of parental counseling. Pediatrics 2000;106:483-488.

49. Marcy SM: New guidelines on acute otitis media: An overview of their key principles for practice. Cleveland Clin J Med 2004;71(Suppl 4):S3-S4.

50. Harrison CJ: How will the new guideline for managing otitis media work in your practice? Contemp Pediatrics 2004; 21:24.

51. Marchetti F, Ronfani L, Nibali SC, Tamburlini G: Delayed prescription may reduce the use of antibiotics for acute otitis media. Arch Pediatr Adolesc Med 2005;159:679-684.

52. Rosenfeld RM: Diagnostic certainty for acute otitis media. Int J Pediatr Otorhinolaryngol 2002;64:89-95.

53. American Academy of Pediatrics: Clinical practice guideline—otitis media with effusion. Pediatrics 2004;113: 1413-1429.

54. Finitzo T, Friel-Patti S, Chinn K, Brown O: Tympanometry and otoscopy prior to myringotomy: Issues in diagnosis of otitis media. Int J Pediatr Otorhinolaryngol 1992;24:101-110.

55. Rosenfeld RM, Culpepper L, Doyle KJ, et al: American Academy of Pediatrics Subcommittee on Otitis Media with Effusion; American Academy of Family Physicians; American Academy of Otolaryngology—Head and Neck Surgery: Clinical practice guideline: Otitis media with effusion. Otolaryngol Head Neck Surg 2004;130(Suppl 5):S95-S118.

56. Carlson LH, Carlson RD: Diagnosis. In Rosenfeld RM, Bluestone CD (eds): Evidence-Based Otitis Media, 2nd ed. Hamilton, Ontario, BC Decker, 2003, pp 136-146.

57. Rosenfeld RM, Culpepper L, Doyle KJ, et al: Clinical practice guideline: Otitis media with effusion. Otolaryngol Head Neck Surg 2004;130:S95-S118.

58. Rosenfeld RM, Casselbrant ML, Hannley MT: Implications of the AHRQ evidence report on acute otitis media. Otolaryngol Head Neck Surg 2001;125:440-448, discussion, 439.

59. Rosenfeld RM, Kay D: Natural history of untreated otitis media. Laryngoscope 2003;113:1645-1657.

60. Rosenfeld RM: Otitis, antibiotics and the greater good. Pediatrics 2004;114:1333-1335.

61. Rosenfeld RM: Observation option toolkit for acute otitis media. Int J Pediatr Otorhinolaryngol 2001;58:1-8.

62. Dagan R, Johnson CE, McLinn S: Bacteriologic and clinical efficacy of amoxicillin/clavulanate vs. azithromycin in acute otitis media. Pediatr Infect Dis J 2000;20:829-837.

63. Hoberman A, Paradise JL, Reynolds EA, Urkin J: Efficacy of Auralgan for treating ear pain in children. Arch Pediatr Adolesc Med 1997;151:675-678.

64. Spiegelblatt L, Laine-Ammara G, Pless IB, Guyver A: The use of alternative medicine by children. Pediatrics 1994;94:811-814.

65. Roberts JE, Rosenfeld RM, Zeisel SA: Otitis media and speech language: A meta-analysis of prospective studies. Pediatrics 2004;113(Pt 1):E238-E248.

66. Rosenfeld RM, Bluestone CD: Clinical pathway for otitis media with effusion. In Rosenfeld RM, Bluestone CD (eds): Evidence-Based Otitis Media, 2nd ed. Hamilton, Ontario, BC Decker, 2003, pp 303-324.

67. Engelhard D, Cohen D, Strauss N, et al: Randomised study of myringotomy amoxycillin/clavulanate or both for acute otitis media in infants. Lancet 1989;5:141-143.

68. Rosenfeld RM: Clinical pathway for acute otitis media. In Rosenfeld RM, Bluestone CD (eds): Evidence-Based Otitis Media, 2nd ed. Hamilton, Ontario, BC Decker, 2003, pp 280-302.

69. Kay DJ, Nelson M, Rosenfeld RM: Meta-analysis of tympanostomy tube sequelae. Otolaryngol Head Neck Surg 2001;124:374-380.

70. Paradise JL, Bluestone CD, Rogers KD, et al: Efficacy of adenoidectomy for recurrent otitis media in children previously treated with tympanostomy-tube placement: Results of parallel randomized and nonrandomized trials. JAMA 1990;263:2066-2073.

Chronic Disorders of the Middle Ear and Mastoid

ERIC D. BAUM, MD

WILLIAM P. POTSIC, MD

In an era of widely available antibiotics, only a small percentage of cases of otitis media lead to more serious problems. Complications of otitis media still occur, however, and both the original infection and any extension or exacerbation can progress to various chronic disorders of the middle ear and mastoid. Otitis media is discussed in detail in Chapter 5 and acute complications are discussed in Chapter 7. This chapter discusses chronic conditions affecting the middle ear and mastoid, most of which are sequelae of otitis media.

BACKGROUND AND EPIDEMIOLOGY

Because chronic middle ear disease is usually the result of persistence and/or progression of acute otitis media, the risk factor profiles of the two disease categories overlap significantly.[1] Well-studied risk factors for otitis media include craniofacial deformity, cleft palate, immune deficiency, daycare attendance, and cigarette smoke exposure (Box 6-1).[2] Some of these patient characteristics, such as immune deficiency[3] and cleft palate,[4] are associated with a substantially higher likelihood of chronic middle ear disease as well, but the contribution of other risk factors from this list is less apparent.[1]

The decreasing use of antibiotics in the treatment of otitis media, often as part of a coordinated effort to avoid the emergence of resistant pathogens in the community, may contribute to an increase in the number of children in whom otitis media progresses to chronic middle ear disease.[5] It has been postulated that other factors, including the use of vaccines and societal changes regarding daycare attendance, may alter the incidence of acute otitis media and otitis media with effusion in children.[2] It is unclear whether this will translate into a difference in the epidemiology of chronic middle ear disease as well.[6]

SPECIFIC DISORDERS

Eustachian Tube Dysfunction

Eustachian tube dysfunction (ETD) is an important pathophysiologic factor in many cases of chronic middle ear disease, and it can also be considered one of those chronic conditions.[7] Under normal conditions, the eustachian tube equalizes the pressure of the middle ear–mastoid system with the external environment through intermittent active contraction of the tensor veli palatini muscle. The middle ear and mastoid provide an air cushion that, when combined with the normally closed eustachian tube, effectively prevents the reflux of nasopharyngeal contents into the middle ear space.[8]

ETD can manifest as either a tube that does not open effectively or one that does not close effectively. In the first case, a poorly opening tube prevents pressure equalization between the middle ear space and the ambient environment, leading to progressive gas absorption and negative pressure in the middle ear space. This impairs emptying of middle ear secretions and predisposes to otitis media by providing a favorable environment for bacterial growth.[9] The latter condition, known as a patulous eustachian tube, allows reflux of the nonsterile

Box 6-1 Risk Factors for Otitis Media in Children[1,2]

Specific ethnic groups—Native Americans, Eskimos, Aborigines
Cleft palate
Craniofacial syndromes—Down, Crouzon's, Apert's, Turner's, Pierre Robin
Immune disorders—acquired immunodeficiency syndrome (AIDS), severe combined immunodeficiency (SCID), X-linked agammaglobulinemia, many others
Ciliary dyskinesias—Kartagener's syndrome, cystic fibrosis
Daycare attendance
Male gender
Family history of middle ear disease
Lower socioeconomic status
Allergy
Exposure to cigarette smoke
Bottle-feeding in lieu of breast-feeding

Adapted from Forsen J: Chronic diseases of the middle ear and mastoid. In Wetmore RF, Muntz HR, McGill TJI (eds): Pediatric Otolaryngology: Principles and Practice Pathways. New York, Thieme, 2000, pp 281-304; and Casselbrant ML, Mandel EM: Risk factors for otitis media. In Alper CM, Bluestone CD, Casselbrant ML, et al (eds): Advanced Therapy of Otitis Media. Hamilton, Ontario, BC Decker, 2004, pp 26-31.

nasopharyngeal contents into the middle ear space, also predisposing to infection.[10] A similar phenomenon can occur when the middle ear–mastoid air cushion cannot be maintained because of a tympanic membrane perforation.[11]

Obstruction of the eustachian tube can be functional, as in the case of cleft palate, in which maldevelopment leads to ineffective tensor veli palatini contraction.[12] It can also be caused by a physical blockage anywhere in the system, including a middle ear mass (cholesteatoma or tumor), nasopharyngeal mass (large adenoid pad or tumor), or blocked or stenotic eustachian tube.[1] Even in the absence of any apparent anatomic or functional abnormality, ETD in young children is common. There are various overlapping theories that attempt to explain the phenomenon, but normal dimensions, compliance, and overall function are frequently not realized until children reach the age of 7 years.[8]

Symptomatically, ETD is manifested primarily by other middle ear disease. Patients with ETD are less able to clear fluid from the middle ear space, predisposing them to recurrent acute otitis media, persistent middle ear effusion with its attendant conductive hearing loss, and tympanic membrane retraction.[11] Occasionally, patients without signs of otitis media on examination will complain of symptoms suggestive of it (e.g., hearing loss, otalgia, tinnitus). In these cases, and especially when the patient also complains of autophony (hearing one's own breathing and vocalization in the ear), ETD is the likely diagnosis.[10,13]

Perhaps most importantly, ETD can cause atelectasis of the middle ear with ossicular erosion and cholesteatoma formation.[7] Atelectasis occurs because persistent negative middle ear pressure (caused by failure of the eustachian tube to open intermittently and equalize air pressure with the ambient environment) eventually draws all or part of the tympanic membrane medially. This persistent negative pressure may cause the tympanic membrane to form a retraction pocket.

Retraction pockets often occur in the posterosuperior quadrant and can lead to destruction of the ossicles and progressive conductive hearing loss. More centrally, the eardrum can collapse against and attach to the promontory. A retraction pocket can harbor desquamated debris, eventually leading to middle ear and mastoid cholesteatoma formation.[14]

Middle ear atelectasis caused by persistent ETD is common; one report has noted that between 10% and 52% of patients who had previously required myringotomy tubes for serous otitis media develop the condition.[15] Patients with a history of ETD should be followed closely and for an extended period to avoid such complications.[16]

ETD that leads to significant or progressive middle ear atelectasis must be addressed to avoid permanent changes. Tympanostomy tube insertion provides a mechanism for pressure equalization and can prevent ossicular erosion and adhesive otitis media.[17] Even with appropriate ventilation, the diseased tympanic membrane may have stretched and become flaccid over time, predisposing to recurrent atelectasis. In these cases, patients may require insertion of a longer-lasting ventilation tube[18] or cartilage tympanoplasty, which reconstructs the eardrum using stiffer material.[19] Research continues into less invasive surgical solutions to this problem.[20]

Tympanic Membrane Perforation

Perforation of the tympanic membrane (TM) should be classified as acute or chronic (present for longer than 3 months), and the location and size of the defect should always be recorded. Associated conditions, including a history of middle ear infection, prior surgery, and the presence of active drainage, should also be noted. There are many possible causes, each with a different impact on treatment decisions.

The most common cause of TM perforation is acute otitis media, occurring in up to 30% of patients with acute ear infections.[21] Accumulation of fluid and multiple inflammatory mediators in the fixed space of the middle ear eventually causes spontaneous rupture of and discharge through a weak point in the membrane. Purulent drainage in the canal is seen on examination, and patients will occasionally note an abrupt resolution of otalgia at the onset of drainage. Perforations of this type are generally small and heal spontaneously, sometimes in just a few days.[22] The purulent discharge can cause otitis externa, for which treatment with oral and topical antibiotics is indicated.[21]

In rare cases, perforations of this type do not close on their own. Infections with *Streptococcus pyogenes* can lead to central or even complete TM necrosis.[23] Classically, middle ear infections caused by *Mycobacterium tuberculosis* were said to show chronic drainage through multiple pinpoint perforations[22]; more recent studies have suggested that this unusual appearance is unlikely and that a central perforation with chronic drainage is typically seen.[24]

Acute perforation may also be the result of trauma. Deep insertion of a foreign body (e.g., cotton cleaning swab, hairpin) into the external auditory canal will typically result in a breach of the posterior portion of the eardrum. A slap to the side of the head can momentarily seal a column of air in the ear canal, resulting in rupture of the membrane at a natural weak spot.[1] Extremely rapid changes in atmospheric pressure, which can occur during air travel or diving, cannot be adequately equalized by the eustachian tube. This phenomenon may also cause tympanic membrane perforation.[25]

Patients with acute traumatic perforations must be evaluated carefully for signs of middle and inner ear damage. They may suffer from conductive and/or sensorineural hearing loss, vertigo, tinnitus, or a sensation of aural fullness.[22] Drainage of blood or clear fluid may signal damage to soft tissues of the ear canal, middle ear, skull base, or otic capsule. All patients should undergo microscopic examination and complete audiometry.[26] Although larger perforations are associated with greater amounts of conductive hearing loss, an air-bone gap larger than 35 dB is suspicious for ossicular injury.[27]

The inverted edges of a traumatic perforation should be gently folded out to avoid squamous ingrowth toward the middle ear, which can result in cholesteatoma formation. If the ear is kept dry, even a fairly large traumatic perforation will generally close spontaneously, although it may take many months. Conservative treatment is generally successful, and usually consists of no more than keeping water out of the ear canal and treating any signs of infection or drainage promptly.[28]

The most common cause of chronic TM perforation in children is the prior placement of pressure-equalizing tubes (PETs). Published rates of persistent perforation after PET placement vary widely and many factors influence the likelihood that the TM will not heal—patient age, eustachian tube dysfunction, chronic infection, and presence of cholesteatoma. Certain types and sizes of tubes increase the risk of a persistent perforation, as does a longer time in which the tube had been in place.[16] T-tubes, for example, are purposely designed to stay in place for 2 to 3 years, and have been reported to leave persistent perforations in their wake from 9% to 30% of the time.[29]

In these cases, the risk of requiring an additional surgical procedure to repair the drum must be weighed against the potential need for tube reinsertion if retraction, hearing loss, or serous otitis media recur before the eustachian tube matures.[1] This is why the timing of repair is controversial. Based on the understanding that the eustachian tube functionally matures in almost all patients by the age of 7 years, many practitioners have recommended waiting until at least that age,[30] although others have noted that repair is frequently successful, even in younger children.[31] It may be useful to monitor the contralateral eardrum; if the nonperforated side shows signs of good eustachian tube function for an extended period, closure of the perforated eardrum is reasonable.

The question then arises as to whether certain perforations should be closed at all. On one hand, a small dry hole can prevent retraction and cholesteatoma, may contribute a negligible amount of hearing loss, and may obviate the need for repeated tympanostomy tube placement. Conversely, such a perforation increases the incidence of nasopharyngeal reflux up the eustachian tube (by obliterating the middle ear-mastoid air cushion) and may allow for squamous ingrowth, thus increasing the risk of cholesteatoma.[7] Moreover, physicians' recommendations to avoid water exposure may substantially limit children's activities.[32] These conflicting issues, especially in the context of a growing patient, guarantee that the timing and indications for perforation repair will remain a matter of judgment.[1]

As noted, most perforations of the TM close with no treatment, and the initial management includes avoiding further injury, keeping the ear dry, treating any infectious episodes, and monitoring the healing process. By definition, chronic perforations that have not resolved despite appropriate watchful waiting require surgical repair.

There are an astonishing number of reliable techniques available to repair the TM,[33] and choosing among them depends on many variables, including surgeon preference, size and location of the perforation, and associated procedures to be performed (e.g., ossiculoplasty, mastoidectomy). Appropriate operations span a large spectrum, from removal of the edges of the perforation and temporary placement of a tiny piece of paper[34] all the way to total TM reconstruction with foreign materials.[35]

Chronic Suppurative Otitis Media

Chronic suppurative otitis media (CSOM) describes persistent inflammation of the middle ear and mastoid mucosa, with ongoing purulent drainage through a perforation in the TM or tympanostomy tube.[7] This condition is more common in certain populations, including Native Americans and Eskimos, caused by a congenital predisposition to a patulous eustachian tube. A patulous eustachian tube allows nasopharyngeal contents to reflux into the middle ear, and this phenomenon is enhanced by a hole in the TM. Thus, CSOM can represent a vicious cycle, in which further contamination of the middle ear with the nonsterile contents of the external auditory canal and nasopharynx can help perpetuate chronic infection and drainage.[1] Tympanostomy tube insertion alone, even in the absence of active infection, can precipitate otorrhea up to 50% of the time[36] and leads to persistent CSOM in 3.6% of patients.[37]

Clinically, CSOM may be associated with a visible aural polyp and perforation of the TM of any size. Pain and fever are not typical and, if present, should prompt an investigation for another intratemporal infectious process.[7] Cholesteatoma and foreign bodies (including tympanostomy tubes) can help perpetuate CSOM, and biofilm formation may have a role in persistence of the process.[38] The drainage in CSOM is frequently polymicrobial, although *Pseudomonas* species are most commonly cultured.[39]

The mainstay of initial diagnosis and treatment in CSOM is microscopic examination of the TM and middle ear. Débridement of squamous debris and fluid from the ear canal may be required for adequate visualization. Signs of cholesteatoma (e.g., visible white mass, significant eardrum retraction) should prompt a thorough investigation, including a computed topography (CT) scan.[1] Meticulous attention to keeping the canal clean and dry is the cornerstone of successful treatment, although it is less effective alone than when combined with ototopical agents.[40]

Culture-directed therapy should be used, but many choices of nonototoxic ear drops are effective and can be started before laboratory results are available (Table 6-1).[41] It should be noted that older topical agents may contain ototoxic antimicrobial agents, including aminoglycosides (e.g., neomycin, gentamicin) and polymixins. Fluoroquinolone preparations, which have not been shown to cause inner ear damage, are preferred.

With consistent evacuation of debris from the canal and application of topical agents, most patients will experience a rapid decrease in drainage within a few days. If not, the addition of systemic antibiotics should be considered. Despite the frequent presence of *Pseudomonas*, many clinicians find success using antimicrobials active against bacteria typically associated with acute otitis media (including amoxicillin and amoxicillin-clavulanate), probably because these organisms also contribute to the infection.[1]

Table 6-1 Ototopical Therapy for Chronic Suppurative Otitis Media

Generic Name	Trade Name
Acetic acid (2%) solution	VōSol Otic
Acetic acid (2%) solution, hydrocortisone	VōSol HC Otic
Acetic acid (2%) in aqueous aluminum acetate	Otic Domeboro
Ciprofloxacin	Ciloxan ophthalmic
Ciprofloxacin, hydrocortisone	Cipro HC Otic
Ciprofloxacin, dexamethasone	Ciprodex
Colistin, neomycin, thonzonium, hydrocortisone	Cortisporin-TC
Neomycin, polymyxin B, hydrocortisone	Pediotic suspension
Ofloxacin	Floxin Otic
Gentamicin	Garamycin ophthalmic
Tobramycin, dexamethasone, chlorobutanol	TobraDex ophthalmic

Adapted from Bluestone CD: Suppurative complications. In Rosenfeld RM, Bluestone CD (eds): Evidence-Based Otitis Media, 2nd ed. Hamilton, Ontario, BC Decker, 2003, pp 482-504.

In many culture-positive cases, however, a systemic antipseudomonal drug will be required. No U.S. Food and Drug Administration (FDA)-approved oral agent for children is available that is reliably active against *Pseudomonas* species, although fluoroquinolones have been shown to be safe and effective for this indication.[42] A recent study of 867 children treated with gatifloxacin for recalcitrant otitis media has reported no cases of permanent arthropathy; this study included almost 200 patients younger than 2 years.[43] Another report has estimated that over 9000 children have been treated with fluoroquinolones in the previous 5 years without significant joint problems, although this report included few, if any, patients younger than 12 months.[44]

Topical agents and oral antibiotics will successfully clear the infection in about 90% of patients[45,46] but, in the remainder, intravenous antibiotics must be considered. Both empirical and culture-directed therapy usually dictate the use of an extended-coverage, antipseudomonal penicillin (e.g., piperacillin, ticarcillin-tazobactam) or a third-generation cephalosporin (e.g., ceftazidime).[41] Drainage can be eliminated in most patients with this regimen, but in one long-term follow-up study, almost 25% of patients ultimately required tympanomastoid surgery to permanently eradicate CSOM.[47] Older recommendations have suggested an intravenous aminoglycoside (e.g., gentamicin, tobramycin, amikacin) because of their activity against *Staphylococcus aureus* and gram-negative organisms, but the significant risk of nephrotoxicity and ototoxicity and the requirement for frequent serum monitoring makes them less attractive, especially because excellent alternatives are now available.[48]

Box 6-2 Risk Factors for Persistent Chronic Suppurative Otitis Media

- Exposures
  - Water
  - Cigarette smoke
- Daycare attendance
- Gastroesophageal reflux disease
- Anatomic obstruction
  - Adenoid hypertrophy
  - Craniofacial anomaly
  - Nasopharyngeal mass
  - Infectious or inflammatory
- Nasal foreign body
- Cholesteatoma
- Chronic adenoiditis
- Myringotomy tube
- Biofilm formation in the middle ear and mastoid
- Other—immunodeficiency, ciliary dysmotility

From Forsen J: Chronic diseases of the middle ear and mastoid. In Wetmore RF, Muntz HR, McGill TJI (eds): Pediatric Otolaryngology: Principles and Practice Pathways. New York, Thieme, 2000, pp 281-304.

Failure of maximal medical therapy mandates tympanomastoidectomy with tympanoplasty, although medical therapy before, during, and after surgery may improve the ultimate outcome. Preoperative planning should include a CT scan of the temporal bones.[49,50] The goals of surgery include eradication of any infectious nidus (e.g., diseased air cells and mucosa, occult cholesteatoma, osteitic bone, infected granulation tissue), establishment of reliable communication between the middle ear and mastoid, and reconstitution of the TM. Although it is not always possible, maintenance of an intact external auditory canal is an important goal. By keeping the mastoid cavity separated from the outside world, the incidence of persistent infection and drainage, even after surgery, can be minimized.

Various factors affect long-term success, but the presence of *Pseudomonas* and the persistence of diseased bone and soft tissue are often cited as important causes of surgical failure.[1] A complete list of factors that can perpetuate CSOM and make it harder to eradicate is presented in Box 6-2. Prompt treatment of recurrent drainage before chronic infection is reestablished aids long-term success.[41] Diligent débridement and judicious use of powerful topical agents resolves most cases of CSOM without surgery,[51] but operative intervention has a high success rate when it is required.[52,53]

Cholesteatoma

Cholesteatoma, more correctly referred to as keratoma, is a skin-lined mass filled with squamous debris found in the middle ear or mastoid spaces. In congenital cholesteatoma, patients without a history of significant ear disease or perforation of the TM are found to have squamous growth in the middle ear space, presumably from inappropriate or incomplete migration of precursor cells during embryologic development.[54] In primary acquired cholesteatoma, progressive retraction of the TM leads to ingrowth of a debris-filled pocket into the middle ear space. In secondary acquired cholesteatoma, prior infection or perforation allows ingress of squamous elements through a defect in the TM.[55]

As with other chronic ear disorders, the prevalence of cholesteatoma varies among populations. Although found to be present in 3 children/100,000 population in one study of the general population,[56] it was estimated to be present in 9.2% of cleft palate patients in another study.[1]

Cholesteatoma causes damage to the middle ear, mastoid, and surrounding structures in various ways.[57] As an expansile mass, it causes bone loss (including ossicular bone) through pressure resorption.[58] In addition, the subepithelial layer produces enzymes that destroy bone.[59] The sac can also become colonized with bacteria, acting as an ongoing source of infection. Any or all of these mechanisms can lead to further intratemporal or intracranial complications, primarily caused by direct extension of infection into nearby structures.[60] Although cholesteatoma in children and adults is similar on a molecular level, the disease process generally behaves more aggressively in the younger age group, a finding that may be the result of anatomic and physiologic differences in the vicinity of the squamous growth.[60]

Except in the unusual case in which cholesteatoma is obviously visible on examination, no pathognomonic symptoms or signs denote its presence. In many cases, cholesteatoma remains completely asymptomatic for a long time. A number of patients, especially children, do not notice the mild and insidious progression of conductive hearing loss associated with progressive TM retraction and ossicular erosion. In a recent retrospective review, more than 50% of patients with cholesteatoma presented with chronic otorrhea, recurrent acute otitis media, conductive hearing loss, or some combination of these three findings.[61]

When present, more dramatic symptoms such as otalgia, dizziness, or sensorineural hearing loss should prompt an urgent search for other complications of otitis media, and cholesteatoma will often be found lurking in these patients. In any suspected case, complete otomicroscopic examination is mandatory. If such a procedure, which must include removal of any crusts or drainage that obscure the examiner's vision, is not tolerated by the patient, arrangements for appropriate sedation or anesthesia must be made.[14]

Under the microscope or otoscope, cholesteatoma is often suspected when an aural polyp, obvious squamous debris, or middle ear granulation tissue is seen through a persistent perforation. The patient may have typical signs of CSOM but has had a poor response to medical treatment. TM perforation may or may not be detectable. Deep retraction pockets may not always be reliably differentiated from frank perforation with squamous ingrowth.

If cholesteatoma is suspected, CT can help confirm the diagnosis, although many pathologic entities share similar imaging characteristics. More importantly, it can help plan the surgical approach and alert the clinician to existing or impending complications, including erosion of the structures of the middle and inner ear or mastoid, or anterior petrous bone involvement, and can help define the location and involvement of the facial nerve.[62] Magnetic resonance imaging has a limited role in the diagnosis and management of cholesteatoma.[63]

The range of surgical approaches for cholesteatoma removal varies widely, and the choice of operation depends on location and extent of disease, residual hearing, patient comorbidities, and hearing status of the contralateral ear.[17] The primary goal is eradication of all squamous epithelial cells, because even minimal amounts of residual debris can lead to recurrence. The secondary goal of surgery is preservation of hearing.[64,65]

Tympanosclerosis

Postinflammatory calcification of collagen-containing structures in the middle ear is known as tympanosclerosis.[66] In 90% of patients, it manifests primarily as visible white plaques in the lamina propria of the tympanic membrane, a condition known as myringosclerosis.[67] The pathophysiology is not well elucidated,[68] although it is known to involve various common inflammatory mediators[69] and may involve a process similar to that of arteriosclerosis.[70] The overwhelming risk factor for tympanosclerosis in children is a history of chronic otitis media with effusion or recurrent acute otitis media requiring tympanostomy tube insertion, with over 50% of such patients showing permanent myringosclerotic plaques on examination.[71]

Tympanosclerosis is rarely a clinical problem, although it can partially obscure the view of the middle ear on examination and can occasionally be mistaken for visible cholesteatoma. Myringosclerosis changes the vibratory properties of the pars tensa, but conductive hearing loss is usually negligible.[72] In rare cases, however, calcified plaques within the middle ear space can cause fixation of the ossicular chain, resulting in conductive hearing loss.[66] Tympanoplasty for chronic TM perforation is generally successful in tympanosclerotic ears,[73] but in patients in whom the ossicles are fixed, ossiculoplasty is usually required to restore good hearing.[74]

Ossicular Discontinuity and Dysfunction

Efficient conduction of sound and normal hearing depend on an intact, appropriately vibrating middle ear system, starting from the tympanic membrane, progressing through the three ossicles (malleus, incus, and stapes), and including the oval and round windows. The ossicular chain can become discontinuous as a result of head trauma,[75] infection, or cholesteatoma in the middle ear, or iatrogenic removal during surgical treatment for middle ear disease.[76] Although perforation of the TM can cause moderate conductive hearing loss, hearing levels worse than 35 dB should be considered suspicious for ossicular dysfunction. Tympanometric findings are sometimes abnormal in cases of ossicular dysfunction, showing decreased compliance in the setting of fixation and increased compliance with discontinuity.[77] There are other audiologic tests that demonstrate increased reliability compared with conventional tympanometry in this clinical situation, but they are not routinely available.[78]

In addition to audiologic findings, ossicular problems may be suspected on visual examination. A severe retraction pocket caused by eustachian tube dysfunction may lead to obvious erosion of the long process of the incus, which has a more tenuous blood supply than the rest of the ossicular chain. Cholesteatoma or another middle ear mass in the region of the ossicles may have displaced the ossicles from their normal location, although near-normal conductive hearing may be preserved.[79] Radiologic studies may show abnormalities in the ossicular chain,[80] but the accuracy of this diagnostic technique is not known. Not surprisingly, ossicular function is best evaluated directly, during surgical exploration of the middle ear.[1]

As in the case of tympanoplastic closure of a chronic eardrum perforation, reconstruction of a dysfunctional ossicular chain should only be undertaken when the ear is reliably free of infection and cholesteatoma. Recurrent eardrum retraction and repeated bouts of otitis media substantially decrease the long-term success of ossicular reconstruction,[81] but simultaneous placement of a myringotomy tube at surgery may be helpful in keeping the repair functioning and durable.[82] Long-term results are comparable to those in adults.[83]

Labyrinthine Fistula

The fluid-containing cavities of the inner ear, which are responsible for maintaining the normal function of the cochlea and vestibular apparatus, are normally sealed from the middle ear. Abnormal communication between the inner and middle ear spaces can be caused by congenital abnormalities, trauma, or destructive lesions of the temporal bone. Although infections and inflammation of the inner ear are usually the result of extension through an intact round window, the overwhelming majority of frank labyrinthine fistulae are caused by cholesteatoma causing erosion of the bone overlying the lateral semicircular canal.[84]

According to one study,[85] which encompassed almost 14,000 patients who had undergone mastoidectomy, 7% of patients had intraoperative evidence of a labyrinthine fistula, and almost every case involved dehiscence of the lateral semicircular canal. Virtually all patients had cholesteatoma, and approximately two thirds had associated vertigo. Other preoperative findings included diagnosis by preoperative CT scan only 57% of the time, and a positive fistula test result (nystagmus or other vertiginous signs, with air pressure applied to a sealed ear canal) only 50% of the time.[85] These studies included patients of all ages; it is unclear how these findings vary in children.

Because labyrinthine fistula often manifests as a complication of cholesteatoma and associated middle ear disease, appropriate therapy starts with medical and surgical treatment of middle ear infection and drainage.[84] There are many variations of repair technique; ultimately, all involve soft tissue plugging of any abnormal communications between the middle and inner ear spaces.[86,87]

Cholesterol Granuloma

Chronic eustachian tube dysfunction and long-standing otitis media with effusion may lead to the pathologic entity known as cholesterol granuloma. Although the cause is obscure, cholesterol granuloma (CG) is invariably related to poor aeration of the tympanomastoid complex, which results in mucosal gland hypertrophy and collection of a thick brown liquid in the middle ear and mastoid that contains hemosiderin and cholesterol crystals.[88] When seen through an intact eardrum, CG appears dark blue and causes a conductive hearing loss. The differential diagnosis of a blue mass seen through the eardrum is presented in Table 6-2.[89]

Initial conservative treatment with observation and antibiotics is reasonable, because uncomplicated middle ear effusions often resolve without further intervention. Some have advocated myringotomy and evacuation with tube placement as an initial treatment, with the understanding that further surgery will likely be needed if thick material is found.[14] Middle ear exploration and mastoidectomy are necessary for a thorough cleanout.[90] Recurrence is best prevented by establishing good ventilation, which often requires at least a temporary ventilation tube.[14]

Table 6-2 Differential Diagnosis of a Blue Mass in the Middle Ear[89]

Clinical Entity	Comment
Long-standing otitis media with effusion ("glue ear")	More typical findings may be seen in other ear
Dehiscent jugular bulb	Arises from floor of middle ear
Glomus tumor	Possible history of pulsatile tinnitus
Hemotympanum	Likely history of recent trauma
Cholesterol granuloma	History of eustachian tube dysfunction

From Akyildiz AN, Kemaloglu YK: Cholesterol granuloma of the middle ear and mastoid ("blue ear"). In Alper CM, Bluestone CD, Casselbrant ML, et al (eds): Advanced Therapy of Otitis Media. Hamilton, Ontario, BC Decker, 2004, pp 355-358.

SUMMARY

Because otitis media is so common in children, the astute clinician must be aware of the potential for complications. Many chronic disorders of the middle ear and mastoid are caused or exacerbated by functional problems related to immaturity, and an understanding of the anatomy and physiology of the growing child is required. Treatment may include medical therapy (topical or systemic), surgery (ranging from minor to extensive), or some combination, but vigilant follow-up and repeated examination are common to all therapeutic plans. Hearing preservation is an important objective, but establishment and maintenance of a clean, dry, and safe ear are the primary goals.

MAJOR POINTS

Chronic middle ear disease usually occurs in patients with persistent or recurrent acute otitis media.

Eustachian tube dysfunction is extremely common in the growing child. It is an important factor in recurrent otitis media, serous otitis media, tympanic membrane retraction, and acquired cholesteatoma formation.

The differential diagnosis of tympanic membrane perforation is extensive. It may coexist with deeper, more serious pathology (ossicular discontinuity, cholesteatoma). The appropriate workup varies, but must include audiometric testing.

Chronic suppurative otitis media can be difficult to eradicate, occasionally requiring an escalating antimicrobial regimen. Stubborn cases should prompt a search for additional pathology, especially cholesteatoma, which requires surgical treatment.

REFERENCES

1. Forsen J: Chronic diseases of the middle ear and mastoid. In Wetmore RF, Muntz HR, McGill TJI (eds): Pediatric Otolaryngology: Principles and Practice Pathways. New York, Thieme, 2000, pp 281-304.

2. Casselbrant ML, Mandel EM: Risk factors for otitis media. In Alper CM, Bluestone CD, Casselbrant ML, et al (eds): Advanced Therapy of Otitis Media. Hamilton, Ontario, BC Decker, 2004, pp 26-31.

3. Straetemans M, van Heerbeek N, Sanders EA, et al: Immune status and eustachian tube function in recurrence of otitis media with effusion. Arch Otolaryngol Head Neck Surg 2005;131:771-776.

4. Smith TL, DiRuggiero DC, Jones KR: Recovery of eustachian tube function and hearing outcome in patients with cleft palate. Otolaryngol Head Neck Surg 1994; 111:423-429.

5. Pichichero ME: First-line treatment of acute otitis media. In Alper CM, Bluestone CD, Casselbrant ML, et al (eds): Advanced Therapy of Otitis Media. Hamilton, Ontario, BC Decker, 2004, pp 32-38.

6. Daly KA: Epidemiology. In Alper CM, Bluestone CD, Casselbrant ML et al (eds): Advanced Therapy of Otitis Media. Hamilton, Ontario, BC Decker, 2004, pp 21-25.

7. Bluestone CD, Klein JO, Alper CM, et al: Otitis media and eustachian tube dysfunction. In Bluestone CD, Stool S (eds): Pediatric Otolaryngology 4th ed. Philadelphia, WB Saunders, 2003, pp 512-525.

8. Bluestone CD, Doyle WJ: Anatomy and physiology of eustachian tube and middle ear related to otitis media. J Allergy Clin Immunol 1988;81(5 Pt 2):997-1003.

9. Bluestone CD: Eustachian tube function and dysfunction. In Rosenfeld RM, Bluestone CD, (eds): Evidence-Based Otitis Media, 2nd ed. Hamilton, Ontario, BC Decker, 2003, pp 163-179.

10. O'Connor AF, Shea JJ: Autophony and the patulous eustachian tube. Laryngoscope 1981;91(Pt 1):1427-1435.

11. Bluestone CD: Pathogenesis of otitis media: Role of eustachian tube. Pediatr Infect Dis J 1996;15:281-291.

12. Muntz HR: An overview of middle ear disease in cleft palate children. Facial Plast Surg 1993;9:177-180.

13. Bluestone CD: Definitions of otitis media and related diseases. In Alper CM, Bluestone CD, Casselbrant ML, et al (eds): Advanced Therapy of Otitis Media. Hamilton, Ontario, BC Decker, 2004, pp 1-8.

14. Bluestone CD, Klein JO: Intratemporal complications and sequelae of otitis media. In Bluestone CD, Stool S, Alper CM, et al (eds): Pediatric Otolaryngology, 4th ed. Philadelphia, Elsevier, 2003, pp 687-764.

15. Schilder AG: Assessment of complications of the condition and of the treatment of otitis media with effusion. Int J Pediatr Otorhinolaryngol 1999;49(Suppl 1): S247-S251.

16. Kay DJ, Nelson M, Rosenfeld RM: Meta-analysis of tympanostomy tube sequelae. Otolaryngol Head Neck Surg 2001;124:374-380.

17. Chole RA, Choo MJ: Chronic otitis media, mastoiditis, and petrositis. In Cummings CW (ed): Otolaryngology—Head and Neck Surgery, 3rd ed. St. Louis, Mosby, 1998, pp 3026-3046.

18. Duckert LG, Makielski KH, Helms J: Prolonged middle ear ventilation with the cartilage shield T-tube tympanoplasty. Otol Neurotol 2003;24:153-157.

19. Dornhoffer J: Cartilage tympanoplasty: Indications, techniques, and outcomes in a 1,000-patient series. Laryngoscope 2003;113:1844-1856.

20. Ostrowski VB, Bojrab DI: Minimally invasive laser contraction myringoplasty for tympanic membrane atelectasis. Otolaryngol Head Neck Surg 2003;128:711-718.

21. Mandell DL: Acute otitis media with perforation. In Alper CM, Bluestone CD, Casselbrant ML, et al (eds): Advanced Therapy of Otitis Media. Hamilton, Ontario, BC Decker, 2004, pp 52-55.

22. Hellstrom S: Tympanic membrane perforation. In Alper CM, Bluestone CD, Casselbrant ML, et al (eds): Advanced Therapy of Otitis Media. Hamilton, Ontario, BC Decker, 2004, pp 382-386.

23. Hellstrom S, Spratley J, Eriksson PO, Pais-Clemente M: Tympanic membrane vessel revisited: A study in an animal model. Otol Neurotol 2003;24:494-499.

24. Nishiike S, Irifune M, Doi K, et al: Tuberculous otitis media: Clinical aspects of 12 cases. Ann Otol Rhinol Laryngol 2003;112:935-938.

25. Mirza S, Richardson H: Otic barotrauma from air travel. J Laryngol Otol 2005;119:366-370.

26. Gunesh RP, Huber AM: Traumatic perilymphatic fistula. Ann Otol Rhinol Laryngol 2003;112:221-222.

27. Austin DF: Sound conduction of the diseased ear. J Laryngol Otol 1978;92:367-393.

28. Amadasun JE: An observational study of the management of traumatic tympanic membrane perforations. J Laryngol Otol 2002;116:181-184.

29. Saito T, Iwaki E, Kohno Y, et al: Prevention of persistent ear drum perforation after long-term ventilation tube treatment for otitis media with effusion in children. Int J Pediatr Otorhinolaryngol 1996;38:31-39.

30. Vrabec JT, Deskin RW, Grady JJ: Meta-analysis of pediatric tympanoplasty. Arch Otolaryngol Head Neck Surg 1999;125:530-534.

31. Collins WO, Telischi FF, Balkany TJ, Buchman CA: Pediatric tympanoplasty: Effect of contralateral ear status on outcomes. Arch Otolaryngol Head Neck Surg 2003;129:646-651.

32. Sheahan P, O'Dwyer T, Blayney A: Results of type 1 tympanoplasty in children and parental perceptions of outcome of surgery. J Laryngol Otol 2002;116:430-434.

33. Tos M: Approaches, myringoplasty, ossiculoplasty, tympanoplasty. In Tos M (ed): Manual of Middle Ear Surgery. Stuttgart, Thieme, 1993, pp 88-231.

34. Golz A, Goldenberg D, Netzer A, et al: Paper patching for chronic tympanic membrane perforations. Otolaryngol Head Neck Surg 2003;128:565-570.

35. Fishman AJ, Marrinan MS, Huang TC, Kanowitz SJ: Total tympanic membrane reconstruction: AlloDerm versus temporalis fascia. Otolaryngol Head Neck Surg 2005;132:906-915.

36. Mandel EM, Casselbrant ML, Kurs-Lasky M: Acute otorrhea: Bacteriology of a common complication of tympanostomy tubes. Ann Otol Rhinol Laryngol 1994;103: 713-718.

37. McLelland CA: Incidence of complications from use of tympanostomy tubes. Arch Otolaryngol 1980;106:97-99.

38. Saidi IS, Biedlingmaier JF, Whelan P: In vivo resistance to bacterial biofilm formation on tympanostomy tubes as a function of tube material. Otolaryngol Head Neck Surg 1999;120:621-627.

39. Kenna MA, Bluestone CD: Microbiology of chronic suppurative otitis media in children. Pediatr Infect Dis J 1986;5:223-225.

40. Smith AW, Hatcher J, Mackenzie IJ, et al: Randomised controlled trial of treatment of chronic suppurative otitis media in Kenyan schoolchildren. Lancet 1996;348: 1128-1133.

41. Bluestone CD: Suppurative complications. In Rosenfeld RM, Bluestone CD (eds): Evidence-Based Otitis Media, 2nd ed. Hamilton, Ontario, BC Decker, 2003, pp 482-504.

42. Lang R, Goshen S, Raas-Rothschild A, et al: Oral ciprofloxacin in the management of chronic suppurative otitis media without cholesteatoma in children: Preliminary experience in 21 children. Pediatr Infect Dis J 1992;11:925-929.

43. Pichichero ME, Arguedas A, Dagan R, et al: Safety and efficacy of gatifloxacin therapy for children with recurrent acute otitis media (AOM) and/or AOM treatment failure. Clin Infect Dis 2005;41:470-478.

44. Redmond AO: Risk-benefit experience of ciprofloxacin use in pediatric patients in the United Kingdom. Pediatr Infect Dis J 1997;16:147-149; discussion, 60-62.

45. Ah-Tye C, Paradise JL, Colborn DK: Otorrhea in young children after tympanostomy-tube placement for persistent middle-ear effusion: Prevalence, incidence, and duration. Pediatrics 2001;107:1251-1258.

46. Kenna MA, Bluestone CD, Reilly JS, Lusk RP: Medical management of chronic suppurative otitis media without cholesteatoma in children. Laryngoscope 1986;96:146-151.

47. Kenna MA, Rosane BA, Bluestone CD: Medical management of chronic suppurative otitis media without cholesteatoma in children—update 1992. Am J Otol 1993;14:469-473.

48. Fairbanks DNF: Pocket Guide to Antimicrobial Therapy in Otolaryngology—Head and Neck Surgery, 9th ed. Alexandria, Va, American Academy of Otolaryngology–Head and Neck Surgery, 2005, pp 49-51.

49. Banerjee A, Flood LM, Yates P, Clifford K: Computed tomography in suppurative ear disease: Does it influence management? J Laryngol Otol 2003;117:454-458.

50. Flood LM: The role of computerized tomography in the preoperative assessment of chronic suppurative otitis media. Clin Otolaryngol Allied Sci 2003;28:476.

51. Schroeder A, Darrow DH: Management of the draining ear in children. Pediatr Ann 2004;33:843-853.

52. Paparella MM, Froymovich O: Surgical advances in treating otitis media. Ann Otol Rhinol Laryngol Suppl 1994; 163:49-53.

53. Rickers J, Petersen CG, Pedersen CB, Ovesen T: Long-term follow-up evaluation of mastoidectomy in children with non-cholesteatomatous chronic suppurative otitis media. Int J Pediatr Otorhinolaryngol 2006;70:711-715.

54. Kazahaya K, Potsic WP: Congenital cholesteatoma. Curr Opin Otolaryngol Head Neck Surg 2004;12:398-403.

55. Sheehy JL: Acquired cholesteatoma in adults. Otolaryngol Clin North Am 1989;22:967-979.

56. Tos M: Incidence, etiology and pathogenesis of cholesteatoma in children. Adv Otorhinolaryngol 1988;40:110-117.

57. Albino AP, Kimmelman CP, Parisier SC: Cholesteatoma: A molecular and cellular puzzle. Am J Otol 1998;19:7-19.

58. Jung JY, Chole RA: Bone resorption in chronic otitis media: the role of the osteoclast. ORL 2002;64(2):95-107.

59. Chole RA: The molecular biology of bone resorption due to chronic otitis media. Ann N Y Acad Sci 1997;830:95-109.

60. Shohet JA, de Jong AL: The management of pediatric cholesteatoma. Otolaryngol Clin North Am 2002;35:841-851.

61. Semple CW, Mahadevan M, Berkowitz RG: Extensive acquired cholesteatoma in children: When the penny drops. Ann Otol Rhinol Laryngol 2005;114:539-542.

62. El-Bitar MA, Choi SS, Emamian SA, Vezina LG: Congenital middle ear cholesteatoma: Need for early recognition—role of computed tomography scan. Int J Pediatr Otorhinolaryngol 2003;67:231-235.

63. Ayache D, Williams MT, Lejeune D, Corre A: Usefulness of delayed postcontrast magnetic resonance imaging in the detection of residual cholesteatoma after canal wall-up tympanoplasty. Laryngoscope 2005;115:607-610.

64. Karmarkar S, Bhatia S, Saleh E, et al: Cholesteatoma surgery: The individualized technique. Ann Otol Rhinol Laryngol 1995;104:591-595.

65. Dodson EE, Hashisaki GT, Hobgood TC, Lambert PR: Intact canal wall mastoidectomy with tympanoplasty for cholesteatoma in children. Laryngoscope 1998; 108:977-983.

66. Forseni M, Bagger-Sjoback D, Hultcrantz M: A study of inflammatory mediators in the human tympanosclerotic middle ear. Arch Otolaryngol Head Neck Surg 2001;127:559-564.

67. Bhaya MH, Schachern PA, Morizono T, Paparella MM: Pathogenesis of tympanosclerosis. Otolaryngol Head Neck Surg 1993;109(Pt 1):413-420.

68. Jung TT, Hunter LL, Alper CM, et al: Recent advances in otitis media. 9. Complications and sequelae. Ann Otol Rhinol Laryngol 2005;194(Suppl):140-160.

69. Karlidag T, Ilhan N, Kaygusuz I,et al: Comparison of free radicals and antioxidant enzymes in chronic otitis media with and without tympanosclerosis. Laryngoscope 2004;114:85-89.

70. Pirodda A, Ferri GG, Bruzzi C, et al: Possible relationship between tympanosclerosis and atherosclerosis. Acta Otolaryngol 2004;124:574-576.

71. De Beer BA, Schilder AG, Zielhuis GA, Graamans K: Natural course of tympanic membrane pathology related to otitis media and ventilation tubes between ages 8 and 18 years. Otol Neurotol 2005;26:1016-1021.

72. Tos M, Stangerup SE: Hearing loss in tympanosclerosis caused by grommets. Arch Otolaryngol Head Neck Surg 1989;115:931-935.

73. Onal K, Uguz MZ, Kazikdas KC,et al: A multivariate analysis of otological, surgical and patient-related factors in determining success in myringoplasty. Clin Otolaryngol 2005;30:115-120.

74. Bayazit YA, Ozer E, Kara C,et al: An analysis of the single-stage tympanoplasty with over-underlay grafting in tympanosclerosis. Otol Neurotol 2004;25:211-214.

75. Wang LF, Ho KY, Tai CF, Kuo WR: Traumatic ossicular chain discontinuity—report of two cases. Kaohsiung J Med Sci 1999;15:504-509.

76. Batti JS: Ossicular discontinuity/fixation. In Alper CM, Bluestone CD, Casselbrant ML, et al (eds): Advanced Therapy of Otitis Media. Hamilton, Ontario, BC Decker, 2004, pp 414-418.

77. Browning GG, Swan IR, Gatehouse S: The doubtful value of tympanometry in the diagnosis of otosclerosis. J Laryngol Otol 1985;99:545-547.

78. Tabuchi K, Murashita H, Okubo H, et al: Preoperative evaluation of ossicular chain abnormality in patients with conductive deafness without perforation of the tympanic membrane. Arch Otolaryngol Head Neck Surg 2005;131:686-689.

79. Jeng FC, Tsai MH, Brown CJ: Relationship of preoperative findings and ossicular discontinuity in chronic otitis media. Otol Neurotol 2003;24:29-32.

80. Swartz JD, Berger AS, Zwillenberg S, Popky GL: Ossicular erosions in the dry ear: CT diagnosis. Radiology 1987;163:763-765.

81. Schwetschenau EL, Isaacson G: Ossiculoplasty in young children with the Applebaum incudostapedial joint prosthesis. Laryngoscope 1999;109:1621-1625.

82. Chandrasekhar SS, House JW, Devgan U: Pediatric tympanoplasty. A 10-year experience. Arch Otolaryngol Head Neck Surg 1995;121:873-878.

83. Kessler A, Potsic WP, Marsh RR: Total and partial ossicular replacement prostheses in children. Otolaryngol Head Neck Surg 1994;110:302-303.

84. Bluestone CD: Labyrinthitis. In Alper CM, Bluestone CD, Casselbrant ML, et al (eds): Advanced Therapy of Otitis Media. Hamilton, Ontario, BC Decker, 2004, pp 348-354.

85. Copeland BJ, Buchman CA: Management of labyrinthine fistulae in chronic ear surgery. Am J Otolaryngol 2003;24:51-60.

86. Minor LB: Labyrinthine fistulae: Pathobiology and management. Curr Opin Otolaryngol Head Neck Surg 2003;11:340-346.

87. Bluestone CD: Perlilymphatic fistula and eustachian tube surgery. In Bluestone CD, Rosenfeld RM (eds): Surgical Atlas of Pediatric Otolaryngology. Hamilton, Ontario, BC Decker, 2002, pp 123-132.

88. Miura M, Sando I, Orita Y, Hirsch BE: Histopathologic study of the temporal bones and Eustachian tubes of children with cholesterol granuloma. Ann Otol Rhinol Laryngol 2002;111(Pt 1):609-615.

89. Akyildiz AN, Kemaloglu YK: Cholesterol granuloma of the middle ear and mastoid ("blue ear"). In Alper CM, Bluestone CD, Casselbrant ML, et al (eds): Advanced Therapy of Otitis Media. Hamilton, Ontario, BC Decker, 2004, pp 355-358.

90. Maeta M, Saito R, Nakagawa F, Miyahara T: Surgical intervention in middle-ear cholesterol granuloma. J Laryngol Otol 2003;117:344-348.

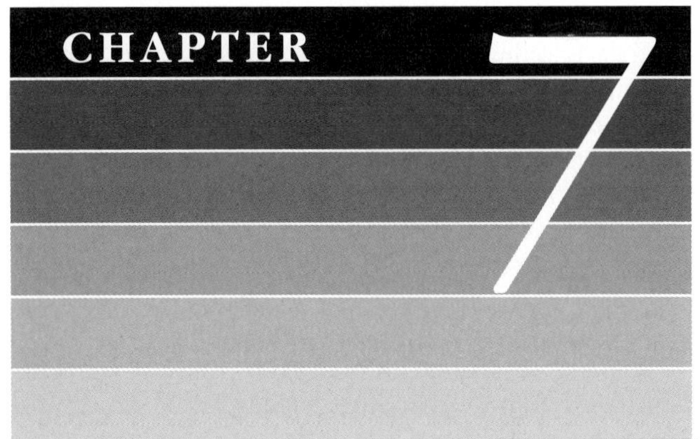

Regional and Intracranial Complications of Acute Otitis Media

IMAN NASERI, MD
STEVEN E. SOBOL, MD

Acute otitis media (AOM) remains one of the most common conditions diagnosed by primary care physicians. It is estimated that 9.3 million episodes of AOM occur annually in children younger than 2 years in the United States.[1] Approximately 50% of all children will have at least one episode of otitis media by their first birthday and 80% by the age of 3 years.[1] Before antibiotics were introduced, the mortality rate from otitis media approached 4%.[2] Today, this number has decreased to virtually zero.

Complications from AOM, although less common than previously seen, can lead to significant morbidity and mortality. They arise when bacteria from the middle ear and mastoid spread through thin bony walls, along preformed pathways, or hematogenously to involve the facial nerve, sigmoid sinus, labyrinth, dura mater, or intracranial structures.[3] Such complications are divided into two main groups—intratemporal (extracranial) and intracranial. Intratemporal complications include mastoiditis, subperiosteal abscess, petrositis, labyrinthitis, and/or facial nerve paralysis. Intracranial complications include epidural, subdural, or parenchymal abscess formation, sigmoid sinus thrombosis, otitic hydrocephalus, and bacterial meningitis. This chapter reviews the pertinent background, key diagnostic, and treatment modalities regarding the complications of otitis media.

BACKGROUND

Clinical Presentation

The child with AOM usually presents to the primary care physician (PCP) with a history of irritability, pulling at the ears, and other symptoms suggestive of an upper respiratory tract infection. Older children may complain of otalgia and hearing loss. The physical examination commonly used in primary care settings may not be sensitive or specific enough to make an accurate diagnosis of AOM.[4] It is imperative that care be taken to remove cerumen and perform pneumatic otoscopy in patients suspected of having AOM. Examination typically reveals an erythematous, bulging, hypomobile tympanic membrane (TM), with fluid in the middle ear space. It is important to differentiate AOM from TM erythema that may be present in the crying child. In the latter case, the TM will have normal mobility with pneumatic otoscopy. It is also critical to differentiate between AOM and otitis media with effusion (OME), which presents with fluid in the middle ear space in the absence of acute infection. Table 7-1 highlights the clinical presentation of AOM.

Both intratemporal and intracranial complications can rapidly lead to life-threatening sequelae, thus making early recognition and management crucial. The clinical evaluation should always include a search for symptoms or signs suggesting complications of AOM, which may include the presence of mastoid tenderness, protrusion of the auricle, unusually severe hearing loss or vertigo, cranial neuropathies, lethargy, and changes in mental status.

Table 7-1 Clinical Presentation of Acute Otitis Media

Symptoms/Signs*	Otologic Examination Findings
Cough, rhinitis (most common symptom)[87]	Bulging and erythematous tympanic membrane, with diminished movement on pneumatic otoscopy
Irritability (may be the only symptom in infants)	Decreased visibility of middle ear landmarks
Fever	
Otalgia	
Decreased hearing	
Otorrhea	

*Usually accompany an ongoing or preceding upper respiratory infection.

Diagnostic Evaluation

When a complication of AOM is suggested by the history and physical examination, imaging studies often provide valuable information and help guide management.[5,6] Computed tomography (CT) of the temporal bone with contrast is often the modality of choice for diagnosing complications of AOM. Findings may include demineralization of the mastoid's bony septations (acute mastoiditis), destruction of bone along the mastoid or zygomatic root cortex with soft tissue fluid collection (subperiosteal abscess), decreased flow within the sigmoid sinus (sinus thrombosis), widening of the ventricles (otitic hydrocephalus), and dehiscence of the tegmen tympani, with or without intracranial abscess formation.

Magnetic resonance imaging (MRI) is used in patients with clinical and CT findings suggestive of intracranial involvement. Although MRI lacks detail on bony structures within the temporal bone, it is superior to CT imaging in demonstrating acute inflammatory changes seen in focal parenchymal lesions, meningeal inflammation, cranial nerve inflammation, and cerebritis. Moreover, protocols that use arterial or venous imaging are helpful in the diagnosis and follow-up of patients with sinus thrombosis. Table 7-2 highlights the imaging findings for the complications of AOM.

When possible, audiologic evaluation should be obtained prior to surgical intervention to assess for

Table 7-2 Imaging Modalities for Acute Otitis Media and Its Complications

	Imaging Modality	
Complication	Computed Tomography (CT)*	Magnetic Resonance Imaging (MRI)
Mastoiditis	Good demonstration of mastoid cells and bony structures; diagnosis obtained by comparing number, thickness, and mineralization of mastoid air cells with contralateral side[88]; acute or chronic mastoiditis suspected if there is erosion or coalescence of bony architecture of mastoid air cells	Bony structures poorly demonstrated
Subperiosteal abscess	Preferred; as good as MRI	More expensive, slightly more sensitive than CT
Petrositis	Usually first-line modality, but supplement with MRI	Good for demonstrating nerve involvement and apical petrositis
Labyrinthitis	Demonstrates bony walls of facial nerve canal and labyrinth or late ossific changes	Good for demonstrating inflammatory changes (e.g., thickening, enhancement) of nerve or membranous labyrinth
Facial nerve involvement	Good for evaluation of facial nerve canal	Only way to demonstrate actual nerve involvement by enhancement
Epidural abscess	Usually first-line modality; good for follow-up if correlation seen with MRI scan	More sensitive acutely; allows earlier detection
Subdural abscess, empyema	Usually first-line modality; good for follow-up if correlation seen with MRI scan	Better than CT in detecting extracerebral fluid collections; may also differentiate between benign and infected tissue because of shortened T1 relaxation times of purulent fluid
Brain abscess	Usually first-line modality; good for follow-up if correlation seen with MRI scan	More sensitive acutely; allows earlier detection
Sigmoid sinus thrombosis	Sensitive but not specific for absence of contrast enhancement in sinus lumen; "delta sign" (circumferential perisinus enhancement)	Hampers diagnosis because of flow-related phenomena†; preferred method is MR angiography

*Noncontrast axial and coronal.
†The presence of a signal void within the sinus excludes a thrombosis.

Box 7-1 Criteria for Obtaining Culture Specimens of Middle Ear Effusion in Patients with Acute Otitis Media (AOM)

Severe intractable pain
Failure to respond to appropriate antibiotic therapy
AOM in certain immunocompromised or nosocomial patients
AOM in neonates
Complications of AOM

conductive and sensorineural hearing loss. This evaluation, however, should not delay definitive management in critically ill patients.

Diagnostic cultures may be helpful in guiding management and should be obtained in patients with AOM with the following criteria (Box 7-1): (1) severe intractable pain; (2) failure to respond to appropriate antibiotic therapy; (3) AOM in certain immunocompromised or nosocomial patients; (4) AOM in neonates; or (5) development of suspected complications. The fastest means of obtaining culture material is by aspirating the middle ear space with a spinal needle attached to a syringe or by using a tympanocentesis apparatus. This may be performed without the need for general anesthesia. When the decision is made to operate, specimens may be obtained through a myringotomy or within the mastoid at the time of general anesthesia.

Medical Management

The usual pathogens in acute otitis media are *Streptococcus pneumoniae*, *Haemophilus influenzae*, and *Moraxella catarrhalis*. Although viruses can also be pathogens in AOM, they are involved in fewer than 10% of such cases. The main concern in the past decade has been the emergence of drug-resistant bacteria, which has led to variations in antibiotic therapy[7] and diagnostic criteria.[8] Table 7-3 highlights the pathogens commonly encountered in otitis media and its complications.

Children with AOM are usually managed in the primary care setting, with the goals of treatment being to eradicate the infection, prevent complications, and provide symptomatic relief. Otolaryngology consultation is not necessary in most cases but should be obtained for the following: (1) continued worsening of symptoms in spite of appropriate antibiotic therapy; (2) recurrent episodes of AOM; (3) persistence of symptoms after multiple courses of antibiotic therapy: (4) comorbid immunodeficiency; (or 5) complications of AOM (Box 7-2). Neurosurgical consultation should be obtained when intracranial complications develop. The goal of management of AOM is to provide appropriate systemic treatment of the likely bacterial pathogens. When complications arise, drainage of the affected ear through a myringotomy or mastoidectomy is often necessary.

The introduction of antibiotics in the 1930s and 1940s has considerably decreased the incidence, morbidity, and mortality from otogenic intratemporal complications.[9] At the start of the 20th century, 50% of

Table 7-3 Microbiology of Otitis Media and Its Complications

Complication	Most Common Pathogen	Second Most Common Pathogen	Third Most Common Pathogen
Acute otitis media (AOM)*	*Streptococcus pneumoniae*	*Haemophilus influenzae*†	*Moraxella catarrhalis*
Chronic suppurative otitis media (CSOM)	*Pseudomonas aeruginosa*	*Staphylococcus aureus*	Coagulase-negative
Acute mastoiditis	*Streptococcus pneumoniae*	*Pseudomonas aeruginosa* and *Streptococcus pyogenes*	*Staphylococcus* *M. catarrhalis*
Subperiosteal abscess	*S. aureus*	*S. pyogenes*	*S. pneumoniae*
Petrositis	*Bacteroides fragilis*	*Proteus mirabilis*	
Labyrinthitis	Same as for AOM		
Facial nerve paralysis	*S. pneumoniae*	*Staphylococcus* sp.	
Epidural abscess	*S. aureus*	*P. aeruginosa*	*Bacteroides fragilis*
Subdural abscess	*Proteus mirabilis*	*P. aeruginosa*	*Staphylococcus* sp.
Brain abscess	*Proteus* sp.‡	*Klebsiella pneumoniae*	*Klebsiella oxytoca*
Sigmoid sinus thrombosis	*S. pneumoniae*	*S. aureus*	Sterile
Bacterial meningitis	*S. pneumoniae*		

*Different from medically refractory AOM, which is commonly seen in complications. The most common bacteriologic studies have shown coagulase-negative staphylococci, *Staphylococcus aureus*, and *Streptococcus pneumoniae*.[89]
†Nontypable strains.
‡Otogenic brain abscesses are usually caused by multiple species of bacteria.[90]

Box 7-2 Criteria for Otolaryngology Consultation for Acute Otitis Media (AOM)

Continued deterioration with appropriate antibiotic therapy
Recurrent episodes of AOM
Persistence of symptoms after multiple courses of antibiotic therapy
Comorbid immunodeficiency
Nosocomial infection
Complications of AOM

patients with otitis media developed acute mastoiditis. This complication decreased to 6% by 1955 and 0.4% by 1959.[10] A decrease from 2.3% to 0.24% has been seen in the incidence of intracranial complications since the introduction of antibiotics.[11] Nevertheless, the morbidity for both types of complications remains significant. With the emergence of resistant strains of bacteria, there has been renewed interest in otogenic complications in recent years. Antonelli and colleagues[12] have demonstrated that there is an increasing incidence rate of acute mastoiditis, mainly attributable to antibiotic-resistant pneumococcus.[12] Hence, the medical management of acute otitis media and its related complications is continuously changing.

Antibiotic management for AOM should involve broad-spectrum agents, accounting for the usual pathogens. Antibiotic choice should provide adequate coverage for the likely bacterial pathogens (*S. pneumoniae*, *H. influenzae*, *M. catarrhalis*), and the physician should be aware of the probability of bacterial resistance within their community. Approximately 44% of *H. influenzae* and almost all *M. catarrhalis* strains have β-lactamase-mediated resistance to penicillin-based antimicrobials in children.[13] As many as 64% of *S. pneumoniae* strains are penicillin-resistant because of altered penicillin-binding proteins.[13] Multiple drug-resistant *S. pneumoniae* strains are also found in substantial numbers of children in daycare settings. Antibiotic choice in children should also be guided by factors that will improve compliance, such as single- or twice-daily dosing and taste.

First-line therapy at most centers is usually amoxicillin or a macrolide antibiotic in penicillin-allergic patients, given their low cost, ease of administration, and low toxicity. Amoxicillin should be given at double the usual dose (80 to 90 mg/kg/day), especially in localities with known *S. pneumoniae* resistance.[14,15] The duration of treatment should be 10 days, with close follow-up if symptoms continue to persist beyond 48 to 72 hours following the initiation of antibiotic therapy.

Second-line antibiotics include amoxicillin clavulanate, second- or third-generation cephalosporins (cefprozil, cefdinir), and macrolides (azithromycin, clarithromycin). These should be considered in patients who live in communities with a high incidence of resistant organisms, those who fail to respond within 48 to 72 hours of commencement of first-line therapy, and those with persistence of symptoms beyond 10 days.[16] Antibiotic choice for patients presenting with complications of AOM should be broad-spectrum agents, given intravenously. Third-generation cephalosporins (cefotaxime, ceftriaxone) in combination with vancomycin provide adequate intracranial penetration, making them a good first-line choice.[16,17] Table 7-4 highlights the antibiotic management of AOM.

Clearance of bacteria from middle ear fluid without the use of antibiotics is evident in studies in which a

Table 7-4 Antibiotics Commonly Used for Acute Otitis Media (AOM) and Its Complications

		Streptococcus pneumoniae				
Antibiotic	**Dosage**	**Sensitive Strain**	**Intermediate Strain**	**Resistant Strain**	***Haemophilus influenzae***	***Moraxella catarrhalis***
First-line Therapy						
Amoxicillin	40-90 mg/kg/day	+++	++	–	++	–
Trimethoprim-sulfamethoxazole	6-12 mg/kg/day (TMP)	++	–	–	++	+
Clarithromycin	15 mg/kg/day	+++	±	–	++	+
Second-line Therapy						
Amoxicillin-clavulanate	25-90 mg/kg/day	+++	+	–	+++	+++
Cefuroxime	30 mg/kg/day	+++	++	–	++	+++
Cefprozil	15 mg/kg/day	+++	++	–	++	+++
Cefdinir	14 mg/kg/day	+++	+	–	+++	+++

+++, Excellent coverage; ++, good coverage; +, fair coverage; –, no significant activity; ±, limited.

Adapted from Brook I, Gooch WM III, Jenkins SG, et al: Medical management of acute bacterial sinusitis. Recommendations of a clinical advisory committee on pediatric and adult sinusitis. Ann Otol Rhinol Laryngol 2000;109(Suppl):2-20.

placebo is used.[18] However, comparative studies have demonstrated that the incidence rate of complications from AOM is higher in countries that tend to manage such cases in children with initial observation rather than prescribing antibiotics.[19]

Surgical Management

Complications of AOM may require drainage of the middle ear and/or mastoid cavity. Myringotomy with tympanostomy tube placement may be adequate for complications including facial nerve paralysis, labyrinthitis, or meningitis, but mastoidectomy is often required in cases of subperiosteal abscess and petrositis. Further surgical management may be necessary for intracranial complications of AOM.

COMPLICATIONS OF ACUTE OTITIS MEDIA

Extracranial and Intratemporal Complications

Acute Mastoiditis

The mastoid cavity is in direct continuity with the middle ear space through the aditus ad antrum mastoideum, creating a large single cavity in which mucosal inflammation may occur and fluid may collect during a bout of AOM. CT during this phase will reveal opacification of the mastoid air cells without destruction of the bony partitions, leading to the often erroneous diagnosis of "mastoiditis." Acute mastoiditis is a clinical diagnosis made when the patient with AOM presents with postauricular erythema, edema, and/or tenderness, with or without anteroinferior protrusion of the pinna and sagging of the posterior external auditory canal. Acute mastoiditis is said to be coalescent in such cases, when the CT findings indicate bony erosion and destruction of the mastoid air cells. This results from increased pressure and osteoclastic activity from the purulent exudates, causing ischemia and reduced blood flow on the thin bony septae of the mastoid cavity.[20]

Although there are no explicit guidelines for the treatment of acute mastoiditis, most practitioners would recommend a course of intravenous antibiotics to cover the most common organisms. In cases in which there is no coalescence noted within the mastoid, antibiotic therapy is usually sufficient, reserving surgical intervention for progression or failure of improvement.

The surgical options for acute mastoiditis include myringotomy, with or without tympanostomy tube placement, and/or simple mastoidectomy. The goal of surgical intervention is to relieve the pressure in the middle ear and mastoid space, in addition to allowing for sampling of the exudate for culture. The indications and timing for both surgical approaches are controversial and practitioner-dependent. In a retrospective study over a 12-year period, Harley and associates demonstrated that there is no statistically significant difference in the cure rates of children treated with antibiotics and myringotomy versus antibiotics with mastoidectomy.[21] Nevertheless, many studies have supported initial myringotomy and insertion of a ventilation tube, along with antibiotics and mastoidectomy, if there is no clinical improvement over a 48-hour period.[22] Circumstances that would warrant an earlier mastoidectomy include a suspected cholesteatoma and other intratemporal or intracranial complications.[23]

Subperiosteal Abscess

The most frequent complication of acute mastoiditis is the development of a subperiosteal abscess.[24-26] Abscess formation most commonly occurs along the lateral surface of the mastoid cortex, manifesting with increased protrusion of the auricle, postauricular fluctuance, effacement of the postauricular crease, and CT demonstrating erosion of the mastoid cortex, with adjacent soft tissue abscess formation (Figs. 7-1 and 7-2). The tympanic membrane may be normal in appearance.[27,28] Other tests may also be of little additional value, because the leukocyte count and erythrocyte sedimentation rate may be normal.[29,30] Erosion may also occur at the level of the zygomatic root or through the mastoid tip, resulting in adjacent neck abscess formation. The latter complication is also called Bezold's abscess (named after Friedrich Bezold, a professor of otology at the University of Munich). In describing the physiology in the late 1880s, he noted that the thickness of the superficial mastoid air cells, coupled with the purulent secretions in the mastoid cavity, can cause perforations through the bony walls of the cells into the soft tissues surrounding the temporal bone.[31] Holt and Young also corroborated these findings through their research, almost a century later.[32]

Management of a subperiosteal abscess includes intravenous antibiotics directed toward the most common pathogens—*Staphylococcus aureus*, *Streptococcus pyogenes*, and *S. pneumoniae*.[33] Simple mastoidectomy with or without myringotomy should be strongly considered in all cases in which an abscess is encountered. Drainage through the neck may also be necessary in cases of Bezold's abscess formation.

Petrositis (Gradenigo's Syndrome)

In 1907, Giuseppe Conte Gradenigo, an Italian otologist, described a syndrome with the following triad: otitis and possible otorrhea, abducens nerve paralysis, and retrobulbar pain.[34] This condition was characterized by an inflammatory disease involving the petrous portion of the temporal bone (petrositis), ipsilateral paralysis of the abducens nerve, causing lateral gaze deficiency, and severe pain in the area supplied by the ophthalmic

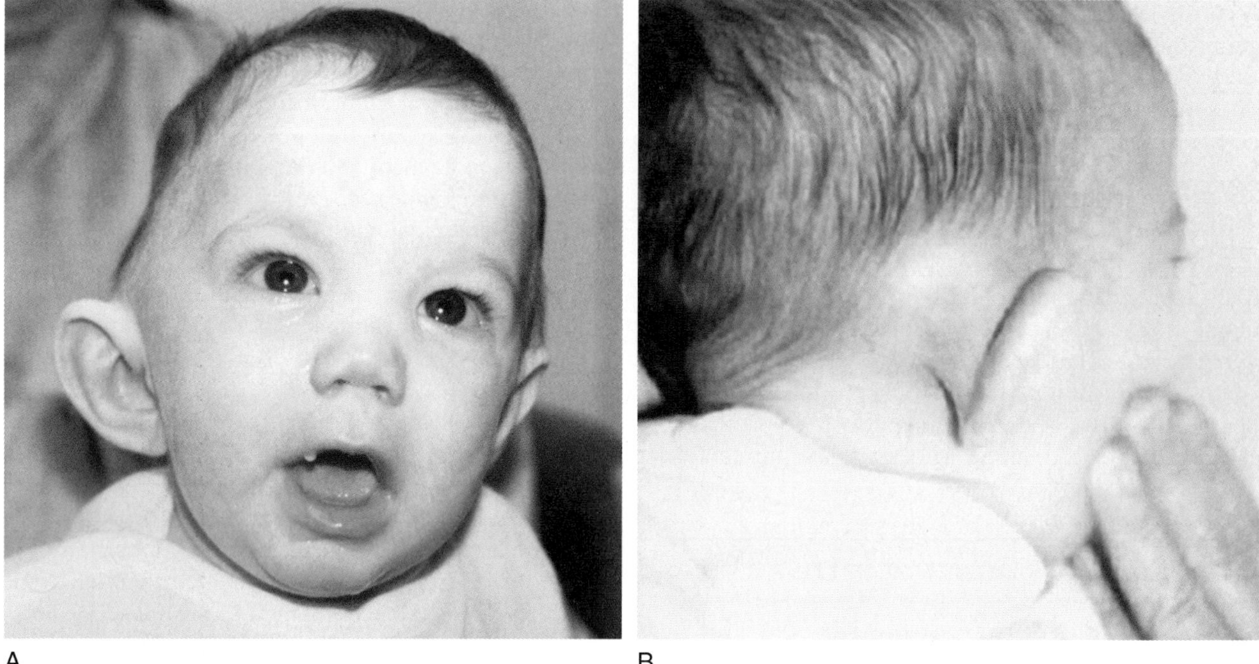

Figure 7-1. Acute mastoiditis with subperiosteal abscess. **A, B,** Note protrusion of the right auricle from the skull with erythema, edema, and effacement of the postauricular crease.

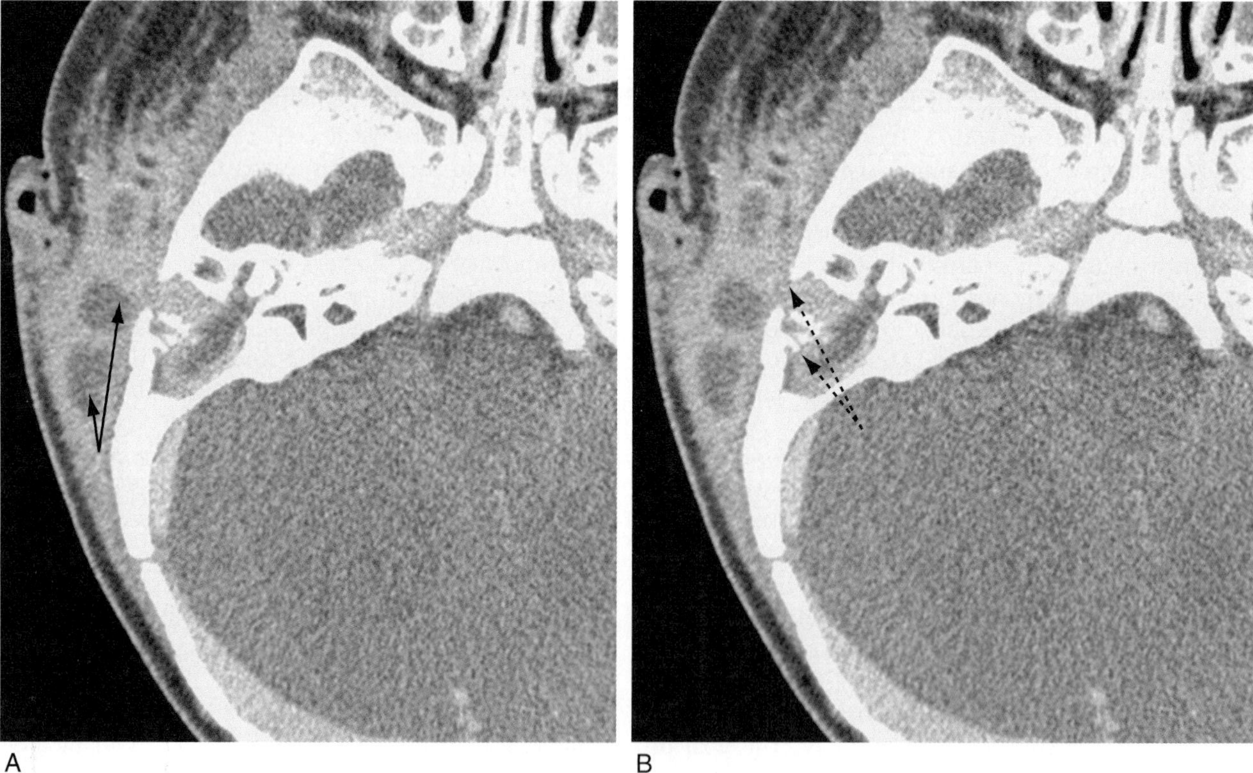

Figure 7-2. Soft tissue (**A**) and bone window (**B**) axial CT scans of the temporal bone demonstrating right acute coalescent mastoiditis with subperiosteal abscess formation. Note the soft tissue edema and abscesses *(**A**, solid arrows)*, as well as the bone destruction within the mastoid *(**B**, dashed arrows)*.

branch of the trigeminal nerve, causing a deep pain perceived behind the eye (retrobulbar pain). After others confirmed the clinical and pathologic findings in their patients, the condition was named Gradenigo's syndrome.[35] Since the advent of antibiotics, the incidence of this condition is low, although modern case reports exist.

Petrositis occurs when infection from the middle ear and mastoid spread to the petrous cells of the temporal bone by vascular canals or bone resorption.[36] The surrounding nerves (cranial nerves V through VII) may then be affected by the local inflammatory process, causing related pain and palsies.[35] The diagnosis is typically made by CT or MRI, usually prompted by high suspicion because of the presence of one or more of the criteria in Gradenigo's triad of symptoms.[37] In the absence of cholesteatoma, which may mimic the clinical picture of acute petrositis, treatment should be analogous to that of acute mastoiditis. Recent case studies have shown a successful outcome with conservative medical management, without the need for mastoidectomy.[38] A high index of suspicion should be maintained in approaching such conditions, because early intervention may prevent intracranial and central nervous system involvement.[39]

Labyrinthitis

Labyrinthitis occurs when the inflammatory process in the middle ear or mastoid spreads to the labyrinth, a structure composed of a delicate membranous network surrounded by an osseous framework. Access to the labyrinthine structures can be through the middle ear by way of the oval and round windows and/or through defects in the bony labyrinth. The typical history is that of an acute onset of sensorineural hearing loss and vertigo in a patient with AOM. No diagnostic tests are necessary when the clinical symptoms appear in the presence of AOM or chronic otitis media.

The two types of labyrinthitis are serous and suppurative. Serous labyrinthitis is caused by disturbance of the tissue-fluid environment within the inner ear,[40] secondary to bacterial toxins, viruses, or products of tissue injury without actual bacterial invasion of the labyrinthine system. Cytotoxic materials from acute or chronic otitis media can spread to the inner ear via the round window, the oval window, or a labyrinthine fistula. Suppurative labyrinthitis is caused by bacterial penetration of the labyrinth.

Serous and suppurative labyrinthitis may not be distinguishable from each other during the acute phase in the presence of an underlying acute or chronic otitis media. Such a distinction can be made more accurately once the acute phase has resolved by gauging the return of vestibulocochlear function.[41] In general, however, patients with serous labyrinthitis usually have milder initial symptoms of audiovestibular dysfunction.[42] Serous labyrinthitis has an excellent prognosis if there are no other intratemporal or intracranial complications. However, most patients do not recover labyrinthine function, and central compensation usually corrects this deficiency.[43] The prognosis for suppurative labyrinthitis is poor in terms of recovery of vestibulocochlear function.

The management of labyrinthitis should be aimed at the underlying otitic infection. Intravenous antibiotic treatment for a course of 10 days is recommended to eliminate the labyrinthine infection and prevent the development of meningitis.[44] Myringotomy should often be employed for drainage and culture of middle ear fluid. Bed rest and labyrinth-suppressing medications may offer some relief of symptoms.[45] Steroid treatment has been shown to reduce subsequent hearing loss in cases with persistent sensorineural hearing loss, despite adequate antibiotic therapy.[46]

Facial Nerve Paralysis

Acute otitis media accounts for 9% to 20% of all cases of facial nerve paralysis in children.[47,48] The course and exposure of the facial nerve in the middle ear place it at an increased risk for inflammatory changes when exposed to toxins. In the setting of acute or chronic otitis media, the natural dehiscences along the horizontal portion of the facial nerve[49] become potential sites where infection can penetrate. The pathophysiology of this phenomenon is believed to involve compression and thrombosis of the microvasculature supplying the facial nerve.[50] The lack of intrinsic nerve involvement makes this damage reversible in almost all cases.

Acute or chronic otitis infection usually precedes the clinical presentation of facial nerve palsy or paralysis by about 5 days.[47] In children, facial nerve paralysis is generally incomplete.[51] In AOM-related facial nerve paralysis, there is generally no facial pain or tic, but only ipsilateral facial muscle weakness.[52]

Management should include broad-spectrum intravenous antibiotic therapy with good meningeal penetration. The most common related organisms isolated are gram-positive cocci.[53] Hence, the use of a third-generation cephalosporin would serve as an appropriate initial antibiotic regimen until more definitive culture and sensitivity results have been obtained. In the setting of an intact tympanic membrane and AOM, the establishment of a proper drainage pathway for the acute middle ear infection by myringotomy is recommended. CT imaging is advocated to exclude other intratemporal involvement, including masked or silent mastoiditis, in which associated clinical signs are absent.[54-56] Initial worsening of facial nerve paralysis is not unlikely during the course of treatment. With conservative treatment, almost all patients with facial nerve palsy regain full functional recovery over a 1- to 2-month period.[57] More aggressive surgical intervention should be reserved for concomitant suppurative complications and clinical regression.[53]

Intracranial Complications

In the preantibiotic era, acute sinusitis and otitis media were the presumed causes of approximately 29% of all suppurative intracranial processes.[58] Intracranial complications of AOM have decreased considerably over the past 80 years.[11,59] Nonetheless, the distribution of specific types of such complications remains similar to that in the preantibiotic era.[21,60] Moreover, mortality from otogenic intracranial complications remains alarmingly high (10% to 20%).[61-64]

A high index of suspicion is essential in the workup of a patient with potential intracranial complications of AOM, because early detection and management may significantly improve their ultimate outcome. A history of headache, seizures, altered mental status, nausea and vomiting, irritability, lethargy, or fluctuating levels of consciousness in a patient with AOM should prompt the physician to explore the possibility of intracranial suppuration. Physical examination should include a complete otologic and neurologic assessment, with specific evaluation for meningismus, focal neurologic deficits, and/or any signs of encephalopathy.[65]

A contrast-enhanced CT scan of the head and temporal bone may demonstrate bony destruction of the tegmen tympani, flow abnormalities within the sigmoid sinus, meningeal enhancement, and/or fluid collections in cases of abscess formation. MRI is now the most specific imaging modality for detection of purulent fluid, especially in the extracerebral space, and its use is often warranted for the initial evaluation and follow-up of patients with otogenic intracranial complications. A lumbar puncture and examination of cerebrospinal fluid are also essential, but only after imaging is performed to exclude a mass effect, to obtain culture material. Initial bacteriologic findings are usually nonspecific, although Hlavin and colleagues[58] found that most operative cultures test positive for bacterial growth. Management of intracranial complications of AOM is specific to the diagnosis and should always include neurosurgical consultation.

Epidural Abscess

An epidural abscess is a pus collection in the space between the dura mater of the brain and overlying bone. It remains one of the most frequent intracranial complications of otitis media.[41] There are a rising number of such infections caused from postcraniotomy surgical wound infections, but complications from otitis media and sinusitis still account for most cases of community-acquired intracranial epidural abscess formation.

The most common bacterial pathogens identified in otogenic epidural abscesses include single or multiple species of *Streptococcus*, *Staphylococcus*, aerobic gram-negative bacilli, and other anaerobes. Therefore, use of broad-spectrum antibiotics with high central nervous system (CNS) penetration used singly or in combination is warranted for coverage of these gram-positive and gram-negative organisms.

If initial improvement is seen with antibiotic treatment alone, close clinical observation is necessary, with the addition of MRI and CT to permit interval comparison. If there is persistent fever and neurologic deterioration, urgent surgical intervention is warranted. Delaying surgical treatment in the presence of such a complication could lead to progression to a subdural empyema, by way of emissary veins through the bone, or to intraparenchymal abscess formation; both have much higher morbidity and mortality.[58,66] Newer approaches in management involve the use of burr holes in drainage of the epidural abscess.[67] In addition, to avoid the morbidity associated with a craniotomy, this approach permits identification of the pathogen involved, allowing for a more targeted antibiotic treatment. If there is lack of resolution, a craniotomy should be performed. In cases in which an epidural abscess is contiguous with mastoiditis, a mastoidectomy approach with decompression of the abscess may avoid the need for neurosurgical intervention.

Subdural Empyema

A subdural empyema is a collection of purulent fluid between the dura mater and arachnoid mater, which has a high mortality rate.[68] This complication has a tendency to spread rapidly through the subdural space, behaving like an expanding lesion limited by specific boundaries (e.g., falx cerebri, tentorium cerebelli, base of the brain, foramen magnum).

Presenting signs and symptoms may include fever, headache, mental status changes, meningismus, and papilledema in advanced cases. CT or MRI is indicated for localization of the abscess. Management should always include neurosurgical evacuation of the abscess collection. Adjunctive medical treatment should include intravenous antibiotics with appropriate CNS penetration, steroids to reduce cerebral edema, and anticonvulsants to prevent seizures. If there is concurrent pyogenic infection of the mastoid or middle ear, a mastoidectomy or ventilation tube placement should be performed after initial neurosurgical stabilization. Prolonging the diagnosis and treatment may lead to formation of an intraparenchymal, commonly cerebellar abscess, which may precipitate central respiratory insufficiency.[69]

Intraparenchymal Brain Abscess

Otogenic brain (cerebral) abscess is the second most common intracranial complication of OM; 25% of all brain abscesses in children are otogenic. Such complications carry a 47.2% mortality rate and a 95% risk of developing epilepsy.[70]

It may result from direct extension through the mastoid bone or internal auditory canal or by retrograde thrombophlebitis through preformed vascular channels.[45] The history is usually remarkable for a recent history of AOM, presence of a low-grade fever, alteration of mental status, focal neurologic signs, seizures, and papilledema in advanced cases. Clinically, these CNS changes may range from indolent to fulminant, thereby making diagnosis difficult. A child presenting with a cerebellar abscess may have nystagmus, ataxia, vomiting, and dysmetria. A temporal lobe abscess may present with headache, ipsilateral aphasia (if the abscess is in the dominant hemisphere), and visual field defects. A sudden worsening of a persisting headache, coupled with new clinical signs of meningismus, may be associated with rupture of a temporal lobe abscess into the lateral ventricle, leading to meningitis.

As with any other intracranial complication of otitis media, a high index of suspicion is needed. Management is similar to that of subdural empyema and should begin with neurosurgical consultation for immediate surgical management. Surgical treatment of the otitis or mastoiditis is ultimately required to eliminate the source of infection, but should be reserved for when the child is neurologically stable.

Sigmoid Sinus Thrombophlebitis

Infections involving the middle ear and mastoid may result in a septic thrombus of the sigmoid sinus. Although the exact mechanism is unknown, the likely cause is by direct extension and thrombosis or by cerebral infarction, leading to tissue congestion and obstruction, and secondarily propagating to thrombosis. In patients with otologic disease, the typical clinical history includes headache, otalgia, and photophobia. The classic presence of a "picket fence" fever has not generally been seen since the advent of antibiotics. Diplopia may be present secondary to abducens neuropathy and should increase the clinical suspicion for this diagnosis. In the 1840s Wilhelm Griesinger, a German psychiatrist and anatomic pathologist, coined the term *Griesinger's sign*, which is swelling and tenderness over the mastoid process caused by thrombosis of the transverse sinus. Sigmoid sinus thrombosis can occur in the presence or absence of other intracranial or intratemporal complications of otitis media. The mortality rate has been reported to range from 13% to 48%.[71-73]

Contrast-enhanced CT scan may demonstrate the absence of flow through the affected sigmoid sinus (Fig. 7-3A). The high sensitivity of MRI, coupled with MR venography, yields a more definitive diagnosis of venous sinus thrombosis (see Fig. 7-3B and C).[74,75] In the young child, transcranial Doppler ultrasonography is an alternative to CT and MRI and is valuable in the evaluation of cerebral venous thrombosis.[76] This noninvasive test is particularly useful in evaluating interval changes when assessing flow and recanalization of the involved sigmoid sinus.

Since the introduction of antibiotics, conservative medical treatment has evolved as the mainstay in the management of sigmoid sinus thrombophlebitis. Initiation of broad-spectrum antibiotics is the most important first step. In the presence of clinical and radiologic indications of underlying middle ear and mastoid involvement, a mastoidectomy is warranted, taking care to decompress the bone overlying the sigmoid sinus. Management of the thrombosis within the sinus by surgical manipulation or anticoagulation is controversial. In general, there is resolution of the thrombosis, with complete recanalization of the sigmoid sinus, within 4 to 6 weeks.[77] Thus, a more conservative approach may minimize the risk of surgical manipulation of the sigmoid sinus and anticoagulation.[78-80]

Otitic Hydrocephalus

In 1931, Sir Charles Putnam Symonds, a British neurologist, described a condition with increased intracranial pressure associated with papilledema, severe headache, and paralysis of the sixth cranial nerve. He found that it occurred in children with a recent history of AOM and coined the term *otitic hydrocephalus*.[81] The pathophysiology is thought to involve a nonobstructing mural thrombus of the transverse sinus, causing retrograde extension and involvement of the sagittal sinus. This is believed to result in obstruction of cerebrospinal fluid absorption by the arachnoid villi.

The usual presenting signs and symptoms are vomiting, giddiness, blurring of vision, diplopia, and transient convulsions. Diagnosis is established by lumbar puncture, after CT scanning to exclude a mass effect, revealing a high cerebrospinal fluid (CSF) opening pressure (higher than 200 mm H_2O) and normal cytology to rule out meningitis.[82] MRI is useful in the diagnostic workup, because it demonstrates the presence and location of a thrombus in the dural sinuses.[83] Management should include measures to decrease the intracranial CSF pressure, such as by the use of diuretics, steroids, or repeated lumbar puncture with drainage. Treatment of the intratemporal infection should involve intravenous antibiotics and specific management of coexisting complications.

Bacterial Meningitis

Otogenic bacterial meningitis is the most common intracranial complication of AOM (accounting for 46% of complications in one series) and is the leading cause of deafness in children.[84] Hematogenous dissemination from AOM is thought to be the most likely cause of this complication.[85,86] Additionally, congenital or acquired defects involving the temporal bone, round window, cochlear aqueduct, and modiolus may predispose affected children to a higher risk of developing meningitis.

The classic symptoms of meningitis in children include fever, altered mental status or change in the

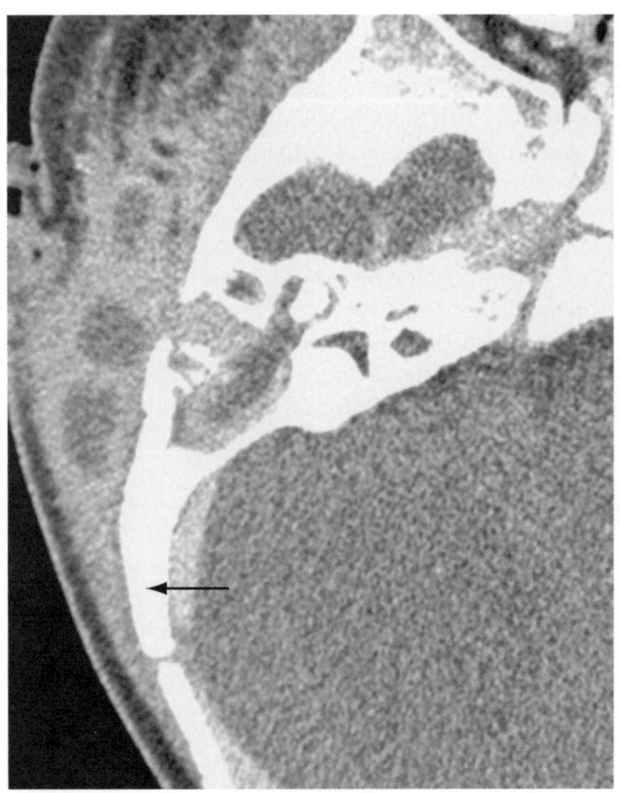

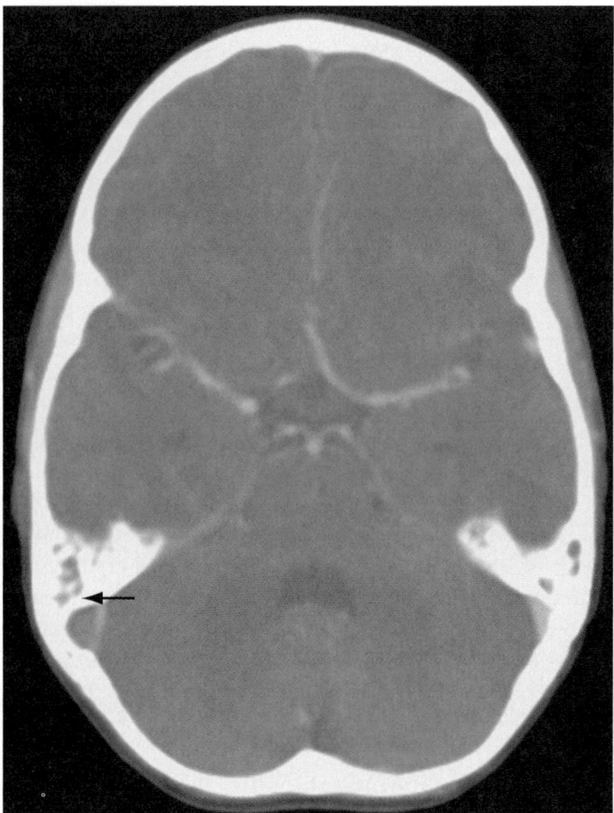

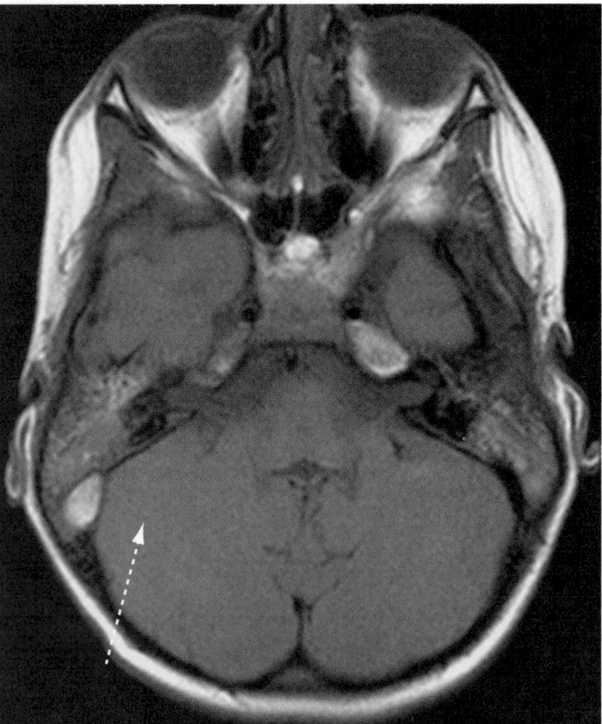

Figure 7-3 **A,** Contrast-enhanced axial CT scan. **B,** Axial T1-weighted MRI scan. **C,** Magnetic resonance venogram (MRV) demonstrating a right sigmoid sinus thrombosis. Note the absence of contrast through the right sigmoid *(arrow)* on the CT scan (**A**). MRI confirms the presence of a thrombus *(**B**, arrow)* and MRV delineates the absence of flow through the right sinus *(**C**, dashed arrow)*.

level of alertness, and poor oral intake. On clinical examination, Kernig's or Brudzinski's sign, papilledema, or isolated cranial neuropathies may be present. Infants may present with bulging fontanelles, hypotonia, or paradoxical irritability. Diagnosis is established by lumbar puncture, which allows measurement of the intrathecal pressure and complete analysis for cell count, glucose, protein, and presence of bacteria. This should be performed after CT or MRI to exclude the presence of other intracranial complications or a tumor, creating mass effect.

In the presence of meningitis, a careful otologic examination is required to assess for the presence of purulent middle ear fluid. If the findings are consistent with suppurative otitis media, a myringotomy with placement of ventilation tubes is indicated as an initial treatment measure in addition to broad-spectrum antibiotics. In the presence of mastoiditis, cortical mastoidectomy should be performed once the patient's neurologic condition has improved.

MAJOR POINTS

AOM is a common condition that is usually managed in the primary care setting with antimicrobial therapy against *S. pneumoniae*, *H. influenzae*, and *M. catarrhalis*, the most common causative organisms.

When properly managed, mortality from the complications of AOM should approach zero.

The complications from SOM can be intratemporal or intracranial.

Imaging studies (CT or MRI) should be performed whenever a complication is suspected

Management of most intratemporal or intracranial complications often requires a combination of intravenous antibiotics and surgery.

REFERENCES

1. American Academy of Pediatrics Subcommittee on Management of Acute Otitis Media: Diagnosis and management of acute otitis media. Pediatrics 2004;113:1451-1465.
2. Kafka MM: Mortality of mastoiditis and cerebral complications with review of 3225 cases of mastoiditis with complications. Laryngoscope 1935;45:790-822.
3. Neely J: Complications of temporal bone infections. In Cummings C (ed): Otolaryngology—Head and Neck Surgery, 2nd ed, vol 4. St. Louis, Mosby, 1993, pp 2840-2864.
4. Pichichero ME, Casey JR: Acute otitis media: Making sense of recent guidelines on antimicrobial treatment. J Fam Pract 2005;54:313-322.
5. Vazquez E, Castellote A, Piqueras J, et al: Imaging of complications of acute mastoiditis in children. Radiographics 2003;23:359-372.
6. Maroldi R, Farina D, Palvarini L, et al: Computed tomography and magnetic resonance imaging of pathologic conditions of the middle ear. Eur J Radiol 2001;40:78-93.
7. Roark R, Petrofski J, Berson E, Berman S: Practice variations among pediatricians and family physicians in the management of otitis media. Arch Pediatr Adolesc Med 1995;149:839-844.
8. Lyon JL, Ashton A, Turner B, Magill M: Variation in the diagnosis of upper respiratory tract infections and otitis media in an urgent medical care practice. Arch Fam Med 1998;7:249-254.
9. Haddad J Jr: Treatment of acute otitis media and its complications. Otolaryngol Clin North Am 1994;27:431-441.
10. Spiegel JH, Lustig LR, Lee KC, et al: Contemporary presentation and management of a spectrum of mastoid abscesses. Laryngoscope 1998;108:822-828.
11. Prellner K, Rydell R: Acute mastoiditis. Influence of antibiotic treatment on the bacterial spectrum. Acta Otolaryngol (Stockh) 1986;102:52-56.
12. Antonelli PJ, Dhanani N, Giannoni CM, Kubilis PS: Impact of resistant pneumococcus on rates of acute mastoiditis. Otolaryngol Head Neck Surg 1999;121:190-194.
13. Slack CL, Dahn KA, Abzug MJ, Chan KH: Antibiotic-resistant bacteria in pediatric chronic sinusitis. Pediatr Infect Dis J 2001;20:247-250.
14. Brooks I, Gooch WM 3rd, Jenkins SG, et al: Medical management of acute bacterial sinusitis. Recommendations of a clinical advisory committee on pediatric and adult sinusitis. Ann Otol Rhinol Laryngol Suppl 2000;182:2-20.
15. Conrad DA, Jenson HB: Management of acute bacterial rhinosinusitis. Curr Opin Pediatr 2002;14:86-90.
16. Sobol SE SM, Tewfik TL: Acute sinusitis: Medical management. Emedicine Textbook of Otolaryngology and Facial Plastic Surgery. Available at http://www.emedicine.com/ent/topic337.htm
17. Manning S: Medical Management of Infectious and Inflammatory Disease, 3rd ed. St. Louis, Mosby, 1998.
18. Klein JO: Otitis media. Clin Infect Dis 1994;19:823-833.
19. Van Zuijlen DA, Schilder AG, Van Balen FA, Hoes AW: National differences in incidence of acute mastoiditis: Relationship to prescribing patterns of antibiotics for acute otitis media?. Pediatr Infect Dis J 2001;20:140-144.
20. Alford BR, Pratt FE: Intracranial complications from otitis media. Tex Med 1966;62:66-70.
21. Harley EH, Sdralis T, Berkowitz RG: Acute mastoiditis in children: A 12-year retrospective study. Otolaryngol Head Neck Surg 1997;116:26-30.
22. Nadal D, Herrmann P, Baumann A, Fanconi A: Acute mastoiditis: Clinical, microbiological, and therapeutic aspects. Eur J Pediatr 1990;149:560-564.
23. Taylor MF, Berkowitz RG: Indications for mastoidectomy in acute mastoiditis in children. Ann Otol Rhinol Laryngol 2004;113:69-72.
24. Gliklich RE, Eavey RD, Iannuzzi RA, Camacho AE: A contemporary analysis of acute mastoiditis. Arch Otolaryngol Head Neck Surg 1996;122:135-139.

25. Khafif A, Halperin D, Hochman I, et al: Acute mastoiditis: A 10-year review. Am J Otolaryngol 1998;19:170-173.
26. Luntz M, Brodsky A, Nusem S, et al: Acute mastoiditis—the antibiotic era: A multicenter study. Int J Pediatr Otorhinolaryngol 2001;57:1-9.
27. Martin-Hirsch DP, Habashi S, Page R, Hinton AE: Latent mastoiditis: No room for complacency. J Laryngol Otol 1991;105:767-768.
28. Wickham MH, Marven SS, Narula AA: Three "silent" mastoid abscesses. Br J Clin Pract 1990;44:242-243.
29. Liston SL: Ambroise Pare and the king's mastoiditis. Am J Surg 1994;167:440-442.
30. Smouha EE, Levenson MJ, Anand VK, Parisier SC: Modern presentations of Bezold's abscess. Arch Otolaryngol Head Neck Surg 1989;115:1126-1129.
31. Bezold F, Siebenmann F: Lecture XIX: Empyema of the Mastoid Process in Acute Inflammation of the Middle Ear. Chicago, EH Colegrove, 1908.
32. Holt GR, Young WC: Acute coalescent mastoiditis. Otolaryngol Head Neck Surg 1981;89:317-321.
33. Migirov L, Kronenberg J: Bacteriology of mastoid subperiosteal abscess in children. Acta Otolaryngol (Stockh) 2004;124:23-25.
34. Gradenigo G: Über Paralyse des Nervus Abducens Ototischen Urspungs. Arch Ohren-Nasen Kehlkopfheilk 1907;74:249.
35. Gillanders DA: Gradenigo's syndrome revisited. J Otolaryngol 1983;12:169-174.
36. Stamm AC, Pinto JA, Coser PL, Marigo C: Nonspecific necrotizing petrositis: An unusual complication of otitis in children. Laryngoscope 1984;94:1218-1222.
37. Murakami T, Tsubaki J, Tahara Y, Nagashima T: Gradenigo's syndrome: CT and MRI findings. Pediatr Radiol 1996;26:684-685.
38. Burston BJ, Pretorius PM, Ramsden JD: Gradenigo's syndrome: Successful conservative treatment in adult and paediatric patients. J Laryngol Otol 2005;119:325-329.
39. Trimis G, Mostrou G, Lourida A, et al: Petrositis and cerebellar abscess complicating chronic otitis media. J Paediatr Child Health 2003;39:635-636.
40. Schuknecht H: Pathology of the Ear, 2nd ed. Philadelphia, Lea and Febiger, 1993.
41. Ludman H: Complications of Suppurative Otitis Media, 5th ed. London, Butterworths, 1987.
42. Jang CH: A case of tympanogenic labyrinthitis complicated by acute otitis media. Yonsei Med J 2005;46:161-165.
43. Glasscock ME: Aural complications of otitis media. In Glasscock ME, Shambaugh GE (eds): Glasscock and Shambaugh's Surgery of the Ear, 4th ed. Philadelphia, WB Saunders, 1990, pp 276-294.
44. Harker LA, Shelton C: Acute Suppurative Labyrinthitis. In Cummings C (ed) Otolaryngology: Head and Neck Surgery, 5th ed. Philadelphia, Mosby, 2005, pp 3030–3031.
45. Jacobs IN: Regional and intracranial complications of otitis media. In Wetmore R (ed): Pediatric Otolaryngology. New York, Thieme, 2000, pp 305-326.
46. Rappaport JM, Bhatt SM, Burkard RF, et al: Prevention of hearing loss in experimental pneumococcal meningitis by administration of dexamethasone and ketorolac. J Infect Dis 1999;179:264-268.
47. Popovtzer A, Raveh E, Bahar G, et al: Facial palsy associated with acute otitis media. Otolaryngol Head Neck Surg 2005;132:327-329.
48. Hof E: Facial palsy of infectious origin in children. In Fisch U (ed): Facial Nerve Surgery. Birmingham, UK, Aesculapius, 1977, pp 414-418.
49. Todd NW, Heindel NH, PerLee JH: Bony anatomy of the anterior epitympanic space. J Otorhinolaryngol 1994;56: 146-153.
50. Graham M: The pathophysiology of otologic facial paralysis. Presented at the 3rd International Symposium on Facial Nerve Surgery, Amstelveen, The Netherlands, 1977.
51. House JW, Brackmann DE: Facial nerve grading system. Otolaryngol Head Neck Surg 1985;93:146-147.
52. Harker LA, Shelton C: Facial nerve paralysis. In Cummings C (ed): Otolaryngology: Head and Neck Surgery, 5th ed. Philadelphia, Mosby, 2005, pp 3029-3030.
53. Zapalac JS, Billings KR, Schwade ND, Roland PS: Suppurative complications of acute otitis media in the era of antibiotic resistance. Arch Otolaryngol Head Neck Surg 2002;128:660-663.
54. Lee ES, Chae SW, Lim HH, et al: Clinical experiences with acute mastoiditis—1988 through 1998. Ear Nose Throat J 2000;79:884-888.
55. Spratley J, Silveira H, Alvarez I, Pais-Clemente M: Acute mastoiditis in children: Review of the current status. Int J Pediatr Otorhinolaryngol 2000;56:33-40.
56. Tovi F, Leiberman A: Silent mastoiditis and bilateral simultaneous facial palsy. Int J Pediatr Otorhinolaryngol 1983;5:303-307.
57. Gaio E, Marioni G, de Filippis C, et al: Facial nerve paralysis secondary to acute otitis media in infants and children. J Paediatr Child Health 2004;40:483-486.
58. Hlavin ML, Kaminski HJ, Fenstermaker RA, White RJ: Intracranial suppuration: A modern decade of postoperative subdural empyema and epidural abscess. Neurosurgery 1994;34:974-980; discussion, 980-981.
59. Kangsanarak J, Navacharoen N, Fooanant S, Ruckphaopunt K: Intracranial complications of suppurative otitis media: 13 years' experience. Am J Otol 1995;16:104-109.
60. Samuel J, Fernandes CM, Steinberg JL: Intracranial otogenic complications: A persisting problem. Laryngoscope 1986;96:272-278.
61. Bannister G, Williams B, Smith S: Treatment of subdural empyema. J Neurosurg 1981;55:82-88.
62. Hitchcock E, Andreadis A: Subdural empyema: A review of 29 cases. J Neurol Neurosurg Psychiatry 1964;27:422-434.

63. Pathak A, Sharma BS, Mathuriya SN, et al: Controversies in the management of subdural empyema. A study of 41 cases with review of literature. Acta Neurochir (Wien) 1990;102:25-32.

64. Renaudin JW, Frazee J: Subdural empyema—importance of early diagnosis. Neurosurgery. 1980;7:477-479.

65. Saah D, Elidan J, Gomori M: Intracranial complications of otitis media. Ann Otol Rhinol Laryngol 1997;106(Pt 1): 873-874.

66. Bleck T: Epidural Abscess, 5th ed. New York, Churchill Livingstone, 2000.

67. Heran NS, Steinbok P, Cochrane DD: Conservative neurosurgical management of intracranial epidural abscesses in children. Neurosurgery 2003;53:893-897; discussion, 897-898.

68. Smith HP, Hendrick EB: Subdural empyema and epidural abscess in children. J Neurosurg Mar 1983;58:392-397.

69. Polyzoidis KS, Vranos G, Exarchakos G, et al: Subdural empyema and cerebellar abscess due to chronic otitis media. Int J Clin Pract 2004;58:214-217.

70. Bradley PJ, Manning KP, Shaw MD: Brain abscess secondary to otitis media. J Laryngol Otol 1984;98:1185-1191.

71. Ameri A, Bousser MG: Cerebral venous thrombosis. Neurol Clin 1992;10:87-111.

72. Buccino G, Scoditti U, Patteri I, et al: Neurological and cognitive long-term outcome in patients with cerebral venous sinus thrombosis. Acta Neurol Scand May 2003; 107:330-335.

73. Ferro JM, Lopes MG, Rosas MJ, et al: Long-term prognosis of cerebral vein and dural sinus thrombosis. Results of the VENOPORT study. Cerebrovasc Dis 2002;13:272-278.

74. Connor SE, Jarosz JM: Magnetic resonance imaging of cerebral venous sinus thrombosis. Clin Radiol 2002;57:449-461.

75. Gaudino S, Vadala R, Valentini V, et al: Combined diagnostic and therapeutic imaging in the diagnosis of venous sinus thrombosis in postpartum patients. Rays 2003; 28:147-156.

76. Wardlaw JM, Vaughan GT, Steers AJ, Sellar RJ: Transcranial Doppler ultrasound findings in cerebral venous sinus thrombosis. Case report. J Neurosurg 1994;80:332-335.

77. Agarwal A, Lowry P, Isaacson G: Natural history of sigmoid sinus thrombosis. Ann Otol Rhinol Laryngol 2003; 112(2):191-194.

78. deVeber G, Chan A, Monagle P, et al: Anticoagulation therapy in pediatric patients with sinovenous thrombosis: A cohort study. Arch Neurol 1998;55:1533-1537.

79. Garcia RD, Baker AS, Cunningham MJ, Weber AL: Lateral sinus thrombosis associated with otitis media and mastoiditis in children. Pediatr Infect Dis J 1995;14:617-623.

80. Spandow O, Gothefors L, Fagerlund M, et al: Lateral sinus thrombosis after untreated otitis media. A clinical problem—again? Eur Arch Otorhinolaryngol 2000;257:1-5.

81. Symonds C: Otitic hydrocephalus. Brain 1931;54:55-71.

82. Sennaroglu L, Kaya S, Gursel B, Saatci I: Role of MRI in the diagnosis of otitic hydrocephalus. Am J Otol 1996;17: 784-786.

83. Clemis JD, Jerva MJ: Hydrocephalus following translabyrinthine surgery. J Otolaryngol Aug 1976;5(4): 303-309.

84. Migirov L, Duvdevani S, Kronenberg J: Otogenic intracranial complications: A review of 28 cases. Acta Otolaryngol 2005;125:819-822.

85. Gower D, McGuirt WF: Intracranial complications of acute and chronic infectious ear disease: A problem still with us. Laryngoscope 1983;93:1028-1033.

86. Singh B, Maharaj TJ: Radical mastoidectomy: Its place in otitic intracranial complications. J Laryngol Otol 1993;107:1113-1118.

87. Ruuskanen O, Heikkinen T: Otitis media: Etiology and diagnosis. Pediatr Infect Dis J 1994;13(Suppl 1):S23-S26.

88. Dhooge IJ, Vandenbussche T, Lemmerling M: Value of computed tomography of the temporal bone in acute otomastoiditis. Rev Laryngol Otol Rhinol 1998;119:91-94.

89. Shiao AS, Guo YC, Hsieh ST, Tsai TL: Bacteriology of medically refractory acute otitis media in children: A 9-year retrospective study. Int J Pediatr Otorhinolaryngol 2004;68: 759-765.

90. Lu CH, Chang WN, Lin YC, et al: Bacterial brain abscess: Microbiological features, epidemiological trends and therapeutic outcomes. QJM 2002;95:501-509.

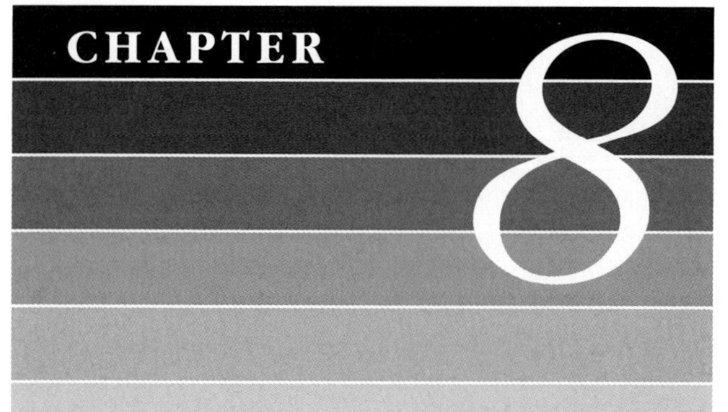

Management of Acute Sinusitis and Its Complications

STEVEN E. SOBOL, MD

DEFINITIONS AND EPIDEMIOLOGY OF ACUTE SINUSITIS

Sinusitis is an inflammatory condition of the paranasal sinuses, usually resulting from bacterial or viral infectious agents. Although there is currently no consensus on the precise definition of the various forms of inflammatory sinus disease, acute sinusitis may be defined as a bacterial or viral infection of the sinuses, of less than 4 weeks' duration, which resolves completely with appropriate treatment, resulting in normalization of the sinus mucosa.[1] Recurrent acute sinusitis is diagnosed when there are four or more episodes of infection per year, with complete resolution between episodes. Sinus inflammation persistent beyond 4 weeks' duration is called subacute sinusitis, whereas chronic sinusitis is defined as the persistence of insidious symptomatology beyond 12 weeks, with or without acute exacerbations.[1]

These various forms of sinusitis are highly prevalent in the North American population. Acute bacterial sinusitis is the fifth most common diagnosis prompting antibiotic administration[2] and accounts for 0.4% of ambulatory diagnoses.[3] The economic burden of acute sinusitis in children is $1.77 billion/year.[4] The focus of this chapter is on acute bacterial sinusitis and its complications in children. See Chapter 9 for a detailed discussion of chronic sinusitis.

PATHOGENESIS

Anatomy and Physiology of the Paranasal Sinuses

The paranasal sinuses are a complex system of air-filled bony cavities, which extend from the skull base down to the alveolar and zygomatic processes (Fig. 8-1). They are composed of four groups of sinuses, being named for the bone in which they are found. The maxillary and ethmoid sinuses are usually present radiologically at birth and continue to develop until early adulthood, whereas the sphenoid sinus usually becomes apparent at about 3 to 7 years of life and the frontal sinus by 6 to 8 years.[5,6] The sinuses share a number of common borders with the orbit, as well as the anterior and middle cranial fossae. These anatomic relationships are important in terms of the pathophysiology of the various pyogenic complications that can arise from acute sinusitis.

The focal point of sinus drainage is through the ostiomeatal complex, located in the middle meatus. The maxillary, frontal, and anterior ethmoid ostia all drain into this anatomic structure.[5] The posterior ethmoids empty into the superior meatus and the sphenoid sinuses into the sphenoethmoidal recess. The paranasal sinuses are lined

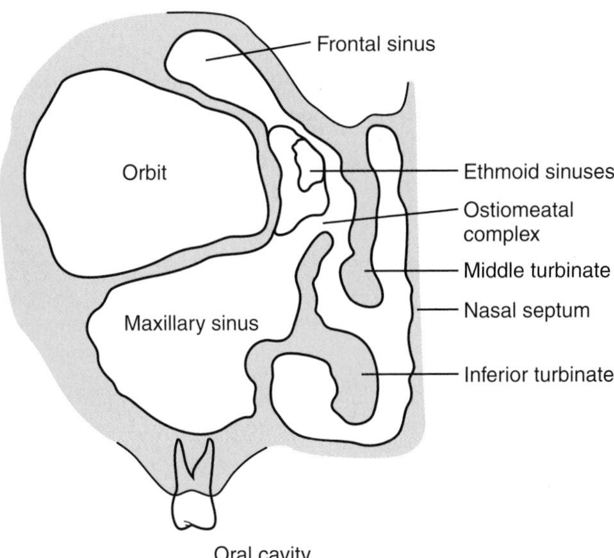

Figure 8-1. Schematic drawing of the paranasal sinus anatomy. The frontal sinus should be absent in a young child. The sphenoid sinus is not shown.

with pseudostratified, ciliated, columnar epithelium that is continuous via their ostia with the lining of the nasal cavity. Cilia are concentrated near and beat in the direction of the natural sinus ostia. Inflammation of the mucosa in the region of the ostia can cause obstruction and ciliary dysfunction, resulting in stasis and accumulation of purulent secretions, with the development of acute sinusitis.

The arterial supply of the paranasal sinuses is from branches of the internal and external carotid arteries, whereas the venous and lymphatic drainage are through the sinus ostia into the venous drainage of the nasal cavity.[7] In addition, venous drainage occurs through valveless vessels corresponding to the arterial supply.[7] Infection of the sinuses may result in retrograde thrombophlebitis of these vessels, resulting in pyogenic intracranial and orbital complications.

The exact function of the paranasal sinuses is not well understood. The possible roles of the sinuses may be to reduce the weight of the skull, act as a pressure dampener, provide humidification and warming of inspired air, serve to cushion trauma, and act to insulate the brain from heat. Other postulated roles have included providing resonance of sound, giving mechanical rigidity to the face, or increasing the olfactory surface area.[8]

Risk Factors

Acute bacterial sinusitis occurs when there is an interruption of the physiologic clearance mechanism of the paranasal sinus system, resulting in obstruction of the ostia, ciliary dysfunction, stasis of secretions, and reduction in the partial pressure of oxygen within the affected sinus cavity.[6] This provides an ideal environment for bacterial growth and the resulting purulent infection that occurs within the normally sterile sinus cavity.

Any condition that causes a blockage of the paranasal sinus ostia can result in acute bacterial sinusitis (Box 8-1). The most common predisposing condition in children is a viral upper respiratory infection (URI).[9] Viral rhinitis may involve the paranasal sinus mucosa in most URIs, resulting in the characteristic symptomatology associated with this self-limiting condition. Although viral URIs are common in young children, only 5% to 10% of cases will have bacterial superinfection requiring antimicrobial treatment.[10] Children in daycare tend to develop more frequent and severe URIs, which may be secondary to bacterial superinfection.[5,11] Other less common factors that can predispose children to obstruction-induced bacterial sinusitis include allergic sinonasal disease, foreign bodies, polyps, tumors, and anatomic variations, such as nasal septal deviation.[12]

Systemic causes of sinus disease in children include cystic fibrosis[13,14] and ciliary motility disorders (e.g., Kartagener's syndrome),[15] which result in decreased mucociliary clearance. Patients with deficiencies in their humoral immune system (agammaglobulinemia, combined variable, IgG, IgA deficiencies) are also predisposed

Box 8-1 Risk Factors Contributing to Acute Sinusitis in Children

OBSTRUCTIVE FACTORS

Viral upper respiratory tract infection
Allergic rhinitis
Nasal foreign body
Anatomic variations (e.g., septal deviation, concha bullosa)
Nasal polyps
Tumors
Nasogastric tube
Nasotracheal tube
Orotracheal tube

NONOBSTRUCTIVE FACTORS

Dental infection
Dental manipulation
Facial trauma
Bacterial inoculation from swimming

PATIENT FACTORS

Immune deficiency
Cystic fibrosis
Ciliary dysmotility

to developing sinusitis.[16,17] Less than 10% of cases of acute sinusitis result from direct inoculation of the sinus with a large amount of bacteria.[18,19] Dental abscesses or procedures, which result in communication between the oral cavity and sinus, can produce sinusitis by this mechanism, as can facial trauma or large inoculations from swimming.[6]

Acute sinusitis in the intensive care population is a distinct entity, occurring in 18% to 32% of patients with prolonged periods of intubation, and is usually diagnosed during the evaluation of unexplained fever.[20] Obstructive causes are usually evident and can include prolonged nasogastric or nasotracheal intubation.[21] Moreover, patients in an intensive care setting are generally debilitated, predisposing them to septic complications, including sinusitis.

Microbiology

Bacterial pathogens that cause acute sinusitis (Box 8-2) are most commonly part of the normal nasal flora, only becoming pathogenic under conditions that bring them into contact with the sinus mucosa (e.g., sneezing, dental procedure) and optimize their growth. The most common bacterial pathogens in acute sinusitis are similar in children and adults[22] and include *Streptococcus pneumoniae* (30% to 40%), *Haemophilus influenzae* (20% to 30%), and *Moraxella catarrhalis* (12% to 20%).[5,23] *Staphylococcus aureus* and *Streptococcus pyogenes* are uncommonly isolated from the sinuses, although group A streptococcal infections may occur concurrently with sinusitis in 15% to 20% of children.[24] Of patients with acute sinusitis, 66% will grow at least one pathogenic bacterial species on sinus aspirates,[25] and 26% to 30% of cases have multiple predominant bacterial species.[22]

Anaerobic organisms are not usually found (less than 10%) in the aspirates of infected sinuses, despite the ample environment available for their growth.[26] The exception is sinusitis resulting from a dental source or in patients with chronic sinus disease, in whom anaerobic organisms are commonly isolated.

Gram-negative organisms including *Pseudomonas aeruginosa* (15.9%), *Escherichia coli* (7.6%), *Proteus mirabilis* (7.2%), *Klebsiella pneumoniae*, and *Enterobacter* species. predominate in nosocomial sinusitis, accounting for 60% of cases. Polymicrobial invasion is seen in 25% to 100% of cultures. The other pathogenic organisms found in nosocomial patients include gram-positive organisms (31%) and fungi (8.5%).[20]

Box 8-2 Microbiology of Acute Sinusitis

MOST COMMON PATHOGENS

Streptococcus pneumoniae
Haemophilus influenzae
Moraxella catarrhalis

LESS COMMON PATHOGENS

Streptococcus pyogenes
Staphylococcus aureus
Gram-negative enteric bacteria
Anaerobes
Fungi

DIAGNOSIS

History

Acute bacterial sinusitis is difficult to diagnose in children because of the similar clinical presentation to common viral URIs. Given this overlap, there is a lack of consensus as to the precise clinical definition of sinusitis in children.[27] No specific clinical symptom or sign is sensitive or specific for acute sinusitis, and the overall clinical impression should be used to guide management. Despite performing an accurate history and physical examination, treatment of presumed acute sinusitis is usually initiated on empirical grounds, leading to overtreatment of common viral colds in 18% to 60% of cases.[28,29] The common presenting complaints in children of fever, nasal discharge, cough, mouth breathing, snoring, bad breath, hyponasal speech, and nasal obstruction are also present in simple URIs and cannot be used solely to make a diagnosis of bacterial sinusitis. A history of purulent secretions, facial pain or pressure over the affected sinus, dental pain, or poor response to nasal decongestants suggests a diagnosis of acute sinusitis in adults but often is difficult to elicit from the young child. Perhaps the most suggestive feature in the history is the duration of symptomatology. The average child has six to eight common colds per year, each lasting on average 7 to 9 days.[30-32] The persistence of symptoms beyond 7 to 10 days is unusual for these patients and strongly suggests a diagnosis of acute bacterial sinusitis. The worsening of symptoms following initial clinical improvement at the end of a viral URI is also predictive of acute sinusitis. As noted earlier, acute sinusitis in the intensive care patient should be suspected in the presence of sepsis of unknown origin.

The complete history in a patient with suspected acute sinusitis should include a review of potential predisposing causes, including the presence of an underlying immunologic dysfunction, allergies, nasal foreign bodies, or recent dental procedure. The history should also include an evaluation for potential complications, including eye pain, diplopia, vision loss, changes in mental status, and focal neurologic complaints.

Box 8-3 Symptoms and Signs of Acute Sinusitis

SYMPTOMS

Duration > 7-10 days
Nasal congestion, obstruction
Facial pain, pressure
Periorbital pain, swelling
Dental pain
Mouth breathing, snoring
Hyponasal speech
Halitosis
Cough
Poor response to nasal decongestants
Fever

SIGNS

Fever
Purulent rhinorrhea
Edema, erythema of nasal mucosa
Tenderness over involved sinus
Periorbital edema

Physical Examination

A complete head and neck physical examination should always be performed in children with suspected acute sinusitis (Box 8-3). Anterior rhinoscopic examination, using an otoscope or nasal speculum, with and without a topical decongestant, is important to assess the status of the nasal mucosa, presence and color of nasal discharge, presence of a foreign body, or anatomic variation. Sinus transillumination and palpation are of little predictive value in children.[12,33] A basic evaluation of ocular and neurologic function is also necessary to rule out potential complications. Adenoid hypertrophy, a common cause of nasal obstruction in young children, should be excluded with a lateral neck radiograph.

Nasal endoscopic examination may reveal the origin of the purulent discharge from the middle meatus and may provide information about the nature of ostiomeatal obstruction. The use of endoscopy may also aid in the diagnosis of acute sinusitis by allowing purulent secretions to be obtained carefully from the sinus ostia for culture.

Radiologic Imaging

As noted, the diagnosis of acute sinusitis in children is often difficult to make on clinical grounds because of the similarity in its clinical presentation to a viral URI. The diagnosis of acute sinusitis is usually based on the constellation of clinical findings and may be overdiagnosed because of the poor predictive value of the history and physical examination. In a child who presents with prolonged URI symptoms (for longer than 7 to 10 days), purulent nasal discharge, and/or significant facial or dental pain, a diagnosis suggestive of acute sinusitis may be made on clinical grounds. Imaging studies are not necessary when the probability of sinusitis is high or low, but may be useful when the diagnosis is in doubt, based on a thorough history and physical examination.[34] Plain sinus radiographs may demonstrate mucosal thickening, air-fluid levels, and sinus opacification. Plain films are limited in their ability to evaluate the ethmoid and sphenoid sinuses and differentiate between inflammatory and neoplastic conditions. Moreover, because children may have asymmetrical sinus development, one should be careful when interpreting sinus radiographs.[6]

Computed tomography (CT) has poor specificity in the evaluation of acute sinusitis, demonstrating sinus air-fluid levels in 87% of individuals with simple upper respiratory tract infections and in 40% of asymptomatic individuals.[19] CT is the modality of choice, however, in specific circumstances, such as in the evaluation of the intensive care patient, when complications are suspected, or in the preoperative evaluation of surgical candidates.[20,35] Moreover, CT is superior to plain films in its ability to evaluate the ethmoid and sphenoid sinuses and to differentiate between inflammatory and neoplastic conditions. Magnetic resonance imaging (MRI) is excellent for evaluating soft tissue disease within the sinuses, but is unnecessary for the evaluation of acute sinusitis.

Role of Sinus Cultures

The gold standard for confirming the diagnosis of acute bacterial sinusitis is to perform a culture of secretions from the involved sinus.[5] Because the nose is colonized with many nonpathogenic species of bacteria, care must be taken when evaluating culture results. A specific organism is considered pathogenic when more than 10^4 colony-forming units/mm^2 of the species is grown on culture.[36] Cultures are not routinely tested in the evaluation of acute sinusitis but should be performed in the intensive care or immunocompromised patient, in children not responding to appropriate medical management, or in patients with complications of sinusitis.[6] Cultures may be obtained in the office using endoscopically directed swabs of the middle meatus or under anesthesia, using various puncture techniques.[6,37,38]

MANAGEMENT

Medical Therapy

Children with acute sinusitis are usually managed in the primary care setting, with the goals of treatment being to eradicate the infection, prevent complications, and

Box 8-4 Reasons for Otolaryngology Consultation

Continued deterioration with appropriate antibiotic therapy
Recurrent episodes of sinusitis
Persistence of symptoms after two courses of antibiotic therapy
Comorbid immunodeficiency
Nosocomial infection
Complications of sinusitis

provide symptomatic relief. Otolaryngologic consultation is not necessary in most cases but should be obtained for continued worsening of symptoms in spite of appropriate antibiotic therapy, recurrent episodes of sinusitis, persistence of symptoms after two courses of antibiotic therapy, comorbid immunodeficiency, nosocomial infection, or complications of sinusitis (Box 8-4). Ophthalmologic or neurosurgical consultation should be obtained when orbital or intracranial complications develop. The goals of management of acute sinusitis include providing adequate drainage of secretions and selecting appropriate systemic treatment of the likely bacterial pathogens.[6]

Ostiomeatal obstruction is the predisposing condition in the pathogenesis of most patients with acute sinusitis. Restoring patency of the affected sinus ostium is of paramount importance when managing these patients and can be achieved by medical and surgical means. α-Adrenergic topical vasoconstrictors, such as phenylephrine hydrochloride or oxymetazoline hydrochloride, provide an excellent local vasoconstrictor effect, but should only be used for 3 to 5 days because of the risk of rebound congestion, vasodilation, and rhinitis medicamentosa when used for longer periods.[5] Oral decongestant therapy has not been found to be more effective than placebo in children with acute sinusitis but may be used for symptomatic relief of common cold symptoms.[9,39]

Other medical agents commonly used in patients with chronic sinusitis are not usually recommended for children with acute infection. These include mucolytic agents such as guaifenesin and saline lavage, which have the theoretical benefit of thinning mucous secretions and improving drainage.[9] Intranasal steroids are the cornerstone of treatment for patients with chronic sinus disease, acting to decrease sinus mucosal inflammation over an extended period. These agents have not been conclusively shown to be of benefit in cases of acute sinusitis.[5] Antihistamines are beneficial for reducing ostiomeatal obstruction in allergic patients with acute sinusitis but are not routinely recommended, because they may complicate drainage by thickening and pooling sinonasal secretions.[5] Another nonsurgical method of improving sinus drainage, such as removal of nasogastric or nasotracheal tubes, should be considered when feasible in the intensive care population.

Antimicrobial Therapy

As mentioned previously, the diagnosis of acute sinusitis is often difficult to make in children. During the winter months, 40% of all pediatrician visits by children aged 1 to 5 years are for cold symptoms.[40] Because only 5% to 10% of URIs are complicated by purulent sinusitis,[10] the decision to use antibiotics should be made judiciously to prevent unnecessary use and the promotion of bacterial resistance. Although 40% of patients with acute sinusitis will recover spontaneously without treatment,[9] it is important to provide adequate systemic antibiotic therapy to prevent potential complications, which can have devastating consequences. Moreover, effective antibiotic therapy often produces a more rapid resolution of symptoms and prevents progression to chronic sinusitis.[5,41]

Antibiotic choice should provide adequate treatment of the likely bacterial pathogens (e.g., *S. pneumoniae, H. influenzae, M. catarrhalis*), and the physician should be aware of the probability of bacterial resistance within the community (see Table 7-4). Approximately 44% of *H. influenzae* and almost all *M. catarrhalis* strains have β-lactamase–mediated resistance to penicillin-based antimicrobials in children.[42] As many as 64% of *S. pneumoniae* strains are penicillin-resistant because of altered penicillin-binding proteins.[42] Multiple drug-resistant *S. pneumoniae* strains are also found in substantial numbers of children in daycare settings. Antibiotic choice in children should also be guided by factors that will improve compliance, such as single- or twice-daily dosing and taste.

First-line therapy at most centers is usually amoxicillin or a macrolide antibiotic in penicillin-allergic patients, given their low cost, ease of administration, and low toxicity. Amoxicillin should be given at double the usual dose (80 to 90 mg/kg/day), especially in areas with known *S. pneumoniae* resistance.[5,43] The duration of treatment should be 10 to 14 days, with close follow-up if symptoms continue to persist beyond 48 to 72 hours following the initiation of antibiotic therapy.

Second-line antibiotics include amoxicillin clavulanate, second- or third-generation cephalosporins (cefprozil, cefdinir), and macrolides (azithromycin, clarithromycin). These should be considered in patients who live in communities with a high incidence of resistant organisms, those who fail to respond within 48 to 72 hours of commencement of first-line therapy, or those with persistence of symptoms beyond 10 to 14 days.[12]

Special consideration to the choice of antibiotics needs to be given in certain circumstances. Intensive care patients with acute sinusitis require adequate intravenous coverage for gram-negative organisms. Aminoglycoside antibiotics are usually the drug of choice for the treatment of such patients because of their excellent gram-negative coverage and sinus penetration.[9] In patients with dental causes of sinusitis or those with foul-smelling discharge, anaerobic coverage is necessary, using clindamycin or amoxicillin with metronidazole. As noted earlier, the selection of antibiotic may need to be based on the culture results of sinus secretions obtained in these special circumstances.

Antibiotic choice for patients presenting with complications of acute sinusitis should be broad spectrum and given intravenously. Third-generation cephalosporins (cefotaxime, ceftriaxone) in combination with vancomycin provide adequate intracranial penetration, making them a good first-line choice.[9,12]

The reader is referred to the article by Brook and colleagues[5] for a comprehensive review of the different antibiotic choices available for the treatment of bacterial sinusitis.

Surgical Therapy

There are a number of surgical techniques that can be used to obtain sinus drainage when medical means have failed. Both endoscopic and nonendoscopic maxillary sinus puncture and irrigation techniques allow for removal of thick, purulent sinus secretions and provide a method of obtaining specimens for culture and sensitivity testing when empirical therapy has failed or when antibiotic choice is limited.[38] These cultures are particularly important in immunocompromised or intensive care patients, in whom sinusitis can be a prominent source of sepsis. In adults, sinus puncture can usually be achieved using local anesthesia, but in children, a general anesthetic is usually necessary.[6] Moreover, maxillary sinus puncture techniques do not address the other sinuses, which may need to be approached by other techniques (e.g., external ethmoidectomy, frontal sinus trephination). Endoscopic techniques are most commonly used to achieve sinus drainage, offering the advantages of being able to open multiple sinuses or to decompress the orbit in case of complications and allowing the surgeon to open the natural ostia of the involved sinuses This provides a more physiologic means of drainage than that possible with nonendoscopic techniques.

COMPLICATIONS

Complications of acute sinusitis are uncommon in appropriately managed children and can be local, orbital, intracranial, and/or systemic (Box 8-5).

Box 8-5 Complications of Acute Sinusitis

LOCAL

Mucus retention cyst
Mucocele
Osteomyelitis

ORBITAL

Periorbital cellulitis
Orbital cellulitis
Subperiosteal abscess
Orbital abscess
Cavernous sinus thrombosis

INTRACRANIAL

Abscess—subdural, epidural, parenchymal
Meningitis
Dural venous sinus thrombosis
Focal neurologic deficits
Seizures
Sepsis

Local Complications

Blockage of the sinus ostium or individual minor salivary glands in the lining mucosa can result in the development of a mucocele or mucus retention cyst, respectively. In the maxillary sinus, mucoceles or mucous retention cysts are usually asymptomatic. Surgical treatment is not necessary for most lesions, which often regress spontaneously over time, but should be considered if they are symptomatic or develop complications.[6] Frontoethmoidal and sphenoethmoidal mucoceles may be associated with cystic fibrosis and have a high potential for bony erosion; these are usually treated surgically.

Osteomyelitis of the frontal bone with overlying soft tissue swelling, Pott's puffy tumor (Fig. 8-2),[6] can advance to form a fistula to the upper eyelid with sequestration of necrotic bone if untreated. This rare local complication of frontal sinusitis should be managed with a combination of systemic antibiotics, surgical drainage of affected sinuses, and débridement of necrotic bone.

Orbital Complications

In the pediatric population, orbital inflammation is the most common complication of acute sinusitis.[48] Infection is thought to spread into the orbital tissues by direct extension in most cases although thrombophlebitis, or infected thromboemboli may spread to the orbit along valveless venous connections in some cases.[49,50] Orbital complications of sinusitis (OCS) can be divided into those that do not penetrate the periorbital septum (preseptal cellulitis) and those that cause inflammation and abscess formation within the orbit (postseptal).[51] In extreme cases, OCS can lead to cavernous sinus thrombosis, blindness, intracranial complications, and death.[51] A classification of OCS, first

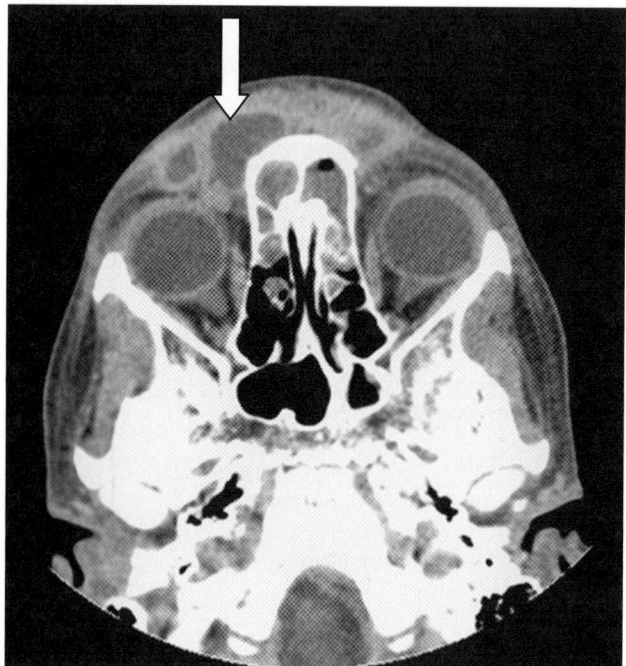

Figure 8-2. Axial contrast-enhanced CT image of the sinuses in a patient with acute sinusitis. Note the soft tissue abscess located superomedially to the orbit on the right side *(arrow)*.

established by Hubert[52] and modified by Chandler (Table 8-1),[49] is commonly used to guide management in children who present to the otolaryngologist.

The physician should be suspicious for OCS in a child with sinusitis who presents with eyelid edema and erythema. The clinical examination should assess for vision loss, proptosis, and ophthalmoplegia. Any deficit in these findings should prompt urgent radiologic evaluation and consultation with both an otolaryngologist and ophthalmologist. In 139 children, Sobol and associates[51] have found that patients with preseptal inflammation (N = 101) uniformly present with eyelid edema and erythema in the absence of ophthalmoplegia and proptosis. Conversely, most patients who present with postseptal complications, including orbital cellulitis (N = 26) and subperiosteal abscess (N = 12), present with ophthalmoplegia and proptosis in addition to erythema and edema.[51]

Computed tomography (CT) (Fig. 8-3) has become the preferred method of radiologic evaluation of OCS in most centers and is recommended when there is any evidence of ophthalmoplegia, proptosis, decreased visual acuity, or lack of response to medical treatment.[50,51] At some institutions, CT is performed in all cases of OCS, including preseptal disease, to exclude an occult postseptal inflammation. CT is excellent for differentiating preseptal from postseptal disease, but is less sensitive at distinguishing between a phlegmon and small abscess. Clary and colleagues[50] have assessed the accuracy of CT and found that it correlates with surgical findings in 84% of cases. Other studies have also reported a good correlation between CT and intraoperative findings,[53] whereas some have reported disparities between the two.[54,55]

Children with OCS should be managed according to the principles outlined earlier for acute sinusitis and should always include intravenous antimicrobial therapy. In cases of preseptal and postseptal cellulites, drainage may be carried out by the medical measures advocated earlier. On the other hand, patients presenting with an intraorbital abscess (Chandler class IV; see Table 8-1) or cavernous sinus thrombosis (Chandler class V) require surgical drainage.[6] Surgery is also advocated if there is inadequate improvement or progression, despite medical therapy, or with loss of visual acuity.[6,51] The role of surgical drainage for a subperiosteal abscess (Chandler class III) is controversial in the literature, with some reports advocating a role for medical management in selected cases.[56-58] Other studies have stressed combined medical and surgical management for all cases of subperiosteal abscess.[59,60]

Surgical drainage can be achieved by open or endoscopic techniques. Endoscopic techniques offer the

Table 8-1 Chandler's Classification of Orbital Complications of Sinusitis

Class	Complication	Clinical Signs
I	Inflammatory edema	Eyelid edema and erythema Normal extraocular movement Normal visual acuity
II	Orbital cellulitis	Diffuse edema of orbital contents without discrete abscess formation
III	Subperiosteal abscess	Collection of purulent exudate beneath periosteum of lamina papyracea Displacement of globe downward and laterally
IV	Orbital abscess	Purulent collection within orbit Proptosis, chemosis, ophthalmoplegia, decreased vision
V	Cavernous sinus thrombosis	Bilateral eye findings Prostration and meningismus

Adapted from Chandler JR, Langenbrunner DJ, Stevens ER: The pathogenesis of orbital complications in acute sinusitis. Laryngoscope 1970;80:1414-1428.

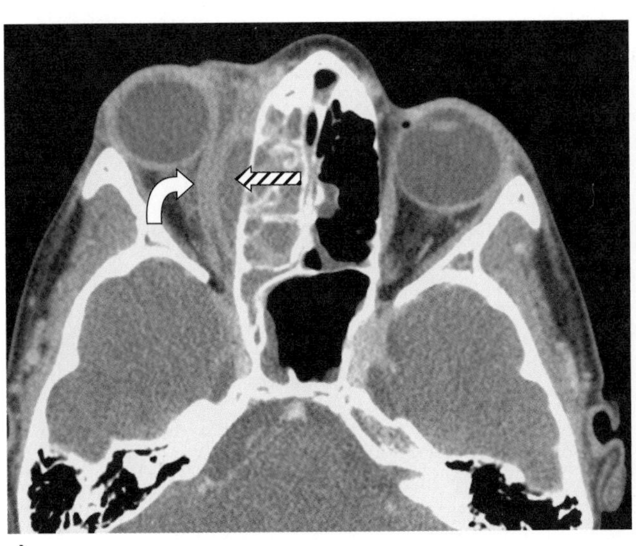

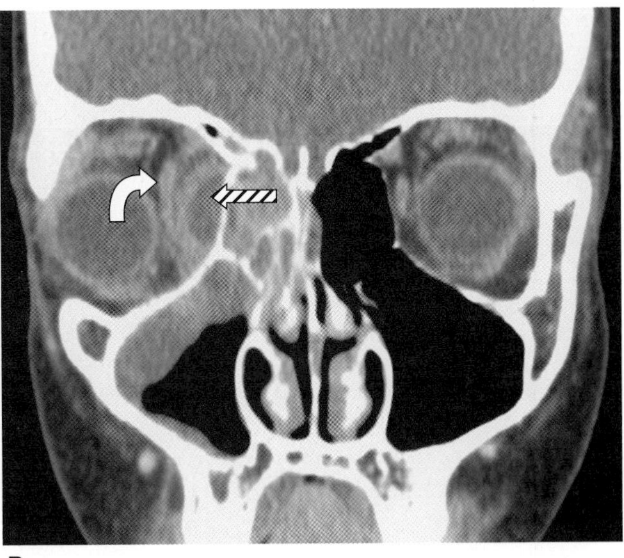

Figure 8-3. Axial (**A**) and coronal (**B**) CT scans of the sinuses and orbits demonstrating a right subperiosteal abscess *(cross-hatched arrows)*. Note the proptosis and bowing of the medial rectus muscle *(solid arrows)* on the right side, which is characteristic of this process.

advantage of accessing multiple sinuses without the need for a facial scar, but may be suboptimal in cases of anterosuperior orbital abscesses. Several studies have found equivalent success rates between open and endoscopic techniques, making endoscopy the initial method of choice for most surgeons.[59,61] When endoscopic techniques fail to drain the abscess sufficiently (e.g., anterior-superior abscess) or are not feasible, external ethmoidectomy is indicated. This technique allows for excellent exposure to both the ethmoid sinuses and the medial orbital contents but requires the use of an external facial (Lynch) incision.

Intracranial Complications

Intracranial complications of acute sinusitis are rare but may occur as a result of direct extension through the posterior frontal sinus wall or through retrograde thrombophlebitis of the ophthalmic veins. Fenton and colleagues[44] found that sinogenic brain abscesses occur most commonly in young males, with *Streptococcus milleri* being the most commonly isolated organism. Jones and associates[45] reported similar findings and also noted that the frontal sinus is the most common source of infection. Intracranial complications of sinusitis include epidural, subdural, or intracerebral abscesses, dural venous sinus thrombosis, and bacterial meningitis. The diagnosis requires a high index of suspicion, because the symptoms and signs may be subtle. Patients may present with unremitting fever, headaches, neck pain and stiffness, change in sensorium, focal neurologic deficits, seizures, or death.[6,46] A CT scan with contrast is indicated as a screening tool when an intracranial complication is suspected. I and my colleagues have found that CT may underestimate the extent of an abscess and fail to differentiate cerebritis from normal brain parenchyma; MRI scans should be obtained on all patients who have a positive screening CT scan (Figs. 8-4 and 8-5).

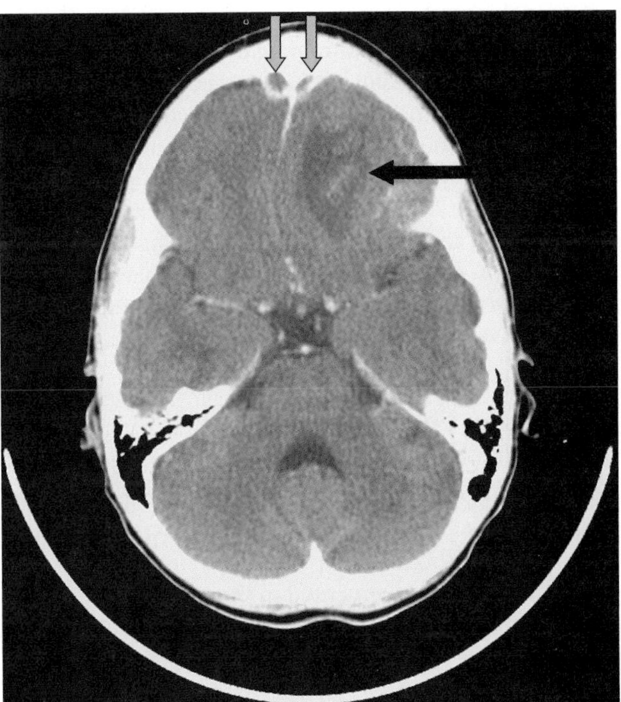

Figure 8-4. Axial contrast-enhanced CT scan of the brain in a patient with acute sinusitis. Note the bilateral epidural abscesses *(gray arrows)* and intraparenchymal cerebritis *(black arrow)* located in the anterior cranial fossa.

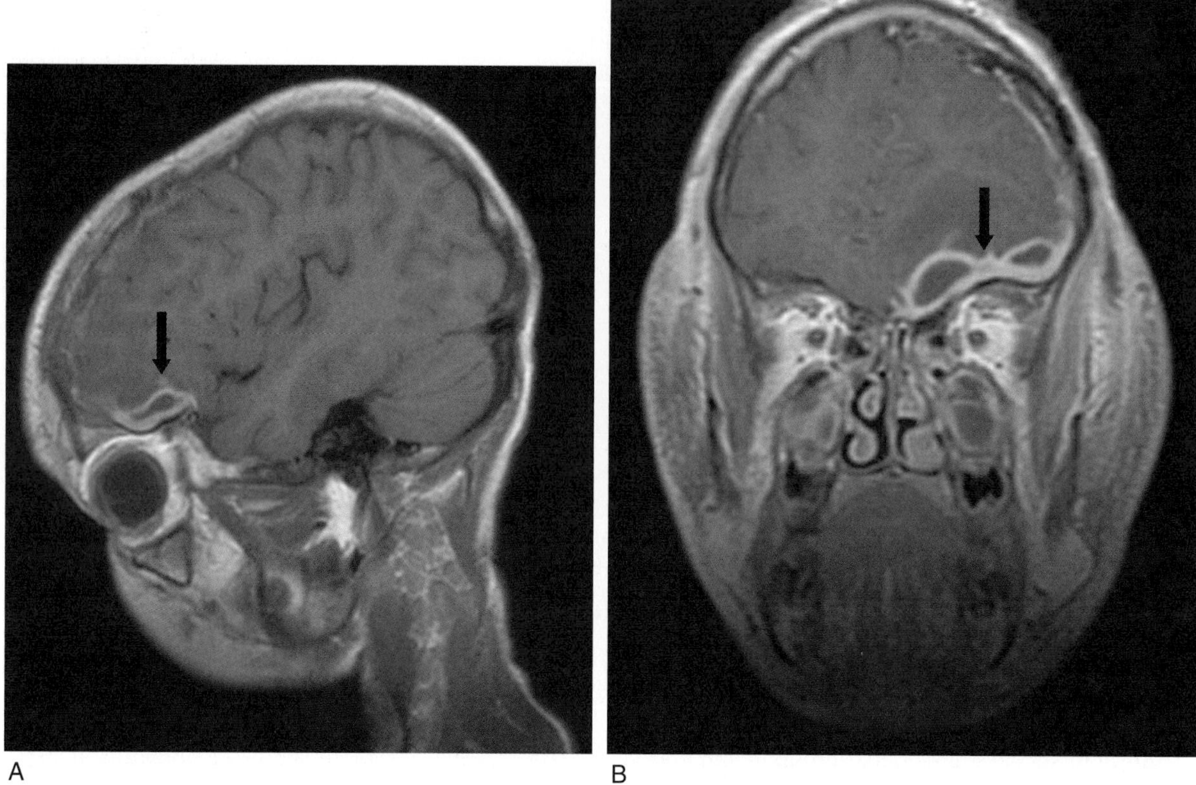

Figure 8-5. Sagittal (**A**) and coronal (**B**) gadolinium-enhanced MR images of the same patient as in Figure 8-4, demonstrating subdural abscesses adjacent to the undersurface of the left frontal lobe *(arrows)*.

The management of intracranial complications should include broad-spectrum antibiotics and surgical drainage of the affected sinus(es), with aggressive neurosurgical treatment of the intracranial component. We obtain postoperative MRI scans on patients prior to discharge to confirm the absence of subclinical intracranial abscess recollection. Gianonni and co-workers have reviewed 12 cases of sinogenic intracranial complications and found a 100% survival rate, although three patients had significant neurologic sequelae.[47]

Systemic Complications

Acute sinusitis can result in sepsis and multisystem organ failure, usually in the intensive care population, by seeding of the blood and various organ systems. Reports of bacteremia, thoracic empyema, and nosocomial pneumonia have been documented in the literature, and mortality in this group can be as high as 11%.[12]

SUMMARY

Acute sinusitis complicates 1% to 5% of all upper respiratory tract infections in children. The usual pathogens are *Streptococcus pneumoniae, Haemophilus influenzae,* and *Moraxella catarrhalis*. The clinical presentation is similar to that of a viral URI, and making the diagnosis requires a high index of suspicion. Management should always include 10 to 14 days of antimicrobial therapy directed toward the most common pathogens and should incorporate vasoconstrictor sprays to enhance sinus drainage. The potential for serious complications of acute sinusitis in children is real and underscores the need to be vigilant in management of these patients.

MAJOR POINTS

Acute sinusitis may be defined as a bacterial or viral infection of the sinuses of less than 4 weeks' duration. It may complicate 5% to 10% of all upper respiratory tract infections in children.

Differentiation from viral URI on clinical presentation is often difficult. Prolonged URI symptoms (longer than 7 to 10 days), purulent nasal discharge, and/or significant facial or dental pain strongly suggests the diagnosis of acute sinusitis.

MAJOR POINTS—cont'd

Diagnostic imaging is usually not indicated to establish the diagnosis of acute sinusitis and should be reserved for evaluation of the intensive care patient, when complications are suspected, or in the preoperative evaluation of surgical candidates.

Cultures are not routinely obtained in the evaluation of acute sinusitis but should be assayed in the intensive care or immunocompromised patient, children not responding to appropriate medical management, or patients with complications of sinusitis.

The goals of management are to reestablish sinus drainage to treat the usual pathogens—*Streptococcus pneumoniae, Haemophilus influenzae*, and *Moraxella catarrhalis*. Intensive care patients with acute sinusitis require adequate intravenous antibiotic coverage for gram-negative organisms.

Management should initially include systemic antibiotic therapy and topical decongestion of the sinuses. Surgical drainage of the affected sinus is indicated when medical management fails, in selected immunocompromised patients, and in patients in whom complications are present.

Orbital complications are the most common complication in children and must be treated aggressively to prevent possible intracranial spread and loss of vision.

Intracranial complications of sinusitis are rare and require urgent management by the otolaryngologist and neurosurgeon when diagnosed.

REFERENCES

1. Poole MD: A focus on acute sinusitis in adults: Changes in disease management. Am J Med 1999;106:38S-47S.
2. McCaig LF, Hughes JM: Trends in antimicrobial drug prescribing among office-based physicians in the United States. JAMA 1995;273:214-219.
3. Agency for Health Care Policy and Research Evidence Report: Diagnosis and Treatment of Acute Bacterial Rhinosinusitis. Rockville, Md, Agency for Health Care Policy and Research, 1999.
4. Ray NF, Baraniuk JN, Thamer M, et al: Healthcare expeditures for sinusitis in 1996. Contributions of asthma, rhinitis, and other airway disorders. J Allergy Clin Imunol 1999;103:408-414.
5. Brook I, Gooch WM III, Jenkins SG, et al: Medical management of acute bacterial sinusitis. Recommendations of a clinical advisory committee on pediatric and adult sinusitis. Ann Otol Rhinol Laryngol 2000;109(Suppl):2-20.
6. Johnson JT, Ferguson BJ: Infection. In Cummings CW, Fredrickson JM, Harker LA, et al (eds): Otolaryngology—Head and Neck Surgery, 3rd ed. St. Louis, Mosby, 1998, pp 1107-1118.
7. Graney DO, Rice DH: Anatomy. In Cummings CW, Fredrickson JM, Harker LA, et al (eds): Otolaryngology—Head and Neck Surgery, 3rd ed. St. Louis, Mosby, 1998, pp 1059-1064.
8. Blanton PL, Biggs NL: Eighteen hundred years of controversy: The paranasal sinuses. Am J Anat 1969;124:135-147.
9. Manning SC. Medical Management of Infectious and Inflammatory Disease. In Cummings CW, Fredrickson JM, Harker LA, et al (eds): Otolaryngology—Head and and Neck Surgery, 3rd ed. St. Louis, Mosby, 1998, pp 1135-1144.
10. Wald ER: Sinusitis. Pediatr Ann 1998;27:811-818.
11. Wald ER, Guerra N, Byers C: Frequency and severity of infections in day care: Three-year follow-up. J Pediatr 1991;118:509-514.
12. Sobol SE, Schloss MD, Tewfik TL: Acute sinusitis, medical management. In Meyers A (ed): Emedicine Textbook of Otolaryngology and Facial Plastic Surgery, July 2001. Available at http://www.emedicine.com/ENT/Topic337.htm.
13. Hui Y, Gaffney R, Crysdale WS: Sinusitis in patients with cystic fibrosis. Eur Arch Otolaryngol 1995;252:191-196.
14. Ramsey B, Richardson MA: Impact of sinusitis in cystic fibrosis. J Allergy Clin Immunol 1992;90:547-552.
15. Karja J, Nuutinen J: Immotile cilia syndrome in children. Int J Pediatr Otrhinolaryngol 1983;5:275-279.
16. Shapiro GG, Virant FS, Furukawa CT, et al: Immunologic defects in patients with refractory sinusitis. Pediatrics 1991;87:311.
17. Kurono Y, Fujiyoshi T, Mogi G: Secretory IgA and bacterial adherence to nasal mucosal cells. Ann Otol Rhinol Laryngol 1989;98:273-277.
18. Axelsson A, Brorson IE: Correlation between bacteriologic findings in the nose and maxillary sinus in acute maxillary sinusitis. Laryngoscope 1973;83:2003-2011.
19. Gwaltney JM Jr., Phillips CD, Miller RD, et al: Computed tomographic study of the common cold. N Engl J Med 1994;330:25-30.
20. Talmor M, Li P, Barie PS: Acute paranasal sinusitis in critically ill patients: Guidelines for prevention, diagnosis, and treatment. Clin Infectious Disease 1997;25:1441-1446.
21. Rouby JJ, Laurent P, Gosnach M: Risk factors and clinical relevance of nosocomial maxillary sinusitis in the critically ill. Am J Respir Crit Care Med 1994;150:776-783.
22. Wald ER: Microbiology of acute and chronic sinusitis in children and adults. Am J Med Sci 1998;316:13-20.
23. Ahuja GS, Thompson J: What role for antibiotics in otitis media and sinusitis? Postgrad Med 1998;104:93-99, 103-104.
24. Wald ER: Expanded role of group A streptococci in children with upper respiratory infections. Pediatr Infect Dis J 1999;18:663-665.
25. Penttila M, Savolainen S, Kiukaanniemi HM, et al: Bacterial findings in acute maxillary sinusitis-European study. Acta Otolaryngol Suppl 1997;529:165-168.
26. Gwaltney JM Jr., Scheld WM, Sande MA, et al: The microbial etiology and antimicrobial therapy of adults with acute community-acquired sinusitis: A fifteen-year experience at

the University of Virginia and review of other selected studies. J Allergy Clin Immunol 1992;90:457-462.

27. Jones NS: Current concepts in the management of paediatric rhinosinusitis. J Laryngol Otol 1999;113:1-9.

28. Mainous AG III, Hueston WWJ, Clark JR: Antibiotics and upper respiratory infection: Do some folks think that there is a cure for the common cold? J Fam Pract 1996;42:357-361.

29. Hamm RM, Hicks RJ, Bemben DA: Antibiotics and respiratory infections: Are patients more satisfied when expectations are met? J Fam Pract 1996;43:56-62.

30. Taylor JA, Weber W, Standish L, et al: Efficacy and safety of echinacea in treating upper respiratory tract infections in children: A randomized controlled trial. JAMA 2003;290:2761-2898.

31. Wald ER, Guerra N, Byers C: Upper respiratory tract infections in young children: Duration and frequency of complications. Pediatrics 1991;87:129-133.

32. Bishai WR: Issues in the management of bacterial sinusitis. Otolaryngol Head Neck Surg 2002;127(Suppl):S3-S9.

33. Lusk RP, Stankiewicz JA: Pediatric rhinosinusitis. Otolaryngol Head Neck Surg 1997;117 (Suppl):S53-S57.

34. Low DE, Desrosiers M, McSherry J, et al: A practical guide for the diagnosis and treatment of acute sinusitis. CMAJ 1997;156(Suppl):S1-S14.

35. Zinreich SJ, Kennedy DW, Rosenbaum AE, et al: Paranasal sinuses: CT imaging requirements for endoscopic surgery. Radiology 1987;163:769-775.

36. Wald ER, Milmoe GJ, Bowen AD, et al: Acute maxillary sinusitis in children. N Engl J Med 1981;304:749-754.

37. Eibling DE: Maxillary sinus: Irrigation techniques. In Myers EN (ed): Operative Otolaryngology Head and Neck Surgery. Philadelphia, WB Saunders, 1997, pp 81-85.

38. Sobol SE, Schloss MD, Tewfik TL: Acute Sinusitis, Surgical Management. In Meyers A (ed): Emedicine Textbook of Otolaryngology and Facial Plastic Surgery, July 2001. Available at http://www.emedicine.com/ENT/Topic340.htm.

39. McCormick DP, John SD, Swischuk LE, et al: A double-blind, placebo-controlled trial of decongestant-antihistamine for the treatment of sinusitis in children. Clin Pediatr (Phila) 1996;35:457-460.

40. Aitkin M, Taylor JA: Prevalence of clinical sinusitis in young children followed up by primary care pediatricians. Arch Pediatr Adolesc Med 1998;152:244-248.

41. Gwaltney JM Jr: State-of-the-art: acute community-acquired sinusitis. Clin Infect Dis 1996;23:1209-1223.

42. Slack CL, Dahn KA, Abzug MJ, Chan KH: Antibiotic-resistant bacteria in pediatric chronic sinusitis. Pediatr Infect Dis J 2001;20:247-250.

43. Conrad DA, Jenson HB: Management of acute bacterial rhinosinusitis. Curr Opin Pediatr 2002;14:86-90.

44. Fenton JE, Smyth DA, Viani LG, Walsh MA: Sinogenic brain abscess. Am J Rhinol 1999;13:299-302.

45. Jones RL, Violaris NS, Chavda SV, et al: Intracranial complications of sinusitis: The need for aggressive management. J Laryngol Otol 1995;109:1061-1062.

46. Clayman GL, Adams GL, Paugh DR, et al: Intracranial complications of paranasal sinusitis: A combined institutional review. Laryngoscope 1991:101:234-239.

47. Giannoni CM, Stewart MG, Alford EL: Intracranial complications of sinusitis. Laryngoscope 1997;107:863-867.

48. Hirsh M, Lifshitz T: Computerized tomography in the diagnosis and treatment of orbital cellulitis. Pediatr Radiol 1988;18:302-305.

49. Chandler JR, Langenbrunner DJ, Stevens ER: The pathogenesis of orbital complications in acute sinusitis. Laryngoscope 1970;80:1414-1428.

50. Clary RA, Cunningham MJ, Eavey RD: Orbital complications of acute sinusitis: Comparison of computed tomography scan and surgical findings. Ann Otol Rhinol Laryngol 1992;101:598-600.

51. Sobol SE, Marchand J, Tewfik TL, et al: Orbital complications of sinusitis in children. J Otolaryngol 2002;31:131-136.

52. Hubert L: Orbital infections because of nasal sinusitis. N Y State J Med 1937;37:1559-1563.

53. Eustus H, Armstrong DC, Buncic JR, et al: Staging of orbital cellulitis in children: Computerized tomography characteristics and treatment guidelines. Pediatr Ophthalmol Strabismus 1986;23:246-251.

54. Catalano RA, Smoot CN: Subperiosteal orbital masses in children with orbital cellulitis: Time for a reevaluation? J Pediatr Ophthalmol Strabismus 1990;27:141-142.

55. Patt BS, Manning SC: Blindness resulting from orbital complications of sinusitis. Otolaryngol Head Neck Surg 1991;104:789-795.

56. Goodwin WJ Jr: Orbital complications of ethmoiditis. Otolaryngol Clin North Am 1985;18:139-147.

57. Rubin SE, Rubin LG, Zito J, et al: Medical management of orbital subperiosteal abscess in children. J Pediatr Ophthalmol Strabismus 1989;26:21-27.

58. Souliere CR, Antoine GA, Martin MP, et al: Selective non-surgical management of subperiosteal abscess of the orbit: Computerized tomography and clinical course as an indication for surgical drainage. Int J Pediatr Otorhinolaryngol 1990;19:109-119.

59. Arjmand EM, Lusk RP, Muntz HR: Pediatric sinusitis and subperiosteal orbital abscess formation: Diagnosis and treatment. Otolaryngol Head Neck Surg 1993;109: 886-894.

60. Shahin J, Gullane PJ, Dayal VS: Orbital complications of acute sinusitis. J Otolaryngol 1987;16:23-27.

61. Froehlich P, Pransky SM, Fontaine P, et al: Minimal endoscopic approach to subperiosteal orbital abscess. Arch Otolaryngol Head Neck Surg 1997;123:280-282.

CHAPTER 9

Diagnosis and Management of Chronic Sinusitis

LAWRENCE W. C. TOM, MD

Sinusitis is the most common chronic illness for all age groups in the United States.[1] The exact incidence of sinusitis in children is unknown, but because children develop upper respiratory tract infections (URIs) more frequently than adults, it is likely that the prevalence of sinusitis is higher in children.

Acute sinusitis most commonly occurs following upper respiratory tract infections. Children have six to eight upper respiratory infections per year, and 5% to 10% will develop acute sinusitis.[2] This high prevalence may result from immature immune systems, smaller nasal passages, and closer interactions in group settings, such as daycare. Acute sinusitis should be suspected when the signs of a URI persist beyond 10 days. They include low-grade fever, irritability, rhinorrhea, daytime cough, which may worsen at night, halitosis, facial pain, and headache. Treatment consists primarily of antibiotics.

Recurrent acute sinusitis in children is defined by the occurrence of more than four episodes of acute sinusitis in a year. These episodes resolve with medical therapy, and the patient is asymptomatic between episodes.

Subacute sinusitis represents a continuum between acute and chronic sinusitis and is defined as the persistence of symptoms lasting longer than 6 weeks but less than 12 weeks. Treatment is similar to that of acute sinusitis.

Chronic sinusitis represents a more complex and poorly understood condition. It may represent a heterogeneous group of conditions resulting from a wide range of processes. It is defined as the persistence of signs and symptoms of inflammation of one or more of the paranasal sinuses persisting beyond 12 weeks, or the occurrence of six or more episodes of acute sinusitis per year corroborated by computed tomography (CT) findings. Bacteria, fungus, bacterial superantigens, biofilms, and osteitis may play roles in the development and persistence of chronic sinusitis. The cause appears to be multifactorial, and there is no consensus regarding the best treatment. There is, however, no mistaking its negative impact on the quality of life. Patients, parents, and physicians are frequently frustrated about the lingering symptoms. Children with chronic sinusitis may have more pain and greater limitation of physical activities compared with children with asthma, rheumatoid arthritis, and other chronic disorders.[3]

PATHOGENESIS

Normal sinus pathology requires mucociliary clearance of normal sinus mucus through patent ostia. Normal mucus is produced in a well-ventilated sinus, and cilia direct the mucus toward and through the natural ostia into the nose.

The causes of sinusitis are multifactorial, but ultimately mucostasis occurs. It develops when one or more of the following conditions are present: ostial obstruction, mucociliary dysfunction, reduction in the number of cilia, or increased production or change in viscosity of the mucus.[4,5] Once one of these conditions occurs, it may initiate a cycle of events that lead to sinusitis (Fig. 9-1). Ostial obstruction, primarily of the ostiomeatal complex, the area between the middle and inferior turbinates where the maxillary, anterior ethmoid, and frontal sinuses drain, is the most common of these conditions.

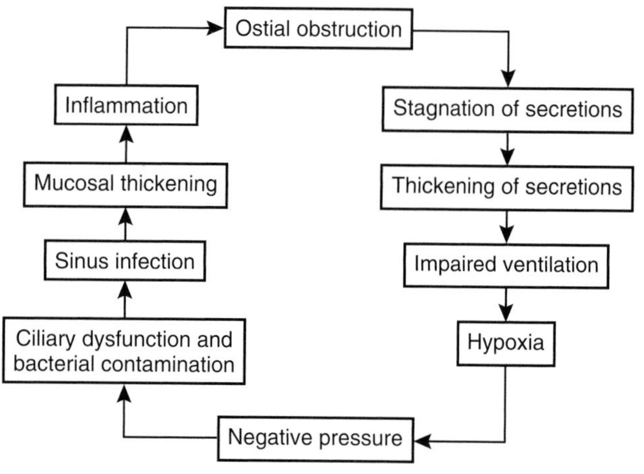

Figure 9-1. Sinusitis cycle.

Box 9-1 Systemic Predisposing Factors for Sinusitis

Upper respiratory infections
Allergies
Immunodeficiencies
IgA and IgG subclass deficiencies
Antibody formation defects
Hypogammaglobulinemia of infancy
Acquired immunodeficiencies—immunosuppressive medications, acquired immunodeficiency syndrome (AIDS)
Cystic fibrosis
Primary ciliary dyskinesias

This obstruction causes mucostasis and impaired sinus ventilation. Oxygen is absorbed within the sinus, and negative intrasinal pressure develops. Hypoxia causes ciliary dysfunction, and the negative pressure draws bacteria-contaminated nasal and nasopharyngeal secretions into the sinuses. Bacteria proliferate within the stagnant mucus, and infection may occur. Infection causes inflammation, alters the sinus mucosa and production and character of the mucus, and adversely affects the cilia. With the resolution of infection, the mucosa returns to normal. If infections recur or persist, irreversible damage to the sinus mucosa may develop. This damage may result from actual infection or the subsequent inflammatory response triggered by the infection.[6] In addition to the mucosa, the underlying bone may also become involved, with both infection and inflammation. This chronic osteitis may play a significant role in the persistence of the mucosal disease.[7]

PREDISPOSING FACTORS

There are many predisposing factors for sinusitis. Management of these factors leads to prevention or resolution of the disease, whereas inability to identify them will probably result in treatment failures. These factors can be divided into systemic and local conditions. Systemic conditions include URIs, allergies, immunodeficiencies, cystic fibrosis (CF), and primary mucociliary dyskinesia (Box 9-1). Structural anomalies, adenoid hypertrophy or infection, trauma, gastroesophageal reflux (GER), and irritants are the most common local factors (Box 9-2).

Viral URIs are the most common predisposing conditions for pediatric chronic sinusitis. Because of the smaller anatomy of the sinuses and nasal cavity and the immaturity of the immune system, children are naturally more susceptible to URIs. The rise in daycare attendance has also contributed to an increase in URIs.[8] Children experience between six and eight URIs per year compared with two or three in adults. During a URI, nasal secretions containing viruses, bacteria, and inflammatory mediators enter the sinuses, where they produce inflammation and/or infection. This inhibits mucociliary clearance and causes mucosal edema, with the potential to develop ostial obstruction. Although most URIs resolve spontaneously without sequelae, sinusitis develops in 5% to 10% of patients.[4] Repeat infections may lead to permanent mucosal injury and even scar formation.[5]

Allergic rhinitis is another common predisposing condition for chronic pediatric sinusitis. There is a 50% incidence of positive allergic skin tests in children with sinusitis, and patients with allergies and sinusitis have more severe CT abnormalities compared with patients without allergies.[9,10] The allergic response causes mucosal swelling and increases the viscosity of mucus, thereby impeding mucociliary transport. Because family history is an excellent prognostic indicator for pediatric allergies, all children with suspected chronic sinusitis must be questioned about a family history of allergies. Children should be examined for signs and symptoms of sinusitis, and an allergy evaluation should be done in any child with significant sinus disease.

Box 9-2 Local Predisposing Factors for Sinusitis

Structural factors—nasal septal deviation, nasal polyps, concha bullosa, tumors, foreign bodies, choanal atresia
Adenoid hypertrophy, chronic adenoiditis
Trauma
Gastroesophageal reflux
Irritants—second-hand tobacco smoke, pollution, topical decongestants

Children have a physiologic immaturity in their immune systems. By 2 years of age, the immune system is developed to 50% of the adult level, and it reaches the adult level by 10 years. Young children are more prone to URIs, but the incidence of URIs diminishes with age. Immunodeficiency disorders should be suspected if a child has recurrent episodes of URI, sinusitis, otitis media, or pneumonia. The most common deficiencies in children with chronic sinusitis are immunoglobulin A and G (IgA and IgG) subclass deficiencies, defects in specific antibody formation, and hypogammaglobulinemia of infancy.[11] If an immunodeficiency is considered likely, quantitative immunoglobulin levels and specific antibody responses to diphtheria and tetanus toxoid and pneumococcal vaccine are determined. The diagnosis of an acquired immunodeficiency may be more apparent in children receiving immunosuppressive medications or those with acquired immunodeficiency syndrome (AIDS).

Cystic fibrosis, an autosomal recessive disorder of the exocrine mucous glands, is caused by defects in region q31 of chromosome 7 and is characterized by the production of thick, inspissated mucus. It is associated with chronic endobronchial infections, gastrointestinal malabsorption, and chronic sinusitis. In CF, the nasal mucus is 30 to 60 times thicker than normal,[12] which results in mucostasis and subsequent ostial obstruction. The classic nasal sign of CF is the appearance of nasal polyps. Ten percent to 30% of CF patients present with polyps, whereas 70% of children with polyps will have CF. This disease should be suspected in any child with nasal polyps or with both sinusitis and associated pulmonary or gastrointestinal conditions. A sweat chloride test or genetic testing may help establish the diagnosis.

Primary ciliary dyskinesias are rare, but chronic sinusitis is a common manifestation of these conditions. Structural and functional ciliary anomalies impair mucociliary transport. Structural abnormalities include immotile cilia syndrome and Kartagener's syndrome; these are diagnosed by electron microscopic examination of the cilia from nasal turbinate or tracheal mucosa. Low ciliary beat frequency and ciliary beat disorientation are examples of functional abnormalities that can be assessed with a saccharin mucociliary clearance test.[13]

Structural abnormalities may facilitate the development of chronic sinusitis. They cause obstruction of the ostiomeatal complex by direct blockage of the ostia or indirectly by altering the normal nasal laminar airflow. Septal deviation, concha bullosa, paradoxical middle turbinate, tumors, foreign bodies, polyps, choanal atresia, craniofacial anomalies, encephaloceles, and meningomyeloceles have all been implicated as predisposing factors for chronic sinusitis.

Adenoid tissue may affect the sinuses in several ways and must be assessed in any child with chronic sinusitis. Enlarged adenoids may obstruct the nasopharynx, disrupting the laminar airflow. Obstruction may causes stasis of secretions. Regardless of the size, adenoid tissue may act as a reservoir for bacterial pathogens.[14,15]

Gastroesophageal reflux may predispose affected children to sinusitis, but the exact incidence is unknown. Inflammation results from the reflux of gastric contents into the nasopharynx and nose and may lead to ostial obstruction. Studies have shown that GER is more prevalent in children with chronic sinusitis and that symptoms of sinusitis may abate with reflux treatment.[16,17] An evaluation for GER should be considered in any patient who fails aggressive medical therapy.

Irritants adversely affect the nasal mucosa, thicken mucus, and alter ciliary function. The most obvious of these is second-hand tobacco smoke. Others include pollution and topical decongestants. If they are present, these factors must be eliminated from the patient's environment.

MICROBIOLOGY

It is well accepted that acute sinusitis is caused primarily by *Streptococcus pneumoniae, Haemophilus influenzae,* and *Moraxella catarrhalis*. The role of bacterial pathogens in chronic sinusitis is less clear. It is even hypothesized that bacterial infection plays only a minor role in many cases of pediatric chronic sinusitis.[18] Bacteria may incite the initial event, but it is the subsequent inflammatory response, rather than the actual infection, that is responsible for the chronicity of the disease.[6]

Studies to determine the causative organisms have been limited by poor patient cooperation, variable definitions of chronic sinusitis, nonsterile technique, concurrent use of antibiotics, and lack of quantitation of results.[4] The findings of these studies have varied significantly. Isolated organisms have included those responsible for acute sinusitis, alpha-hemolytic streptococci, *Staphylococcus aureus*, *Staphylococcus epidermidis*, *Streptococcus viridans*, normal respiratory flora, and anaerobes.[19-22] With no consensus regarding the most relevant organisms, it is best to consider chronic sinusitis as a polymicrobial infection.

Certain systemic diseases have been associated with specific microbial agents. Children with CF have a high incidence of sinus infections caused by *Pseudomonas* species, whereas fungal agents are common pathogens in immunocompromised children with chronic sinusitis. Invasive fungal organisms must be suspected in severely immunocompromised children.

DIAGNOSIS

The diagnosis of chronic sinusitis is more difficult and challenging in children than in adults. There is no single test that definitively diagnoses chronic sinusitis. A working diagnosis is established by the history and physical examination and may be confirmed by imaging studies.

History

Children are often poor historians and are unable to communicate the presence and severity of symptoms. The signs and symptoms of chronic sinusitis lack specificity and vary with time and age. The most common symptoms are nasal congestion, rhinorrhea, cough, postnasal discharge, headache, facial pain, low-grade fever, irritability, and halitosis. All are found in many other diseases and conditions. Although chronic sinusitis may be manifested by only one symptom, it is more likely to occur when a combination of these symptoms is present. A detailed history of the symptoms, including severity, character, timing, duration, and associated symptoms, must be obtained. It is helpful to ask parents to monitor and document the symptoms as objectively as possible.

The nasal congestion associated with chronic sinusitis usually alternates between each nasal cavity and is associated with rhinorrhea and postnasal discharge.[18] With URIs, enlarged or infected adenoids, and allergies, the congestion is often bilateral. Unilateral obstruction would suggest an anatomic abnormality, tumor, or foreign body.

Purulent rhinorrhea accompanied by other symptoms suggests sinusitis. The presence of isolated, clear rhinorrhea, however, does not. Allergic rhinitis and URIs are more likely causes.

The cough in sinusitis usually occurs during the day but is worse at night. This cough often causes sleep disturbances. A dry, nonproductive cough without a nocturnal component suggests causes other than sinusitis.

There are a number of causes of headaches and facial pain, but sinusitis causes fewer headaches than is commonly thought by many physicians and patients.[23] The location of the headache varies, depending on the involved sinus. In the absence of other signs and symptoms, headache alone is unlikely to be caused by sinusitis. Tension and migraine headaches are more likely causes.[24]

Children have many reasons to be irritable. Irritability associated with sinusitis may be secondary to facial pain, discomfort, or the adverse affects of nasal obstruction, such as sleep disturbances and fatigue.

Physical Examination

The physical findings may help confirm the impression of chronic sinusitis or identify a predisposing factor. In children, the value of the examination is dependent on the degree of cooperation. In young children, it may be limited to anterior rhinoscopy, using an otoscope. In older children, a rigid endoscopic examination may be possible.

During rhinoscopy, crusting and the quality and quantity of secretions should be noted. Nasal crusting is often mistaken as a sign of chronic sinusitis. It is a nonspecific sign associated with many conditions and rarely occurs in children with chronic sinusitis.[5] Clear or white rhinorrhea may be found in children with allergies, vasomotor rhinitis, and viral URIs. Purulent rhinorrhea may be secondary to foreign bodies, choanal atresia, and chronic adenoiditis, as well as sinusitis.

The patency of the nose should be assessed, along with the septum, mucosa, and turbinates. If the child is cooperative, topical vasoconstrictors and anesthetics help facilitate the examination. Polyps, foreign bodies, tumors, congenital masses, and severe septal deviations can obstruct the nose. Erythematous mucosa may be secondary to inflammation or the use of topical steroid nasal sprays.[25] Pale boggy mucosa and edematous purple-bluish turbinates are often seen in patients with allergic rhinitis. An enlarged or paradoxical middle turbinate may block the ostiomeatal complex.

Every effort should be made to visualize the middle meatus. This can be performed using an otoscope, but better visualization is obtained with an endoscope. The middle meatus is examined for narrowing, polyps, and discharge. Purulent discharge from the middle meatus is diagnostic of sinusitis, but its absence does not exclude chronic sinusitis.

A flexible endoscope allows assessment of the nasopharynx and larynx. Obstructing or infected adenoid tissue may predispose to sinusitis and cause signs and symptoms mimicking those of sinusitis. Laryngeal inflammation and granulation are manifestations of GER.

The oral cavity should be examined. Postnasal discharge, mucosal inflammation, and lymphoid hyperplasia of the posterior pharyngeal walls ("cobblestoning") are frequently observed in children with chronic sinusitis.[11]

Imaging Studies

With the nonspecific signs and symptoms of chronic sinusitis and the difficulties in obtaining a precise history and examination in children, radiographic imaging plays a significant role in the diagnosis of pediatric chronic sinusitis. CT scans are a useful guide, but in children the results must be interpreted judiciously. Because many asymptomatic children have incidental radiographic abnormalities, it is important not to overemphasize these findings. Conversely, a symptomatic child may have normal sinus CT findings (Fig. 9-2). The CT findings should be evaluated in conjunction with the clinical presentation.

Although plain radiographs may aid in the diagnosis of acute sinusitis, they provide little diagnostic information regarding chronic sinusitis. Plain films do not demonstrate sinus anatomy well and provide an inaccurate

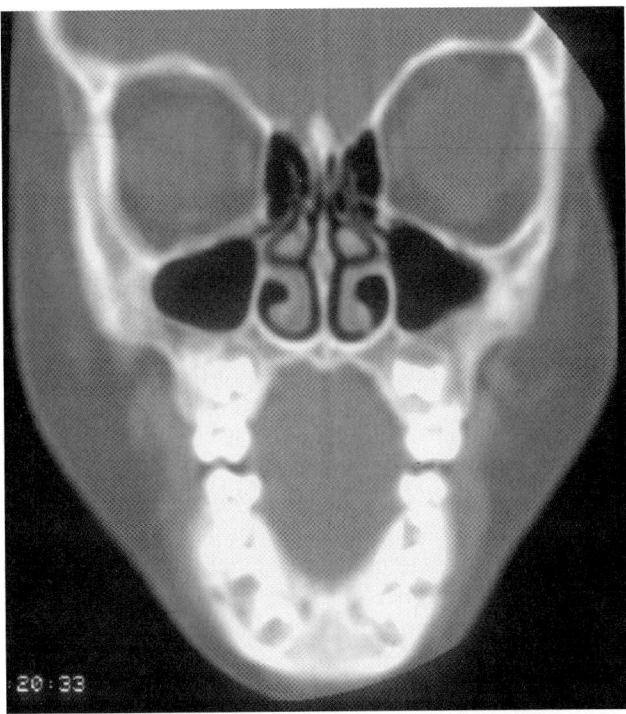

Figure 9-2. Normal sinus CT scan. This coronal sinus CT scan demonstrates normal maxillary and ethmoid sinuses.

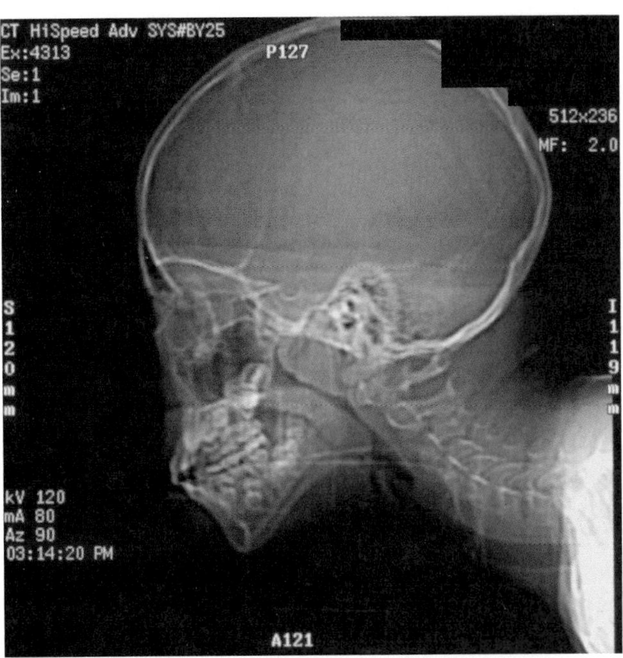

Figure 9-3. Enlarged adenoid. In this CT scan, the adenoid is enlarged and obstructs the nasopharynx.

representation of chronic sinus disease.[26,27] Plain films should not be obtained for the evaluation of pediatric sinusitis. The limited information that can be gained from them does not appear to justify the radiation exposure.[18]

CT scanning, specifically the coronal view, is the diagnostic study of choice for chronic sinusitis. It provides excellent resolution of the bony anatomy, surrounding structures, and mucosa. Because the adenoid plays a significant role in the cause and management of chronic sinusitis, both the adenoid and sinuses should be evaluated when reviewing the CT. The adenoid can be best demonstrated on the CT survey film (Fig. 9-3).

CT demonstrates superior accuracy for the diagnosis of chronic pediatric sinusitis, with excellent specificity and sensitivity.[28] The correlation between the clinical and CT diagnosis has ranged from 64% to 93%.[26,27,29] Sinus CT is not recommended for all cases of chronic sinusitis. It is performed for the following circumstances: to rule out sinus involvement, to monitor symptomatic patients after therapy, and to assess the anatomy for possible surgery. When performing CT to monitor therapy, timing is critical. It should be done 2 to 3 weeks after a trial of maximal medical therapy, consisting of 4 to 6 weeks of an oral antibiotic and nasal steroid and saline sprays.

The presence of positive CT findings in children does not necessarily establish the diagnosis of chronic sinusitis. Incidental CT findings of sinusitis, such as mucosal thickening and opacification, have been reported to be as high as 41% to 70% in asymptomatic children, with the incidence being higher in children younger than 2 year.[20,30,31] Positive CT findings may also persist for up to 2 weeks after resolution of an URI.[32] In these cases, management decisions should be based on the clinical presentation.

A less common but equally difficult situation occurs when a symptomatic child has a normal CT scan. This discrepancy may relate to the timing of the CT.[25] CT should be repeated 2 to 3 weeks after the cessation of therapy. If the CT scan remains normal, the physician should search for other conditions that may masquerade as chronic sinusitis.

Magnetic resonance imaging (MRI) is not recommended for the routine diagnosis of chronic sinusitis. An MRI scan does not demonstrate bony anatomy and cannot be used to assess the anatomy prior to any surgery. It provides excellent display of soft tissue and, compared with CT, MRI tends to overemphasize mucosal pathology, leading to a higher false-positive rate for sinus disease.[33] The greatest value of MRI is in the evaluation of intracranial and orbital complications of sinusitis and fungal sinusitis, and in distinguishing mucoceles from other lesions.

MANAGEMENT

As with any chronic condition, patients, parents, and physicians frequently are frustrated by the persistence of symptoms. An important and necessary aspect of management is counseling. All involved parties must be thoroughly informed about the nature of the disease and should be given realistic expectations regarding therapeutic modalities.

The initial management of chronic sinusitis is the identification and treatment of any predisposing factors. If possible, children should be removed from daycare or placed in smaller centers. If they have been identified, allergies, immunodeficiencies, and GER should be treated. Cigarette smoke must be eliminated from the child's environment.

There have been varied recommendations for the treatment of pediatric chronic sinusitis, ranging from observation (no therapy) to endoscopic sinus surgery. Advocates of watchful waiting have noted that spontaneous resolution of chronic sinusitis is the norm in children, especially younger ones, but this may be the least acceptable option.[34,35] Most practitioners initially treat chronic sinusitis medically, reserving surgery for treatment failures.

Medical Therapy

The primary goals of medical therapy are the reduction of inflammation, reestablishment of ostial patency, and restoration of ventilation and drainage. Most pediatric otolaryngologists use a combination of nasal steroids, saline nasal sprays, and oral antibiotics as their initial medical therapy and have reported that more than 50% of their patients respond successfully.[36] Although this treatment regimen has been widely accepted, it is based on empirical impressions rather than on well-controlled clinical studies.

The key to medical therapy is a prolonged course (4 to 6 weeks) of a broad-spectrum β-lactamase–resistant antibiotic with anaerobic coverage. Amoxicillin-clavulanate and a second-generation cephalosporin (excluding cefaclor) are good initial choices. For children allergic to penicillin or a cephalosporin, clarithromycin and clindamycin are good alternatives.

Topical intranasal steroids are an important adjunct to antibiotics. They inhibit early- and late-phase inflammatory responses and IgE-mediated release of histamine, reducing mucosal edema and hyperactivity and helping prevent ostial occlusion and improve mucociliary clearance. Mometasone (Nasonex) is approved for use in children 2 years and older, whereas fluticasone (Flonase) is approved for children 4 years and older. Both have a higher topical potency, receptor binding affinity, and receptor binding half-life compared with other available nasal steroids.

Topical nasal irrigations help cleanse the nose mechanically, but it is mandatory that large volumes be used. The irrigations facilitate the removal of secretions, crusts, and debris and improve mucociliary clearance by rehydrating mucosal secretions.[5] Hypertonic saline appears to be better than isotonic saline because it will also reduce edema, promoting mucociliary clearance and ostial patency.[2]

As an alternative to endoscopic sinus surgery in patients who have not responded to this standard medical therapy, the use of intravenous antibiotics with selective adenoidectomy has been proposed.[37] It has been recommended that these children undergo maxillary sinus puncture, irrigation, culture, and placement of a central venous catheter for intravenous access. Adenoidectomy may be performed on selected children at the discretion of the surgeon. An antibiotic, chosen based on the culture results, is administered intravenously for 1 to 4 weeks, followed by oral antibiotics for 8 weeks. Although the 89% success rate is impressive, the percentage of improvement based on the adenoidectomy alone has not been determined. The great majority of pediatric otolaryngologists do not recommend intravenous antibiotics as medical treatment for pediatric chronic sinusitis.[36]

Surgery

Surgery for pediatric chronic sinusitis is indicated in children who fail medical therapy and have CT evidence of sinusitis (Fig. 9-4). Procedures are performed to correct predisposing anatomic abnormalities, such as a deviated

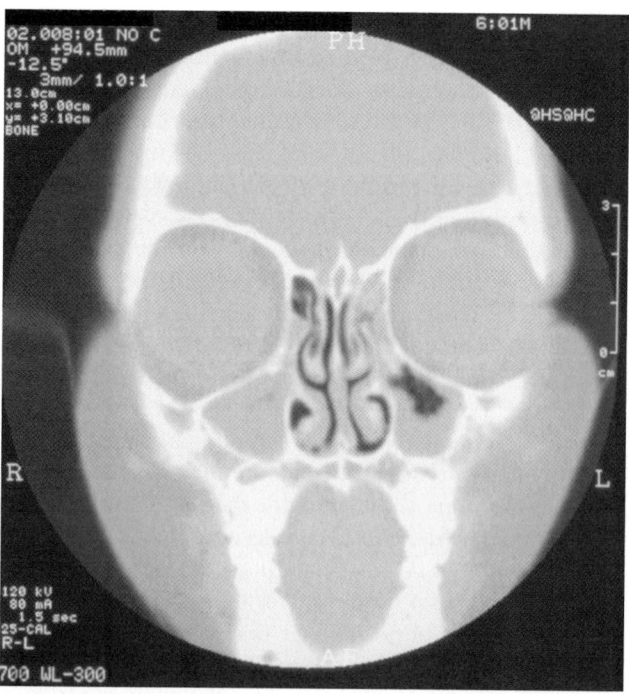

Figure 9-4. Abnormal sinus CT scan. This coronal sinus CT shows opacification of the right maxillary and left ethmoid sinuses and mucosal thickening of the left maxillary sinus.

nasal septum, nasal polyp, concha bullosa, or choanal atresia, remove adenoid tissue, and open, drain, and restore ventilation to the sinuses.

The role of adenoidectomy in the management of pediatric chronic sinusitis had been controversial, but is now accepted as an initial surgical treatment.[6,38] Adenoidectomy has been reported to improve sinus symptoms in 47% to 58% of cases.[39,40] Most pediatric otolaryngologists routinely perform adenoidectomy for the treatment of chronic sinusitis, with most adenoidectomies being performed prior to any sinus surgery.[36] Comparing the potential complications of adenoidectomy with those of sinus surgery, this approach is highly recommended.

Similar to the treatment of adenoidectomy for otitis media, the adenoid does not have to be enlarged to improve symptoms. Relief of symptoms is probably related to the reduction of the bacterial reservoir of infected or colonized tissue and relief of nasal obstruction and stasis of secretions. If an adenoidectomy is performed as the initial surgical procedure, a minimum of 3 months should elapse before endoscopic sinus surgery is performed.[41]

Formerly, maxillary aspiration, with irrigation and inferior meatal antrostomy, had been used to treat chronic sinusitis, but these procedures are rarely used now. Maxillary sinus aspiration with cultures may be performed in conjunction with other procedures, such as adenoidectomy as a diagnostic rather than therapeutic tool.

Endoscopic sinus surgery is indicated for children with persistent signs and symptoms, despite maximal medical therapy, and with CT evidence of sinusitis. The role of endoscopic surgery for children continues to evolve, and several trends have developed in the past 3 to 5 years. Pediatric otolaryngologists have more stringent criteria for surgery and, as a result, endoscopic sinus surgery is being performed less frequently.[6,36] Instead of extensive surgical dissection, surgery has become more limited and conservative, with an emphasis on preservation of normal tissue. The most common procedure is now maxillary antrostomy with anterior ethmoidectomy.

Endoscopic sinus surgery is a safe and effective option for the management of pediatric chronic sinusitis. Its goal is the restoration of normal sinus physiology by alleviating ostiomeatal obstruction and reestablishing sinus ventilation. A meta-analysis of several studies has suggested an improvement rate of 88%, with surgery appearing to be less successful in children younger than 3 years.[42,43] Improvement, however, does not mean a cure, and many children continue to have symptoms. Revision surgery is not uncommon. Most pediatric otolaryngologists have reported a revision rate of less than 25%, with a majority of these reporting less than 10%.[36] Prior to surgery, it is mandatory to address parental expectations and emphasize the need for continued management, even after initial surgery.[1]

Complications of endoscopic sinus surgery are low (approximately 2%) and include bleeding, formation of synechiae, orbital hematoma, eye muscle injury, blindness, cerebrospinal fluid rhinorrhea, and meningitis.[44] There had also been a concern regarding potential adverse effects of endoscopic sinus surgery on midfacial growth in young children, but it has been reported that this concern is not valid.[45]

SUMMARY

Chronic pediatric sinusitis is a complex, poorly understood condition that has a significant negative impact on the quality of life of many children. The correct diagnosis may be difficult, because the signs and symptoms of chronic sinusitis are nonspecific and overlap those of many other conditions. Primary management includes identification and treatment of any predisposing factors, patient and parent counseling, and medical therapy. Surgery is reserved for children who have failed aggressive medical therapy and have CT evidence of significant disease.

MAJOR POINTS

- Chronic sinusitis is a complex, poorly understood condition.
- Signs and symptoms are varied and nonspecific.
- It is imperative to identify and manage predisposing factors.
- Computed tomography is the diagnostic study of choice
- Medical therapy consisting of antibiotics and steroid and saline nasal sprays is the primary treatment.
- Endoscopic sinus surgery is reserved for symptomatic children who have failed medical therapy and have CT evidence of sinusitis.

REFERENCES

1. Lieu JEC, Piccirillo JF, Lusk RP: Prognostic staging system and therapeutic effectiveness for recurrent or chronic sinusitis in children. Otolaryngol Head Neck Surg 2003;129:222-232.
2. Lieser JD, Derkay CS: Pediatric sinusitis: When do we operate? Curr Opin Otolaryngol Head Neck Surg 2005;13:60-66.
3. Cunningham MJ, Chiu EJ, Landgraf JM, et al: The health impact of chronic recurrent rhinosinusitis in children. Arch Otolaryngol Head Neck Surg 2000;126:1363-1368.
4. Wald ER: Chronic sinusitis in children. J Pediatr 1995; 127:339-347.

5. Muntz HR: Diagnosis and management of chronic sinusitis. In Wetmore RF, Muntz HR, McGill TJ, et al (eds): Pediatric Otolaryngology: Principles and Practice Pathways. New York, Thieme, 2000, pp 475-485.
6. Baroody FM: Pediatric sinusitis. Arch Otolaryngol Head Neck Surg 2001;127:1099-1101.
7. Kennedy DW, Senior BA, Gannon FH, et al: Histology and histomorphometry of ethmoid bone in chronic rhinosinusitis. Laryngoscope 1998;108:502-507.
8. Carron J, Derkay CS: Pediatric rhinosinusitis: Is it a surgical disease? Curr Opin Otolaryngol Head Neck Surg 2001;9:61-66.
9. Slavin RG: Resistant rhinosinusitis: What to do when usual measures fail. Allergy Asthma Proc 2003;24:303-306.
10. Ramadan HH, Fornelli R, Ortiz AO, et al: Correlation of allergy and severity of sinus disease. Am J Rhinol 1999;13:345-347.
11. Madgy DN, Haupert MS: Management of pediatric rhinosinusitis. Curr Opin Otolaryngol Head Neck Surg 2000;8:469-476.
12. Nishioka GJ, Cook PR: Paranasal sinus disease in patients with cystic fibrosis. Otolaryngol Clin North Am 1996;29:193-205.
13. Stanley P, MacWilliams L, Greenstone M, et al: Efficacy of a saccharine test for screening to detect abnormal mucociliary clearance. Br J Dis Chest 1984;78:62-65.
14. Lee D, Rosenfeld RM: Sinonasal symptoms and adenoid bacteriology. Otolaryngol Head Neck Surg 1997;116:301-307.
15. Bernstein J, Dryja D, Murphy T: Molecular typing of paired bacterial isolates from the adenoid and lateral nasal wall of the nose in children undergoing adenoidectomy: Implications in acute rhinosinusitis. Otolaryngol Head Neck Surg 2001;125:593-597.
16. Barbero GJ: Gastroesophageal reflux and upper airway disease. Otolaryngol Clin North Am 1996;29:28-38.
17. Bothwell MR, Parsons DS, Talbot A, et al: Outcome of reflux therapy on pediatric chronic sinusitis. Otolaryngol Head Neck Surg 1999;121:255-262.
18. Meltzer EO, Hamilos DL, Hadley JA, et al: Rhinosinusitis: Establishing definitions for clinical research and patient care. Otolaryngol Head Neck Surg 2004;131:s1-s61.
19. Brook I: Bacteriologic features of chronic sinusitis in children. JAMA 1981;246:967-969.
20. Tinkelman DG, Silk HJ: Clinical and bacteriologic features of chronic sinusitis in children. Am J Dis Child 1989;143:938-941.
21. Muntz HR, Lusk RP: Bacteriology of the ethmoid bullae in children with chronic sinusitis. Arch Otolaryngol Head Neck Surg 1991;117:179-181.
22. Orobello PW, Park RI, Belcher LJ, et al: Microbiology of chronic sinusitis in children. Arch Otolaryngol Head Neck Surg 1991;117:980-983.
23. Pincus RL, Lucente FE: Facial pain and headache. In Bluestone CD, Stool SE, Kenna MA (eds): Pediatric Otolaryngology. Philadelphia, WB Saunders, 1996, pp 787-792.
24. Tepper SJ: New thoughts on sinus headache. Allergy Asthma Proc 2004;25:95-96.
25. Arjmand EM, Lusk RP: Management of recurrent and chronic sinusitis in children. Am J Otolaryngol 1995;16:367-382.
26. McAlister WH, Lusk RP, Muntz HR: Comparison of plain radiographs and coronal CT scans in infants and children with recurrent sinusitis. AJR Am J Roentgenol 1989;153: 1259-1264.
27. Lazar RH, Younis RT, Pavey LS: Comparison of plain radiographs, coronal CT, and intraoperative findings in children with chronic sinusitis. Otolaryngol Head Neck Surg 1992;107:29-34.
28. Bhattacharyya N, Jones DT, Hill M, et al: The diagnostic accuracy of computed tomography in pediatric chronic sinusitis. Arch Otolaryngol Head Neck Surg 2004;130:1029-1032.
29. van der Veken PJ, Clement PA, Buisseret T, et al: CT scan study of the incidence of sinus involvement and nasal anatomic variations in 196 children. Rhinology 1990;28:177-184.
30. Diament MJ, Senac MO, Gilsanz V, et al: Prevalence of incidental paranasal sinuses opacification in pediatric patients: A CT study. J Comput Assist Tomogr 1987;11:426-431.
31. Lesserson JA, Kieserman SP, Finn DG: The radiographic incidence of chronic sinus disease in the pediatric population. Laryngoscope 1994;104:159-166.
32. Glasier CM, Mallory GB, Steele RW: Significance of opacification of the maxillary and ethmoid sinuses in infants. J Pediatr 1989;114:45-50.
33. Zinreich SJM, Kennedy DW, Kumar AL: MR imaging of normal nasal cycle: Comparison with sinus pathology. J Comput Assist Tomogr 1988;12:1014-1019.
34. Clement PAR, Bluestone CD, Gordts F, et al: Management of rhinosinusitis in children. Int J Pediatr Otorhinolaryngol 1999;49:S 95-100.
35. Chan KH, Winslow CP, Levin MJ, et al: Clinical practice guidelines for the management of chronic sinusitis in children. Otolaryngol Head Neck Surg 1999;120:328-334.
36. Sobol SE, Samadi DS, Kazahaya K, et al: Trends in the management of pediatric chronic sinusitis: Survey of the American Society of Pediatric Otolaryngology. Laryngoscope 2005;115:78-80.
37. Don DM, Yellon RF, Casselbrandt ML, et al: Efficacy of a stepwise protocol that includes intravenous antibiotic therapy for the management of chronic sinusitis in children and adolescents. Arch Otolaryngol Head Neck Surg 2001;127:1093-1098.
38. Rosenfeld RM: Pilot study of outcomes in pediatric rhinosinusitis. Arch Otolaryngol Head Neck Surg 1995; 121:729-736.
39. Ramadan HH: Adenoidectomy vs endoscopic sinus surgery for the treatment of pediatric sinusitis. Arch Otolaryngol Head Neck Surg 1999;125:1208-1211.
40. Vandenbery SJ, Heatley DG: Efficacy of adenoidectomy in relieving symptoms of chronic sinusitis in children. Arch Otolaryngol Head Neck Surg 1997;123:675-678.

41. Clinical Indicators Compendium, vol 19. Alexandria, Va, American Academy of Otolaryngology—Head and Neck Surgery Bulletin, 2000, p 34.
42. Herbert RL, Bent JB: Meta-analysis of outcomes of pediatric functional endoscopic sinus surgery. Laryngoscope 1998;108:796-799.
43. Ramadan HH: Relation of age to outcome after endoscopic sinus surgery in children. Arch Otolaryngol Head Neck Surg 2003;129:175-177.
44. Faust RA, Rimell FL: Chronic RS in children. Curr Opin Otolaryngol Head Neck Surg 1996;4:373-377.
45. Bothwell MR, Piccirillo JF, Lusk RP: Long-term outcome of facial growth after functional endoscopic sinus surgery. Otolaryngol Head Neck Surg 2002;126:628-634.

Acute and Chronic Infections of the Oral Cavity and Pharynx

UDAYAN K. SHAH, MD

Infections of the oral cavity and pharynx require an appreciation for the interrelatedness of the aerodigestive structures of the head and neck. A multidisciplinary approach is necessary for the evaluation and management of these common disorders. The importance of understanding these diseases cannot be overestimated, because even though antibiotic use may prevent the more severe presentations, children today are nonetheless still susceptible to respiratory, hematologic, or central nervous system complications of these diseases and to long-term sequelae, such as rheumatic fever. This chapter reviews the typical presentations of oral and pharyngeal infections.

GENERAL CONSIDERATIONS

Oropharyngeal Anatomy

Oropharyngeal anatomy can be conceptualized as a framework covered by drapery. The floor of mouth serves as a theater stage, whereas the posterior pharynx (backstage) is partially hidden on either side and above by the drapery of the soft palate and tonsils. Moving from superior to inferior and anterior to posterior, the hard palate of the maxilla limits the region superiorly and anteriorly, and the skull base and clivus provide the posterior roof (Fig. 10-1). The cervical spine provides the posterior bony border, and the mandible provides the lateral and anterior bony framework. Inferiorly and anteriorly, the hyoid provides suspension of the floor of mouth. The mucosa of the soft palate, retropharynx and oropharynx, and floor of the mouth provide the medial limit. Drainage from the major salivary glands is lateral, from the paired parotid or Stensen's ducts, and inferior, from Wharton's ducts, which drain the submandibular glands. The potential

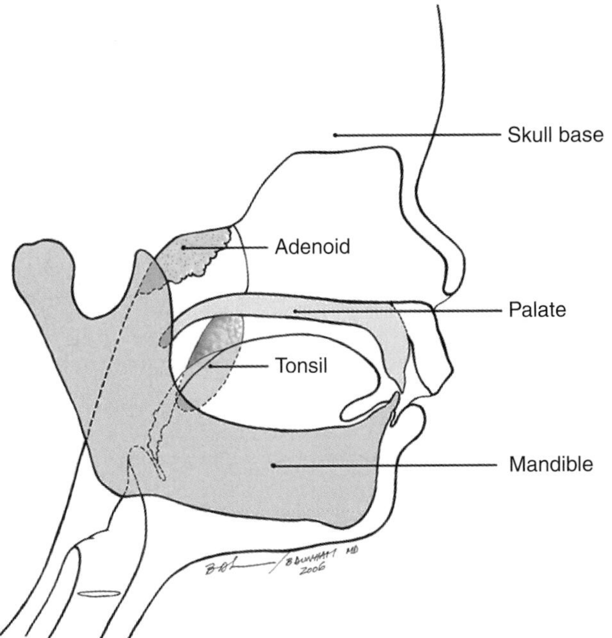

Figure 10-1. Oropharyngeal anatomy. (Courtesy of Brian Dunham, MD, and Eleanor Eve Porges.)

spaces between the deeper retropharyngeal and parapharyngeal fibromuscular layers permit spread of infection from the initial location to regional areas, resulting in airway compromise or thrombosis of major vessels. The spread of infection into the mediastinum may prove fatal.

Lymphoid tissue is present within the mucosa throughout this region, with the largest aggregations present in Waldeyer's tonsillar ring, which surrounds the border between the oral cavity and pharynx. Superiorly, Waldeyer's ring consists of the adenoid or nasopharyngeal tonsil, laterally, the paired palatine tonsils and inferiorly, the lingual tonsil at the tongue base.

Clinical Evaluation

Evaluation of the child suspected of having an infection in the oral cavity or pharynx begins with a thorough history from the child's caretakers, with attention to prodromal symptoms, recent travel and illness contacts, immunization status, degree of activity, airway and swallowing concerns, ability to maintain hydration, and the child's response to supportive and pharmacologic therapy.

Physical Examination

Physical examination should focus on determining the degree of immediate distress—fever, mental status, and adequacy of airway—keeping in mind that a lethargic child may not exhibit severe compromise because of inactivity. Evidence of serous otitis media on otoscopy may indicate inflammation or obstruction in the nasopharynx, affecting the eustachian tubes. Oral examination should note the degree of trismus, state of salivary papillae (Stensen's and Wharton's ducts), lingual papillary color, degree of mucosal dehydration, evidence of posterior pharyngeal secretions, tonsillar size and color, and presence of exudates on the tonsils. Asking the child simply to open her or his mouth without protruding the tongue facilitates examination of the posterior pharynx. Gentle depression of the midportion of the tongue with a tongue depressor allows a better view of the tonsils and posterior pharynx while avoiding precipitation of the gag reflex and allows for an effective examination, even with a degree of trismus (Fig. 10-2). The oral mucosal examination can be accomplished by gently directing the child's head, using one hand on the back of the head while stabilizing the other hand with the tongue depressor against the child's mandible. The tongue depressor can then be walked around the upper and lower alveoli, permitting comfortable and complete evaluation of the mucosa, salivary ducts, gingiva, and dentition. The fingers of the directing hand may be used to milk secretions from the parotid and submandibular glands (Fig. 10-3). Flexible nasopharyngoscopy may be used in selected cases, particularly when the oral airway appears compromised. The neck should be assessed for tenderness, fullness, adenopathy, and range of motion.

Laboratory and Radiologic Studies

Laboratory studies are not always necessary, but for children in whom intravenous therapy or hospitalization

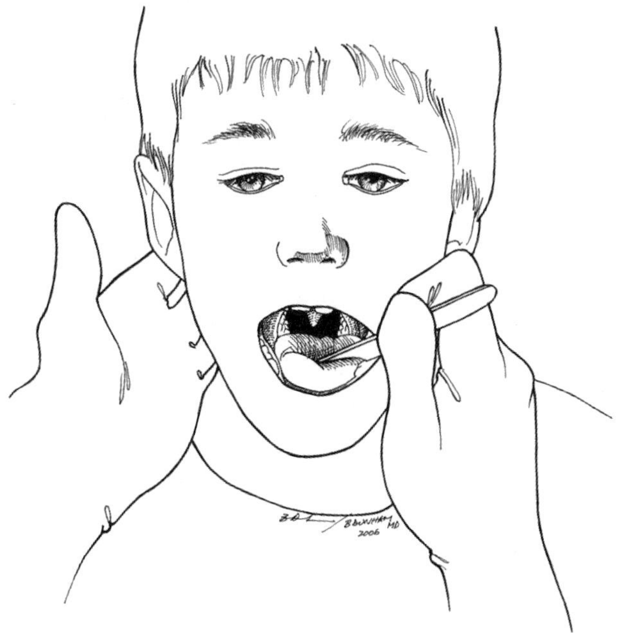

Figure 10-2. Examination of the oropharynx. Oral examination is facilitated by placing the tongue depressor against the middle of the tongue rather than posteriorly, thereby allowing a good examination of the posterior pharynx while avoiding gagging. This technique is usually effective, even in children with trismus.

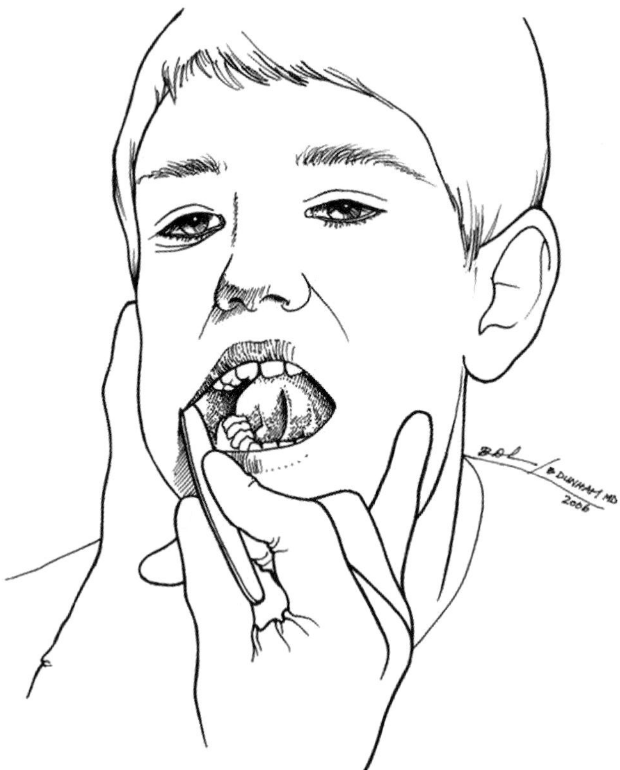

Figure 10-3. Examination of the oral mucosa. The oral mucosal examination is facilitated by gently directing the child's head from a posterior position using one hand while stabilizing the other hand with the tongue depressor against the child's mandible. The tongue depressor can then be "walked" around the upper and lower alveoli, permitting comfortable and complete evaluation of the mucosa, salivary ducts, gingiva, and dentition. The fingers of the directing hand may be used to milk secretions from the parotid and submandibular glands.

is considered, a baseline urinalysis, serum metabolic panel, complete blood count with differential, and assays for serum markers for inflammation (C-reactive protein [CRP] or erythrocyte sedimentation rate [ESR]) may be indicated.

The need for radiographic studies varies by site and extent of presentation, and emerging concern regarding the long-term effects of low-dose diagnostic irradiation has suggested judicious use of plain radiography and computed tomography (CT) studies.[1] Plain radiography has a limited role in the initial assessment of most throat infections and should be reserved for patients in whom fiberoptic nasopharyngolaryngoscopy is not available or possible. Lateral neck radiography may show bulging of the retropharyngeal soft tissues, with resultant airway narrowing.

A contrast-enhanced CT scan (CECT) or an MRI with contrast (MRIC) permits the differentiation of abscess from phlegmon. An abscess is identified by a rim-enhancing fluid collection, whereas a hypolucent area without ring enhancement is defined as phlegmon. In general, MRI with contrast enhancement offers superior tissue detail and diagnostic information, but this benefit must be balanced against the risks involved in this lengthier study, which often requires sedation in a child with a potentially compromised airway. A scan should be considered for children who exhibit clinical worsening or a failure to improve after 24 to 48 hours of antibiotic therapy. Repeat imaging is not necessary for children who are improving clinically, nor is follow-up imaging generally warranted.

Interventional radiologic techniques may have a role with selected abscesses, either for therapeutic drainage or for diagnostic aspiration, to provide material for microbial culture.

VIRAL INFECTIONS OF THE ORAL CAVITY AND PHARYNX

Most pharyngitis in children is viral and is usually caused by adenovirus, influenza A virus, Epstein-Barr virus (EBV), herpes simplex virus, rhinovirus, coronavirus, enterovirus, coxsackievirus, and echovirus.[2] Viral pharyngitis occurs most commonly during colder weather, when more ill contacts are indoors. The hallmarks of viral pharyngitis are a prodrome of fever, fatigue and/or malaise, and arthralgias.

Most children with viral pharyngitis respond well to oral rehydration, rest, antipyretics, and analgesics, specifically acetaminophen or ibuprofen. Aspirin should be avoided because of the risk of Reye's syndrome (acute encephalopathy, hepatic steatosis, and an elevated serum transaminase level). Despite teaching by health care providers and public health initiatives, caretakers may still use aspirin because of a lack of understanding (or inadvertently) in the form of aspirin-containing over-the-counter preparations, or folk or traditional remedies.[3] Gargling with a warm solution of dilute baking soda or salt water may also provide symptomatic relief.

Traditional or folk remedies, such as homeopathy, acupuncture, chiropractic, and medicinal herbs (known as complementary and alternative medicine [CAM]), are used by 1.8%[4] to 21%[5] of families caring for infants or children. Because of this degree of use, and despite the paucity of data on the efficacy and safety of CAM for pediatric pharyngitis, some experiences have been published. Caregivers and families usually appreciate information about potentially dangerous side effects of these treatments.[6-11]

Rhinovirus

The most common viral pathogen of acquired acute pharyngitis is thought to be the rhinovirus, which causes the common cold—a self-limited episode of coryza, rhinorrhea, fever, and malaise, for which supportive care is indicated. Oral antibiotics are not routinely prescribed.

Coxsackievirus

Children afflicted by coxsackievirus A16 infection develop hand-foot-and-mouth disease, in which a viral prodrome of fever, sore throat, and oral and pharyngeal erythema is followed 1 to 2 days later by vesiculopapular skin lesions that are usually but not exclusively seen on the palms and soles. Hand-foot-and-mouth disease often affects children younger than 5 years.[12] It generally resolves in 1 week. Supportive care is indicated, and baking soda baths soothe the rash.

Epstein-Barr Virus

EBV infection most often afflicts children older than 15 years, in whom it manifests as typically infectious mononucleosis (IM).[13] Fever and significant lethargy accompany dysphagia and odynophagia, with resultant dehydration. The physical examination shows enlarged cervical nodes bilaterally, often giving the neck a full appearance. Enlarged erythematous tonsils have gray exudates that can be peeled off without causing bleeding. The tonsillar enlargement contributes to airway obstruction, initially with a "hot potato" voice and loud, stertorous mouth breathing, which may progress to obstructive symptoms at night. Hepatosplenomegaly and enlarged axillary and inguinal lymph nodes may be seen as well. Children often experience a prolonged period of fatigue, which may last for months following initial management.

Clinical diagnosis can be confirmed by laboratory testing, usually by the serum heterophil antibody test (Mono spot). False-negative results are more common in children, especially children younger than 4 years.[13] Specific serologic tests may be required for diagnosis in heterophil-negative children. The serum IgG level against the Epstein-Barr viral capsid antigen (VCA) is high early in IM, whereas IgM anti-VCA antibodies identify recent infection. Serum antibody against EBV nuclear antigen (EBNA) is present weeks to months after infection.[14]

Management of IM begins with hydration, analgesics, antipyretics, and oral or parenteral steroids for airway obstruction. Children should be cautioned against vigorous physical activity, particularly contact sports, until the spleen is no longer palpable, because of concern over splenic rupture. This period of athletic abstinence may be required for 1 month,[13] and complete recovery may take several months.

Antibiotics may be necessary to treat bacterial superinfection of the tonsils, may reduce dysphagia, and therefore may promote the resumption of oral intake.[15] Children with infectious mononucleosis should not receive amoxicillin or ampicillin because of the risk of a drug-induced papular skin rash.[14] The oral antibiotic azithromycin has also been reported to cause a nonspecific skin rash.[16] The rash resolves a few days after discontinuation of the drug and does not preclude its future use.[17] Infectious mononucleosis must therefore be excluded in all children who present with acute pharyngitis, either by history and examination or by serologic testing.

A short course of oral corticosteroid therapy may be considered for children with aerodigestive compromise from acute infectious tonsillar hypertrophy or in children with systemic complications, such as massive splenomegaly, myocarditis, thrombocytopenia, or hemolytic anemia.[13] Corticosteroids may shorten the duration of fever and pharyngitis. Gamma globulin may be helpful in severe cases.

Hospitalization may be required for hydration and for airway observation. Tonsillectomy is rarely necessary to relieve airway obstruction or dysphagia. Post-tonsillectomy hemorrhage may be more likely to occur in children who require surgery during the acute phase of IM.[18,19]

Herpangina

Herpangina is a severe viral pharyngitis that presents with soft palate, tonsillar, and oropharyngeal erythema and with multiple small clear vesicles, which form shallow ulcers on rupture. Herpangina is caused by coxsackievirus A and B, types 1 to 5,[12] and by human enteric echoviruses. Herpangina has an incubation period of 3 to 7 days and usually resolves after several days.

Herpes Simplex Viruses

Herpes simplex virus (HSV) type 1 infection affects the oral mucosa in children in two different ways—via a primary infection, which is usually severe, and via a secondary recurrent infection, with milder presentation and course. Primary herpetic gingivostomatitis most commonly presents in children between 1 and 3 years of age,[12] with edema, erythema, and a sharp prickling sensation of the lips, gingiva, tongue, and palate. Vesicles rupture into ulcers, which then desquamate and form a gray membrane that may crust, coalesce, or develop a secondary bacterial infection. Children with HSV infection may exhibit lymphadenopathy, fever, and flulike symptoms, which may progress to disseminated herpetic infection, skin eruptions, or meningoencephalitis.

Secondary recurrent HSV type 1 (HSV-1) infection may occur in up to 40% of people after primary infection.[12] The activation of the dormant virus from regional neuroganglia may occur during periods of reduced host defenses, especially during periods of fever, stress, excessive sun exposure, or immunodeficiency. Oral antiviral therapy with acyclovir, famciclovir, or valacyclovir may benefit children during acute infection and may reduce the frequency of secondary episodes.[14,20] A topical antibacterial ointment, such as mupirocin (Bactroban), may be used for secondarily infected ulcers.[21] Topical creams containing antiviral agents such as acyclovir and penciclovir may also be prescribed for children.[20,22]

Herpes Zoster

Herpes zoster infection, also known as shingles, is caused by the varicella-zoster, or chickenpox, virus, which lies dormant in dorsal root ganglia until it erupts during a period of immunodeficiency into painful vesicular mucosal or dermal eruptions. These appear in stages and then crust and gradually resolve within 10 days. Because the trigeminal ganglion is affected, dental pain may precede the vesicular eruption by 2 or 3 days.[12] Care is supportive, with hydration and analgesics. Oral acyclovir may be considered in primary varicella infection for children older than 12 years, those with chronic cutaneous or pulmonary disorders, and children receiving long-term salicylate or short, intermittent, or aerosolized corticosteroid therapy.[14] Intravenous antiviral therapy is indicated for immunocompromised children. Systemic primary varicella infection (chickenpox) may manifest with similar oral vesicles. Postexposure vaccination may be offered to susceptible children.[14]

Human Papillomavirus

Human papillomavirus (HPV) types 6, 14, and 22 infect the upper respiratory mucosa. Papillomas form at the junction of ciliated and nonciliated mucosa. Presentation varies by site of disease, with hoarseness or dyspnea suggesting laryngeal papillomas. Painless papillomatous lesions may appear on the soft palate or uvula. Although solitary papillomas are generally treated successfully by excision, recurrent respiratory papilloma (RRP) can be a problematic, progressive, and potentially lethal disorder.

Airway obstruction at the level of the larynx requires surgical treatment, usually a number of times throughout childhood and sometimes into adulthood. Recurrent respiratory papilloma (RRP) may result from progressive spread of papillomas throughout the airway, specifically in the larynx and trachea. Removal of pharyngeal papillomas is intended to reduce the risk of spread into the larynx and beyond. Adolescence may bring about gradual clinical resolution. Adjuvant medical management with chemotherapeutic agents may be offered in some cases. RRP may rarely undergo malignant transformation into adenocarcinoma.

Measles

Measles, caused by an RNA virus, occurs rarely in the United States today. Episodes are attributed to the rare failure to immunize a child, vaccine failure, or importation of the virus from another country. Children exhibit fever, cough, coryza, and conjunctivitis and develop an erythematous maculopapular rash. Yellow-white pinpoint papules against an inflamed buccal mucosa (Koplik's spots) may appear 2 to 4 days before other general symptoms or skin rash appear.[12] Patients are contagious 3 to 5 days before the onset of the skin rash to 4 days after its appearance. The incubation period of 8 to 12 days from exposure to onset of symptoms means that the time from rash in a source case to the next case averages 2 weeks. Treatment is supportive, and intravenous or aerosolized ribavirin has been used to treat children who are severely affected or immunocompromised. Vitamin A has been used to reduce morbidity of measles infection in children who are vitamin A–deficient or when the case fatality rate is historically 1% or higher.[14]

Mumps

Bilateral parotitis is the classic otolaryngologic presentation of this now-rare RNA viral infection, with fewer than 300 cases/year reported since the introduction of the mumps vaccine.[14] Postpubertal boys may suffer from orchitis, which rarely results in infertility. Viral culture from body fluids and antibody titers is diagnostic. Care is supportive.

Aphthous Stomatitis

This recurrent ulcerative lesion of the oral cavity typically is a problem for teenagers. It may be caused by a respiratory virus or an autoimmune or delayed-type hypersensitivity response. Aphthous lesions often occur during times of stress. Treatment is supportive. Topical suspensions containing equal parts of viscous lidocaine and diphenhydramine hydrochloride, and a combination of a mucosal-protective agent such as aluminum-magnesium hydroxide (Maalox), may be used to provide symptomatic relief. Another topical agent that has had some success is a suspension of hydrocortisone, nystatin (Mycostatin), and tetracycline. Topical benzocaine-phenol-alcohol (Anbesol) may also offer short-term symptomatic relief when applied to the ulcers.

BACTERIAL INFECTIONS OF THE ORAL CAVITY

Gingivitis

Most cases of gingivitis in children are associated with poor oral hygiene and plaque. Immunosuppressed or malnourished children may present with acute necrotizing ulcerative gingivitis (ANUG), or Vincent's gingivitis. This potentially severe infection is caused by fusobacteria and spirochetes, and possibly by other organisms.[12,23]

ANUG usually affects children older than 12 years and is identified by friable interdental papillae, necrotic pseudomembranes along the gingival margin, fetor oris (foul-smelling breath), malaise, and fever. Treatment includes oral débridement and rinses with dilute hydrogen peroxide or chlorhexidine; oral antibiotics (e.g., amoxicillin, erythromycin, penicillin) may be helpful for extensive infection.[23]

Ludwig's Angina

Acute infection of the floor of the mouth involving the submandibular or sublingual spaces is known as Ludwig's angina. Presentation includes submandibular fullness and induration, drooling, and a "hot potato" voice and may progress without treatment to airway compromise because of superior displacement of the tongue and infectious spread through adjacent compartments.

The potential for rapidly progressive airway compromise warrants a high index of suspicion and rapid protection of the airway by early institution of intravenous antibiotics, corticosteroids, and possibly airway management, including intubation or tracheotomy. Incision and drainage are usually required for cure.

Bacterial Infection of the Submandibular Glands

Bacterial infection of the submandibular glands usually involves only one gland, and manifests with submandibular swelling, tenderness, and erythema of the submandibular duct lateral to the lingual frenulum. Purulent material may be expressed through these ducts with gentle forward pressure on the submandibular region. Infection is promoted by salivary stasis related to dehydration, inspissated secretions, or ductal obstruction due to sialolithiasis. Streptococcal and staphylococcal bacteria are usually the causative agents. Sialogogues, hydration, warm compresses to the neck, and anti-inflammatory drugs provide symptomatic relief. Oral or intravenous antibiotic therapy, depending on the degree of inflammation and concern over airway obstruction, is usually curative. For infections developing into an abscess, induration of the submandibular skin may precede development of an abscess clearly defined by palpation or imaging. Such abscesses require surgical drainage.

Parotitis

Acute bacterial parotitis is not commonly seen in children and is usually caused by *Staphylococcus aureus*. Diagnosis is made clinically with a history of fever, pain, and drooling, and physical findings that include a bulging, erythematous, and tender cheek, with induration of the overlying skin, trismus, and evidence of pus from Stensen's duct (Fig. 10-4). Recurrent parotitis may indicate a rheumatic or collagen-vascular disease. Concurrent rheumatic complaints such as dry eye and arthralgias warrant laboratory evaluation for autoimmune causes by testing for rheumatoid factor (RF) to diagnose juvenile rheumatoid arthritis and by testing for serum markers, such as SSA and SSB, to diagnose Sjögren's disease.

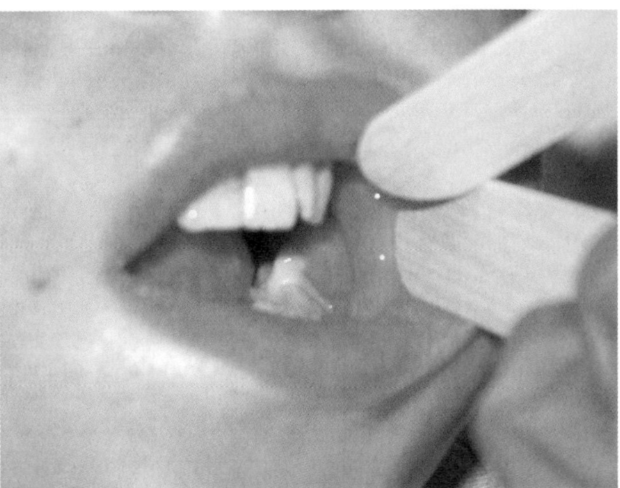

Figure 10-4. Acute parotitis. Pus is seen streaming from the parotid, or Stensen's, duct in this child with acute parotitis.

Hydration, sialogogues, and oral antibiotics can manage most cases of parotitis successfully. When symptoms are refractory or progressive despite oral antibiotics, intravenous antibiotics are begun and CECT or MRIC may be necessary to exclude a mass lesion or abscess. In cases of abscess formation, radiographically guided needle aspiration may offer symptomatic relief, but definitive drainage may require a parotidectomy approach, with identification and protection of the facial nerve.

BACTERIAL INFECTIONS OF THE PHARYNX

Pharyngitis

The most common bacterial pathogen of concern in the pharynx is *Streptococcus pyogenes*, a gram-positive organism that exhibits beta-hemolysis of blood agar by culture and that demonstrates the group A cell wall carbohydrate antigen as defined by Rebecca Lancefield in the 1930s. *S. pyogenes* is therefore referred to simply as group A beta-hemolytic *Streptococcus* (GABHS).[25] More recent techniques have allowed categorization of GABHS by sequencing the 5′-terminal end of the *emm* gene.[26] Other pathogenic bacteria that may cause pharyngitis are *Corynebacterium diphtheriae*, *Neisseria gonorrhoeae*, and *Arcanobacterium haemolyticium*,[13] and commensals such as nontypable *Haemophilus influenzae*,

Streptococcus pneumoniae and *S. viridans*, *Staphylococcus aureus* and *S. epidermidis*, and *Moraxella catarrhalis*.[2]

GABHS causes pharyngitis mostly during the winter and spring, and infection is spread primarily via droplets from respiratory secretions.

Acute, Recurrent, and Chronic Tonsillitis

Acute tonsillitis manifests with fever, throat pain, foul breath, dysphagia and odynophagia, tender cervical adenopathy, and tonsillar erythema and exudates. Acute tonsillar enlargement caused by the infection may result in mouth breathing, disordered nighttime sleep, or sleep apnea. Symptoms may last up to 2 weeks with therapy.

The peak incidence of acute tonsillitis occurs between 5 and 15 years and is rarely seen in children younger than 3 years.[26,27] When several episodes of acute tonsillitis occur in 1 year, the child is said to experience recurrent tonsillitis. The lifetime prevalence of self-reported recurrent tonsillitis in a Norwegian study was noted to be 11.7%[28] and was documented in 12.1% of elementary school children in a Turkish report.[29] A parental history of atopy and of tonsillectomy may be predictive for the development of tonsillitis in children.[28]

Chronic tonsillitis is identified by a 3-month history of sore throat, halitosis, odynophagia, possibly otalgia, and tonsillar inflammation, often with debris within crypts or tonsillar exudates.[30,31] Chronic tonsillitis may also be defined by the presence of tonsilliths, which consist of firm, yellow-white calculi that may be spit out or expressed from the tonsils with a swab. Tonsilliths, as well as softer, cheesy, foul-smelling debris, may accumulate within tonsillar crypts (cryptic tonsillitis).

Carrier State

The carrier state is defined by the presence of GABHS in the pharynx by culture, without evidence of an immunologic response to streptococcal antigens.[32] Between 2.5% and 10.9% of children may be carriers of GABHS.[2,27] In one study from western Pennsylvania, a 27% to 32% prevalence over the course of the school year was seen in children, with a point prevalence per given month of 15.9%. Many children who were carriers were hosts to different organisms, because the bacterial *emm* types changed after an average of 10.8 weeks.[26] In addition, despite living among this reservoir of GABHS carriers, 40% of children were uninfected each school year, perhaps because of their own specific mucosal immunity, local or systemic, or to production of antibacterial peptide. Children are most susceptible to infection from carriers.[27]

Diagnosis

The diagnosis of bacterial pharyngotonsillitis can be made in most cases by symptoms and signs. Sudden onset of sore throat, fever, headache, abdominal pain, and nausea and vomiting are considered characteristic symptoms, whereas characteristic signs are erythema and exudates of the tonsils and pharynx (Fig. 10-5), soft palate petechiae (doughnut lesions), uvular swelling and erythema, anterior cervical adenitis, and a scarlatiniform rash. There is an absence of cough, rhinitis, stridor, hoarseness, conjunctivitis, and diarrhea. Younger children exhibit a less severe febrile response than older children.[33] Lingual swelling and erythema may produce a strawberry tongue, and early in the disease, a white coating of this surface may bring about the so-called white strawberry tongue.[33]

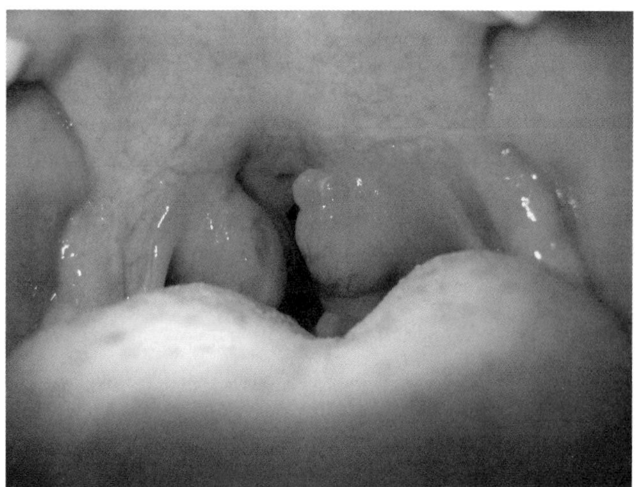

Figure 10-5. Acute tonsillitis.

The scarlet fever rash seen in GABHS is a fine rash, rarely seen in children younger than 3 years, and is caused by an erythrogenic toxin (exotoxin A). Two signs of interest are Pastia's lines and the Rumpel-Leede phenomenon. Pastia's lines (or sign) are the accentuated erythema seen in the flexor skin crease, such as the antecubital or axillary creases. An increase in petechiae distal to the point of application of a tourniquet is known as the Rumpel-Leede phenomenon.[2,13,33]

Laboratory Testing

Tonsillitis is a clinical diagnosis. Testing is indicated when GABHS infection is suspected to determine the need for antibiotic therapy and to avoid unnecessary and potentially harmful antibiotic use.[34] Throat cultures are the gold standard for the diagnosis of GABHS, with identification of the organism by fluorescent antibody testing or disk diffusion testing using bacitracin. Alternatively, the rapid antigen detection test (RADT), also called the rapid strep test, detects the presence of GABHS cell wall carbohydrate from swabbed material and has a high specificity, higher than or equal to 95%. However, its limited sensitivity, only 80% to 90% compared with that of a throat culture, means that a negative RADT result must be followed by a more sensitive throat culture before excluding GABHS infection.[13]

Waiting 24 to 48 hours for throat culture results to return will not diminish the efficacy of antibiotic therapy in preventing rheumatic fever, the major complication of GABHS.[13] Post-therapy culture is usually not necessary, but may be useful for determining antibiotic resistance and for confirming disease resolution. Documentation of culture results is helpful in establishing the frequency and chronology of infections to facilitate future therapeutic decisions.

A complete blood count (CBC) demonstrates leukocytosis, with a predominance of neutrophils. Other acute-phase reactant levels (CRP, ESR) may be elevated. Monospot and serum electrolyte determinations may be indicated. The serum should be examined for antistreptococcal antibodies, such as antistreptolysin O (ASO) and antideoxyribonuclease (anti-DNAse). These titers are useful for documenting prior infection in persons diagnosed with acute rheumatic fever (ARF), glomerulonephritis, or other complications of GABHS pharyngitis. GABHS carriers tend to have higher antibody titers with acute infection than noncarriers.[32]

Management

Acute Viral Tonsillitis

Treatment of acute viral tonsillitis is largely supportive and focuses on maintaining adequate hydration and caloric intake while controlling pain and fever by analgesics, antipyretics, and hydration. Inability to maintain adequate oral caloric and fluid intake may require intravenous therapy and/or hospitalization.

Bacterial tonsillitis requires supportive care as well as oral antibiotics to reduce symptoms of infection and attendant complications. The treatment goals for therapy in GABHS pharyngitis are (1) prevention of ARF, (2) prevention of suppurative complications, (3) abatement of clinical symptoms and signs, (4) reduction in the transmission of GABHS to close contacts, and (5) avoidance of the adverse effects of inappropriate antimicrobial therapy.[2,13] There is no evidence to support the claim that antibiotic therapy reduces the risk of acute post-streptococcal glomerulonephritis (AGN).[13]

Airway obstruction that may accompany acute tonsillitis in children with underlying adenotonsillar hypertrophy may require treatment with a nasal airway, corticosteroids, humidified oxygen, and hospitalization for airway observation.

Antibiotic Therapy. The GABHS organism is generally susceptible to oral penicillin—the antibiotic of choice because of its efficacy, narrow spectrum of antibacterial activity, safety, and low cost. A full 10-day course is necessary to eradicate infection maximally.[13] Other antibiotics proven effective for GABHS pharyngitis are the penicillin congeners (amoxicillin, amoxicillin-clavulanate), cephalosporins, macrolides, clindamycin, vancomycin, rifampin, and metronidazole.[15,35]

Corticosteroid Therapy. Corticosteroids also are indicated for patients with airway obstruction, hemolytic anemia, and cardiac and neurologic disease. A single oral or intramuscular dose of dexamethasone has been shown to provide improved pain relief over placebo when administered to patients 15 years of age and older with acute pharyngitis.[36]

Recurrent and Chronic Tonsillitis

Recurrent tonsillitis may be treated with the same antibiotics as for acute GABHS pharyngitis. If the infection recurs shortly after a course of an oral penicillin agent, treatment with intramuscular (IM) benzathine penicillin G should be considered. A 3- to 6-week course of clindamycin or amoxicillin-clavulanate has been shown to be effective in eradicating GABHS from the pharynx in children suffering from repeated bouts of tonsillitis. Prolonged antibiotics may be attempted for chronic tonsillitis, including cryptic tonsillitis. Oral rinses and mechanical débridement using swabs or irrigation (e.g., using a water pick) are helpful for removal of tonsillar debris.

Carrier State

Antibiotic treatment for the carrier state should be considered when there is a family history of rheumatic fever, a carrier with a history of glomerulonephritis, frequent spread between household contacts ("ping pong" spread), familial anxiety, infectious outbreak within a closed or semiclosed community (e.g., boarding school), outbreak of ARF, or when tonsillectomy is being considered only because of chronic carriage of GABHS. Tonsillectomy may be considered if antibiotic therapy fails to eradicate the carrier status.

Complications

Complications specific to GABHS pharyngitis are scarlet fever, rheumatic fever, septic arthritis, and poststreptococcal glomerulonephritis.

Scarlet fever manifests as a generalized, nonpruritic, macular erythematous rash that is worse on the extremities and spares the face. The resultant strawberry tongue, Pastia's lines, and Rumpel-Leede phenomenon may last up to 1 week and are accompanied by fever and arthralgias. Scarlet fever results from a lysogenic strain[25] of GABHS. Individuals at risk for this rash are those who do not have antitoxin antibodies to the offending exotoxin.

ARF is a nonsuppurative inflammatory reaction related to prior GABHS infection. It is characterized by some combination of septic arthritis, carditis, chorea, erythema marginatum, and subcutaneous nodules. Rheumatic fever follows acute pharyngitis by 2 to 4 weeks and was observed in up to 3% of episodes of streptococcal pharyngitis prior to the development of antibiotics in the mid-20th century. Molecular mimicry between epitopes on GABHS M-protein and cardiac tissue results in immune-mediated valvular endothelial damage.[36] Cardiac valvular vegetations affect the mitral and tricuspid valves, leading to murmurs, persistent relapsing fevers, and valvular stenosis or incompetence, and may be seen within 2 to 3 weeks of onset of infection, whereas chorea and erythema marginatum may be seen as late as 6 months following infection. Diagnosis requires proof of GABHS infection by culture and serologic testing. A throat swab alone does not identify the causative organism, because a positive swab may reflect colonization rather than pathogenicity. Elevated or rising titers of ASO antibodies, anti-DNAse beta, or antihyaluronidase are required to make the diagnosis. Treatment of ARF is with salicylates and corticosteroids. Penicillin does not alter the course of ARF but is given once the diagnosis has been definitively made or if GABHS has been cultured from the pharynx.[25]

In contrast with ARF, which occurs only after pharyngitis, AGN may occur after pharyngitis or cutaneous infection. AGN can occur in up to 10% to 15% of those with pharyngitis. The latent period between infection and nephritis is 1 to 2 weeks after the onset of pharyngitis. AGN is caused by an immunologic reaction between nephritogenic bacterial strains and glomerular basement membrane during the course of pharyngitis or impetigo, resulting in immune complex deposition and in circulating immune complexes.[37] In children, the most common symptoms are edema, oliguria, hypertension, congestive heart failure, and seizures. Urinalysis shows dark or smoky urine with red blood cells (RBCs), RBC casts, white blood cells, and proteinuria. There is an increased level of serum complement and a decreased glomerular filtration rate. Urinalysis is useful in detecting subclinical renal injury by showing proteinuria in children who have suffered from recurrent tonsillitis. Diagnosis requires documentation of GABHS infection, most often by ASO or anti-DNAse beta. Treatment includes hydration, sodium restriction, diuresis, and anticonvulsants.

Septic streptococcal arthritis results in a painful hot joint that contains fluid with bacteria. Arthrocentesis is diagnostic and partially therapeutic. Treatment with intravenous antibiotics for 6 weeks is required to prevent long-term joint complications.

Surgical Options

Surgery is a safe and effective means of treating recurrent and chronic tonsillitis in children.[30] An episode of tonsillitis for the purpose of making a decision about surgery may be defined as acute infection with at least one of the following: fever of at least 38.3°C, cervical adenopathy (larger than 2 cm or tender), tonsillar or pharyngeal exudates, or a positive culture for GABHS.[38] Children had fewer postoperative episodes of tonsillitis when they underwent tonsillectomy for seven or more episodes of tonsillitis in the preceding year, had five or more such episodes in each of the 2 preceding years, or had three or more such episodes in each of the preceding 3 years.[38] Tonsillectomy with or without adenoidectomy is also indicated for chronic or recurrent tonsillitis associated with the streptococcal carrier state that has not responded to antibiotics.

Tonsillectomy for less frequent episodes of tonsillitis is justified by postoperative improvement in upper airway obstruction, reduced time lost from school and work, easing of provider and caretaker concern over antibiotic use, and decreased discomfort experienced by children during infections, particularly related to the severity of episodes (e.g., whether hospitalization was required).[39] Tonsillectomy may also be considered for cryptic tonsillitis when oral rinses and débridement fail to treat foul taste, halitosis, and discomfort adequately.

Adenoidectomy may be performed with tonsillectomy for the surgical management of recurrent or chronic pharyngitis because of concurrent chronic adenoiditis or chronic infection of Waldeyer's ring. However, one study found no additional benefit to adenotonsillectomy over tonsillectomy alone in the surgical treatment of tonsillitis.[38]

Radiotherapy to manage tonsillitis is of historical relevance only. Ionizing radiation was used until the mid-20th century. Children treated in this way have been found to have an increased risk of neoplasia of the thyroid, parathyroid, and salivary glands. Lifelong follow-up to diagnose neoplasia early in these patients is indicated.[40-42]

Peritonsillar Infections

Children may account for approximately one third of all episodes of peritonsillar abscess (PTA).[43] Peritonsillar infection (PTI)—cellulitis, phlegmon, or abscess—involves the potential space surrounding the palatine tonsils and usually manifests with a pointing collection at the superior pole.[44,45]

Although GABHS is the most commonly cultured organism, isolated in approximately one third of cases,[15] it is not the only bacterial pathogen identified. Most PTAs are polymicrobial, with GABHS, *S. aureus*, and *H. influenzae* accounting for most of the aerobic organisms and *Prevotella*, *Porphyromonas*, *Fusobacterium*, and *Peptostreptococcus* strains comprising the common anaerobes.[44]

Diagnosis

The diagnosis of peritonsillar infection is primarily by history and physical examination. Children present with a several-day history of fever, dysphagia, odynophagia, or voice change, with the characteristic "hot potato" voice. Trismus is a strong indicator of a peritonsillar abscess.[44]

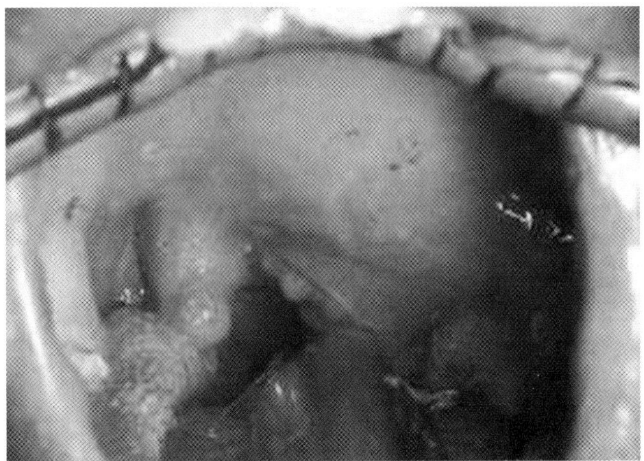

Figure 10-6. Peritonsillar abscess. This causes soft palate bulging above the left tonsil.

Otalgia and neck pain, both usually ipsilateral to the side of the abscess, may be present. Most children have been started on antibiotic therapy prior to the development of a PTA.[44]

Physical examination shows an erythematous bulging of the soft palate above the tonsil, possibly with medial displacement of the tonsil and/or uvula (uvular deviation) (Fig. 10-6). Trismus may limit examination, and the technique described earlier for oral examination is recommended—that is, placing the tongue depressor through whatever degree of mouth opening the patient can offer and displacing the central portion of the tongue only, with gentle downward pressure, as opposed to attempting to force the mandible down and compressing the entire anterior tongue. Cervical adenopathy, typically ipsilateral to the abscess, is also common.

Laboratory evaluation shows a leukocytosis with a propensity to immature cells. A monospot test, as well as a throat culture or rapid strep test, should also be performed. Imaging with CT or MRI scanning with contrast is indicated for unusual presentations (e.g., an inferior pole abscess) or for persistent symptoms despite needle aspiration or surgical drainage.

Management

Treatment aims to resolve discomfort, maintain the airway, and prevent abscess rupture. A ruptured PTA may result in the aspiration of purulence and lead to bronchopneumonia.[44] Aëtius of Amida, a sixth-century Byzantine physician, treated spontaneously draining abscesses with gargles of honey, milk, and herbs or rose extract.[34] Today, oral antibiotics are recommended, including penicillin and its congeners (e.g., amoxicillin-clavulanic acid), cephalosporins, and clindamycin. Hospitalization may be necessary for hydration, analgesia, intravenous antibiotics, and/or airway observation.

Many PTAs require needle aspiration or incision and drainage. Needle aspiration may be performed diagnostically to confirm abscess formation or identify the best point at which to perform incision and drainage, or as a therapeutic measure to relieve symptoms and provide material for microbial culture. Needle aspiration provides relief of pain and may hasten recovery. Although bacterial culture results are not clinically useful in most cases, cultures are valuable when there is a concern over antibiotic resistance (e.g., in immunodeficient children or those who have been recently treated with broad-spectrum antibiotics).[43] CT-guided needle aspiration is indicated when draining a PTA after an unsuccessful surgical attempt and when draining an abscess that is located in an unusual location, such as one that is anticipated to be difficult to reach with standard surgical approaches.

Incision and drainage permit a more complete evacuation than that allowed by needle aspiration. Incision and drainage are performed transorally and are indicated for the older, more cooperative patient, who may more easily permit a longer procedure than that required for needle aspiration. A PTA may be drained in this way using conscious sedation protocols or may require general anesthesia in the operating room because of the child's inability to cooperate. Acute tonsillectomy (quinsy tonsillectomy) may be necessary for relief of obstructive symptoms, a history of recurrent pharyngotonsillitis, or exposure of the abscess. Quinsy tonsillectomy is necessary in approximately one out of three cases of PTA in children.[44,46]

In treating PTA, attention should be paid to the tissue characteristics of tonsillar and peritonsillar tissues. Fleshy, granular, or pale tissue may indicate a neoplasm manifesting as a PTA.[18] In such cases, tissue should be sent for immunohistopathologic evaluation.

Deep Neck Space Infections

Infections of the potential spaces from the skull base to the mediastinum defined by fibromuscular planes are referred to as deep neck space infections. Because of their location and the interconnectedness of potential spaces (highways of infectious spread), deep neck space infections in children may exhibit rapid spread and airway compromise.

Parapharyngeal Space Infections

Children who have an infection of the parapharyngeal space (PPS) infection present with drooling, trismus, dysphagia, odynophagia, and bulging of the lateral pharyngeal wall. Neck stiffness, pain, and torticollis are important signs and symptoms of PPS infections. In contrast with peritonsillar infections, radiologic studies, usually CECT, are required for precise anatomic diagnosis (Fig. 10-7). Sequential radiography may be useful to monitor the efficacy of therapy.

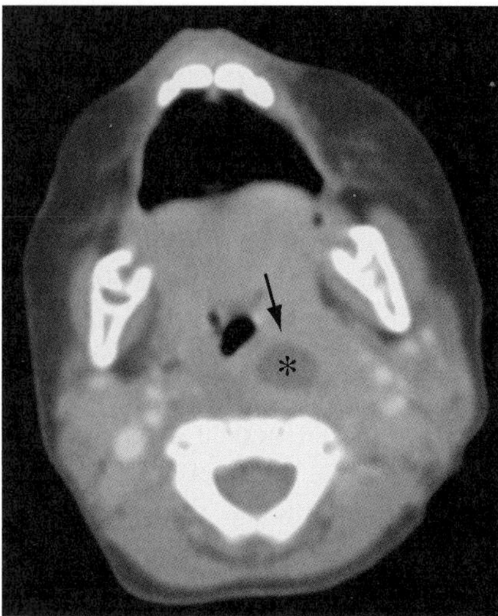

Figure 10-7. Parapharyngeal abscess. A left parapharyngeal abscess *(asterisk)* is shown by a rim-enhancing collection *(arrow points to rim)*, medial to the great vessels on this axial contrast-enhanced computed tomography study. This type of abscess is best drained transorally.

Management of small abscesses or phlegmons of the PPS is by intravenous antibiotics. Antibiotic therapy may need to continue for 2 to 3 weeks and, in some cases, may require placement of an indwelling intravenous catheter for outpatient administration of antibiotics. PPS infections that are extensive or refractory to antibiotics require surgical drainage by the transoral route for lesions medial to the great vessels or transcervically for lesions lateral to the great vessels.

Retropharyngeal Space Infections

Children with infections of the retropharyngeal space present with fever, drooling, neck pain or stiffness, torticollis, and cervical adenitis. Diagnosis is suspected by a bulging of the posterior pharyngeal wall and confirmed by CECT (Fig. 10-8). As with PPS infections, antibiotics are useful for small collections, and surgery is reserved for abscesses that fail to resolve with intravenous antibiotics. Surgical drainage may be performed transorally or externally, depending on the abscess location. Transoral drainage is most straightforward for abscesses above the hyoid, whereas more inferior collections may be better approached via an external transhyoid or lateral route.

FUNGAL INFECTIONS OF THE ORAL CAVITY AND PHARYNX

Candidiasis

Children receiving chronic antibiotic therapy or corticosteroids, and neonates with their transient immunodeficiency, may be afflicted by this oral fungal infection.

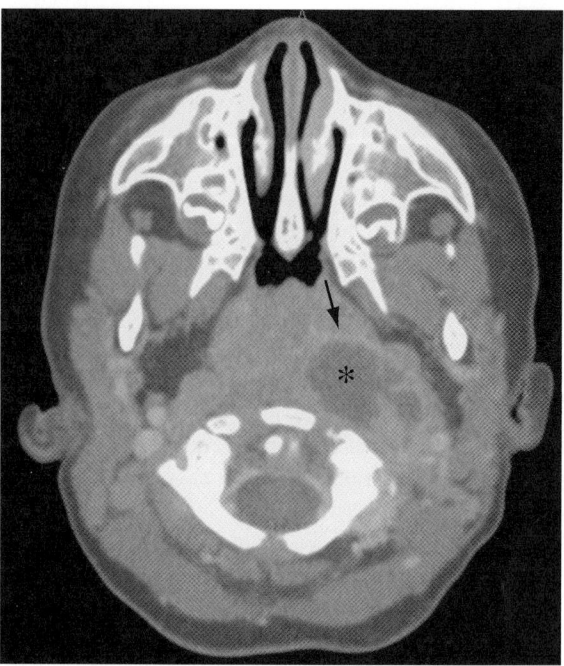

Figure 10-8. Retropharyngeal abscess. This abscess *(asterisk)* is within the rim-enhancing wall *(arrow)* on this contrast-enhanced CT scan.

Candidal infection (thrush, moniliasis) appears as patchy, white, curdlike aggregations on the tongue, palate, or buccal mucosa that may be wiped off with a gauze pad, leaving a raw, painful, bleeding surface. Evidence to date does not suggest that chronic oral candidiasis predisposes to neoplasia.[12] Treatment is with oral nystatin rinses. Swabbing a newborn's mouth with the mother's saliva also has been recommended.[12]

SUMMARY

Infections of the oral cavity and pharynx in children are frequently seen. Accurate diagnosis requires a complete history and thorough physical examination. Radiographic studies are reserved for atypical presentations, infections refractory to initial therapy, or guiding surgical drainage.

Most viral infections are managed by supportive care, including hydration and pain control. Most bacterial infections are initially managed by antibiotics; surgical therapy may be required for chronic infections (e.g., GABHS tonsillitis), regional spread (e.g., PPS infection), or airway obstruction (e.g., Ludwig's angina).

Successful management of these infections requires attention to the nuances of the usually characteristic physical examination findings specific to each infectious diagnosis, awareness of the potential for rapid spread of infection, and a proactive and team-oriented approach to therapy.

MAJOR POINTS

Viral pharyngitis is common in children. Aspirin and aspirin-containing products should not be given, because they may cause Reye's syndrome.
Antibiotic therapy for acute GABHS pharyngitis reduces the risk of rheumatic fever complications.
There are specific criteria for treatment of GABHS carriers.
Radiographic characterization of parapharyngeal and retropharyngeal infections is important for diagnosis and determination of the best surgical approach. Follow-up studies after recovery from the initial episode are not usually indicated.

REFERENCES

1. Berrington de Gonzalez A, Darby S: Risk of cancer from diagnostic X-rays: Estimates for the UK and 14 other countries. Lancet 2004;363:345-351.
2. Wald ER: Commentary: Antibiotic treatment of pharyngitis. Pediatr Rev 2001;22:255-256.
3. Chow EL: Cherry JD, Harrison R, et al: Reassessing Reye syndrome. Arch Pediatr Adolesc Med 2003;157:1241-1242.
4. David MP, Darden PM: Use of complementary and alternative medicine by children in the United States. Arch Pediatr Adolesc Med 2003157: 393-396.
5. Sampson M, Campbell K, Ajiferuke I, Moher D: Randomized controlled trials in pediatric complementary and alternative medicine: Where can they be found? BMC Pediatr 2003;3:1.
6. Harrison H, Fixsen A, Vickers A: A randomized comparison of homeopathic and standard care for the treatment of glue ear in children. Complement Ther Med 1999;7: 132-135.
7. Jacobs J, Springer DA, Crothers DA: Homeopathic treatment of acute otitis media in children: A preliminary randomized placebo-controlled trial. Pediatr Infect Dis J 2001;20:177-183.
8. Riley D, Fischer M, Singh B,et al: Homeopathy and conventional medicine: An outcomes study comparing effectiveness in a primary care setting. J Altern Complement Med 2001;7:149-159.
9. Krause JH, Krause HJ: Patient use of traditional and complementary therapies in treating rhinosinusitis before consulting an otolaryngologist. Laryngoscope 1999;109: 1223-1227.
10. Barnett ED, Levatin JL, Chapman EH, et al: Challenges of evaluating homeopathic treatment of otitis media. Pediatr Infect Dis J 2000;19:273-275.
11. Woolf AD: Herbal remedies and children: Do they work? Are they harmful? Pediatrics 2003;112:240-246.
12. Bhaskar SN: Synopsis of Oral Pathology. St. Louis, Mosby, 1986, pp 94-97, 434-443, 460-461.
13. Bisno AL: Acute pharyngitis. N Engl J Med 2001;344: 205-211.
14. Pickering LK (ed): Red Book: 2006 Report of the Committee on Infectious Diseases, 27th ed. Elk Grove Village, Ill, American Academy of Pediatrics, 2006, pp 361-371, 441-451, 464-468, 711-714.
15. Brook I: The role of anaerobic bacteria in tonsillitis. Int J Pediatr Otorhinolaryngol 2005;69:9-19.
16. Dakdouki GK, Obeid KH, Kanj SS: Azithromycin-induced rash in infectious mononucleosis. Scand J Infect Dis 2002;34:939-941.
17. Geyman JP, Erickson S: The ampicillin rash as a diagnostic and management problem: Case reports and literature review. J Fam Pract 1978;7:493-496.
18. Windfuhr JP, Chen YS, Remmert S: Hemorrhage following tonsillectomy and adenoidectomy in 15,218 patients. Otolaryngol Head Neck Surg 2005;132:281-286.
19. Windfuhr J: Personal communication. August 1, 2005.
20. Raborn GW, Grace MG: Recurrent herpes simplex labialis: Selected therapeutic options. J Can Dent Assoc 2003; 69:498-503.
21. Smitheringale AJ: Acquired diseases of the oral cavity and pharynx. In Wetmore RF, Muntz HR, McGill TJI (eds): Pediatric Otolaryngology. New York, Thieme, 2000, pp 607-618.
22. Raborn GW, Chan KS, Grace MJ: Treatment modalities and medication recommended by health care professionals for treating recurrent herpes labialis. Am Dent Assoc 2004;135:48-54.
23. Miyairi I, Franklin JA, Andreansky M, et al: Acute necrotizing ulcerative gingivitis and bacteremia caused by *Stenotrophomonas maltophilia* in an immunocompromised host. Pediatr Infect Dis J 2005;24:181-183.
24. Sayany Z: Pediatric dental emergencies. In Burg FD, Ingelfinger JR, Polin RA, Gershon AA (eds): Gellis and Kagan's Current Pediatric Therapy, 17th ed. Philadelphia, WB Saunders, 2002, pp 1123-1125.
25. Gallis HA: Streptococcus. In Joklik WK, Willett, HP, Amos DB, Wilfert CM (eds): Zinsser Microbiology, 19th ed. East Norwalk, CT: Appleton & Lange, 1988, pp 357-367.
26. Martin JM, Green M, Barbadora KA, Wald ER: Group A streptococci among school-aged children: Clinical characteristics and the carrier state. Pediatrics 2004;114:1212-1219.
27. Pichichero ME, Casey JR: Defining and dealing with carriers of group A streptococci. Contemp Pediatrics 2003;1:46.
28. Kvestad E, Kvaerner KJ, Roysamb E, et al: Heritability of recurrent tonsillitis. Arch Otolaryngol Head Neck Surg 2005;131:383-387.
29. Kara CO, Ergin H, Kocak G, et al: Prevalence of tonsillar hypertrophy and associated oropharyngeal symptoms in primary school children in Denizeil, Turkey. Int J Pediatr Otorhinolaryngol 2002;66:175-179.

30. Darrow DH, Siemens C: Indications for tonsillectomy and adenoidectomy. Laryngoscope 2002;112(Suppl 100, Pt 2): 6-10.

31. Brodsky L: Tonsil and adenoid disorders. In Gates GA (ed): Current Therapy in Otolaryngology—Head and Neck Surgery, 6th ed. St. Louis, Mosby, 1998, p 414-417.

32. Kaplan EL: The group A streptococcal upper respiratory carrier. In Pechere JC, Kaplan EF (eds): Streptococcal Pharyngitis, vol 3. Basel, Karger, 2004, pp 66-74.

33. Tanz RR: Clinical presentations of pediatric streptococcal pharyngitis in developed countries. In Pechere JC, Kaplan EF (eds): Streptococcal Pharyngitis, vol 3. Basel, Karger, 2004, pp 16-21.

34. Shah UK: Tonsillitis and peritonsillar abscess. Available at http://www.emedicine.com/ ent/topic314.htm.

35. Brook I, Gober AE: Treatment of non-streptococcal tonsillitis with metronidazole. Int J Pediatr Otorhinolaryngol 2005;69:65-68.

36. Wei JL, Kasperbauer JL, Weaver AL, Boggust AJ: Efficacy of single-dose dexamethasone as adjuvant therapy for acute pharyngitis. Laryngoscope 2002;112:97-93.

37. Stevens DL: Virulence factors of *Streptococcus pyogenes*. In Pechere JC, Kaplan EF (eds): Streptococcal Pharyngitis, vol 3. Basel, Karger, 2004, pp 3-15.

38. Paradise JL, Bluestone CD, Colborn DK, et al: Tonsillectomy and adenotonsillectomy for recurrent throat infection in moderately affected children. Pediatrics 2002;110:7-15.

39. Wolfensberger M, Haury J-A, Linder T: Parent satisfaction 1 year after adenotonsillectomy of their children. Int J Pediatr Otorhinolaryngol 2000;56;199-205.

40. Ron E, Lubin JH, Shore RE, et al: Thyroid cancer after exposure to external radiation: A pooled analysis of seven studies. Radiat Res 1995;141:259-277.

41. Schneider AB, Favus MJ, Stachura ME, et al: Salivary gland neoplasms as a late consequence of head and neck irradiation. Ann Intern Med 1977;87:160-164.

42. Cohen J, Gierlowski TC, Schneider AB: A prospective study of hyperparathyroidism in individuals exposed to radiation in childhood. JAMA 1990;264:581-584.

43. Cherukuri S, Benninger MS: Use of bacteriologic studies in the outpatient management of peritonsillar abscess. Laryngoscope 2002;112:18-20.

44. Schraff S, McGin JD, Derkay CS: Peritonsillar abscess in children: A 10-year review of diagnosis and management. Int J Pediatr Otorhinolaryngol 2001;57:213-218.

45. Licameli GR, Grillone GA: Inferior pole peritonsillar abscess. Otolaryngol Head Neck Surg 1998;118:95-99.

46. Bauer PW, Lieu JEC, Suskind DL, Lusk RP: The safety of conscious sedation in peritonsillar abscess drainage. Arch Otolaryngol Head Neck Surg 2001;127:1477-1480.

CHAPTER 11

Infectious and Inflammatory Disorders of the Upper Airway

STEPHEN G. WOLFE, MD
STEVEN D. HANDLER, MD, MBE

Infectious and inflammatory disorders of the pediatric upper airway can lead to potentially life-threatening airway obstruction. Depending on the degree of airway obstruction, it may be necessary to perform the diagnostic evaluation and management simultaneously. Fortunately, with improvements in antibiotics, vaccinations, and techniques for airway management, the morbidity and mortality of acute airway obstruction have greatly decreased. This chapter reviews the signs and symptoms of acute airway obstruction, infectious and inflammatory disorders of the pediatric airway, and evaluation and management of acute airway obstruction.

SIGNS AND SYMPTOMS OF ACUTE AIRWAY OBSTRUCTION

Signs

General Appearance

The general appearance of a patient quickly provides a significant amount of information about his or her respiratory status. Children in respiratory distress may present with tachypnea and signs of air hunger, including restlessness, anxiety, and diaphoresis. To maximize their respiratory status, patients may use accessory muscles of respiration or position themselves in a way to improve their airway, such as the characteristic "tripod position" of patients with supraglottitis. As the airway obstruction progresses or the patient becomes more fatigued, the patient may become cyanotic, obtunded, or unconscious. In these cases, immediate intervention is critical.

Stridor

Stridor is the sound produced by turbulent airflow through the larynx or trachea. An intrinsic or extrinsic lesion narrows the airway, causing turbulent flow and stridor. The timing of the stridor can help localize the site of the lesion narrowing the airway. Inspiratory stridor is usually produced by lesions in the subglottis or glottis that are pulled into and narrow the airway with inspiration. Expiratory stridor is usually produced by abnormalities in the distal trachea and bronchi, which cause increased obstruction with the relatively positive intrathoracic pressure of expiration. Biphasic stridor is usually produced by lesions in the midportion of the trachea.

The frequency of the stridor increases as the airway diameter decreases secondary to the obstruction. Generally, the intensity of the stridor increases with an increase in the pressure gradient across the obstruction and velocity of the airflow. It is important to note that increased intensity does not necessarily correlate with increased obstruction. In fact, the intensity of the stridor may decrease as the obstruction becomes almost complete.

Vocal Changes

Vocal changes are the result of inflammation or obstruction and can manifest as hoarseness, muffling of the voice, and aphonia. Hoarseness is typically caused by inflammation of the mucosa of the larynx and, in particular, the true vocal folds. A muffled voice is characteristic of upper airway obstruction from adenotonsillar hypertrophy. Aphonia is the most ominous sign and may indicate impending respiratory collapse. In addition, patients with respiratory distress may not be able to speak a full sentence without taking multiple breaths.

Drooling

Drooling results from patients being unable to swallow their secretions secondary to pain or edema. It is a common sign of supraglottitis.

Symptoms

Dyspnea

Dyspnea is the most obvious symptom of respiratory distress. The patient may complain of shortness of breath and present with rapid or labored breathing. There may be a positional component to the dyspnea, with certain positions alleviating and others worsening it.

Vocal Symptoms

Patients and families may complain of vocal changes such as hoarseness, muffling of the voice, or aphonia (see "Vocal Changes").

Dysphagia

Depending on the location and severity of the obstruction, patients may complain of difficulty swallowing solids and/or liquids. Patients with adenotonsillar hypertrophy may have difficulty swallowing solid foods but may drink liquids without difficulty. Patients with supraglottitis may not be able to tolerate either liquids or solids or may not even be able to swallow their own saliva, depending on the amount of supraglottic and hypopharyngeal edema.

Other Symptoms

Coughing is usually a nonspecific symptom triggered by inflammation or irritation of the aerodigestive tract. In cases of laryngotracheobronchitis, the cough can assume a barking quality, which is a hallmark of croup. Sore throat is another nonspecific symptom of upper aerodigestive tract inflammation and irritation, which can usually be seen in varying degrees with most of the following disorders.

SPECIFIC DISORDERS

Disorders with Infectious Causes

Laryngotracheobronchitis (Croup)

Laryngotracheobronchitis (LTB), or croup, is a viral upper respiratory tract infection most commonly caused by parainfluenza virus types I, II, and III[1] and influenza virus types A and B. Croup typically affects children between 6 months and 3 years of age, with a peak incidence at 2 years of age.[2] It is the most common cause of upper airway obstruction in patients between 6 months and 6 years of age.[3]

Children with croup typically present with a 2- to 6-day history of an antecedent upper respiratory tract infection that progresses to the characteristic barking cough, biphasic stridor, and hoarseness. Fever and leukocytosis may also be present. The pathophysiology of croup involves symmetrical narrowing of the subglottis secondary to mucosal edema.

The diagnosis of croup is mainly based on history and physical examination. Anteroposterior neck radiographs demonstrating symmetrical subglottic narrowing, the steeple sign (Fig. 11-1), will support the diagnosis; however, radiographic findings are neither sensitive nor specific. Endoscopic evaluation of the larynx, which is usually not indicated, reveals edematous, erythematous, subglottic tissues below the true vocal folds, without significant secretions (Fig. 11-2).

Treatment includes the use of humidified air, nebulized racemic epinephrine, and steroids. The use of humidified air is based on mainly anecdotal evidence and is believed to soothe inflamed mucosa and improve clearance of secretions.[2] Nebulized racemic epinephrine provides a temporary reduction in airway resistance, presumably through α-adrenergic-mediated vasoconstriction within

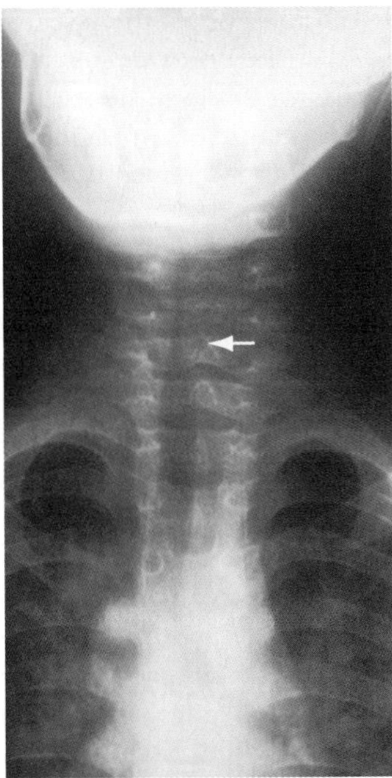

Figure 11-1. Anteroposterior radiograph of the neck region of child with croup. Note the steeple sign *(white arrow)*.

the edematous subglottic mucosa and β-adrenergic-mediated bronchodilation.[3]

Corticosteroids are often used in both the outpatient and inpatient treatment of moderate to severe croup. Although their exact mechanism of action is unknown, corticosteroids may potentially decrease vascular permeability and thus mucosal edema.[4,5] Most clinicians will give severely affected children a single dose of steroids at 0.6 to 1.5 mg/kg dexamethasone equivalent.[2,3]

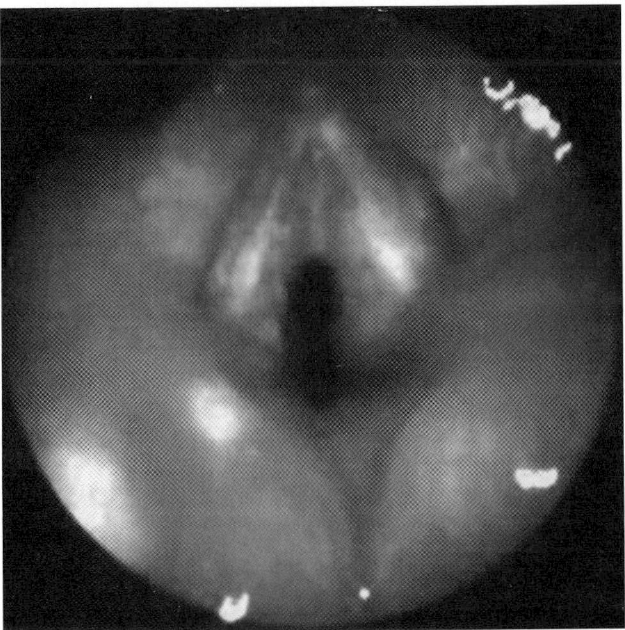

Figure 11-2. Endoscopic view of the airway of a patient with croup.

Intubation and tracheostomy should be avoided, if possible, but are occasionally necessary to secure the child's airway. If intubation is required, an endotracheal tube at least one-half to one size smaller than normal is recommended to minimize the risk of acquired subglottic stenosis.

An endoscopic airway evaluation should be considered in patients with recurrent croup who are younger than 1 year of age, patients with persistent airway symptoms between episodes of croup, patients with severe, atypical, or recurrent croup,[2,3] and patients who respond poorly to therapy. Ideally, endoscopy is performed 3 to 4 weeks after an episode of croup to allow time for resolution of the acute inflammation.

Supraglottitis (Epiglottitis)

Supraglottitis is an acute bacterial infection of the epiglottis and other supraglottic structures (arytenoids and aryepiglottic folds) that can lead to severe acute airway obstruction. The pathogen most commonly identified in supraglottitis is *Haemophilus influenzae* type b (HIB). With the development of the HIB vaccine in the late 1980s and early 1990s, the incidence of pediatric supraglottitis has greatly decreased.[6]

Supraglottitis typically affects children between 2 and 7 years of age. The onset is acute, with signs and symptoms including fever, inspiratory and expiratory stridor, dysphagia, odynophagia, and drooling developing in 2 to 6 hours. Paradoxically, inspiratory stridor may decrease secondary to less air movement as the obstruction becomes more significant or the child becomes more fatigued. Supraglottitis patients appear toxic and often assume the tripod sitting position (leaning forward on their extended arms), using accessory muscles of respiration to facilitate air exchange.

The presumptive diagnosis of supraglottitis is based on the clinical presentation. The physical examination should be limited and the intraoral examination deferred until the patient is in the operating room with the appropriate personnel and equipment. A lateral neck radiograph can be obtained at the patient's bedside to support the diagnosis. The classic radiographic finding is widening of the epiglottis, known as the thumbprint sign (Fig. 11-3). In addition, ballooning of the hypopharynx can be seen as the child tries to inspire through a restricted laryngeal airway.

To confirm the diagnosis, the patient should be transferred to the operating room with an anesthesiologist and an airway surgeon ready to intervene with urgent intubation or tracheostomy, if needed. The patient should be allowed to sit upright while anesthesia is induced. When the patient is anesthetized, direct laryngoscopy and intubation can be performed, usually with an endotracheal tube one size smaller than normal. The characteristic finding on examination is a cherry red, edematous

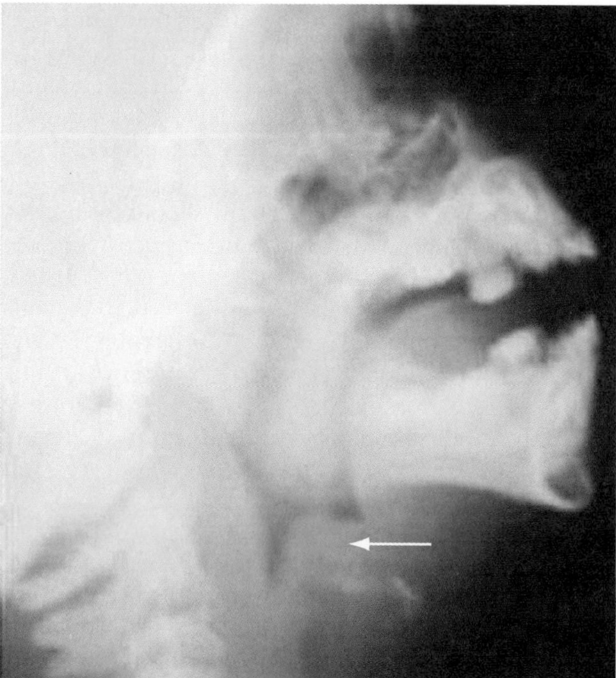

Figure 11-3. Lateral neck radiograph of child with supraglottitis. Note the thumbprint sign *(white arrow)*.

epiglottis (Fig. 11-4). Specimens for supraglottic and blood cultures can be obtained.

Patients with supraglottitis require antibiotics, usually a second- or third-generation cephalosporin such as ceftriaxone or cefuroxime. The antibiotic regimen can later be tailored based on the results of the cultures.

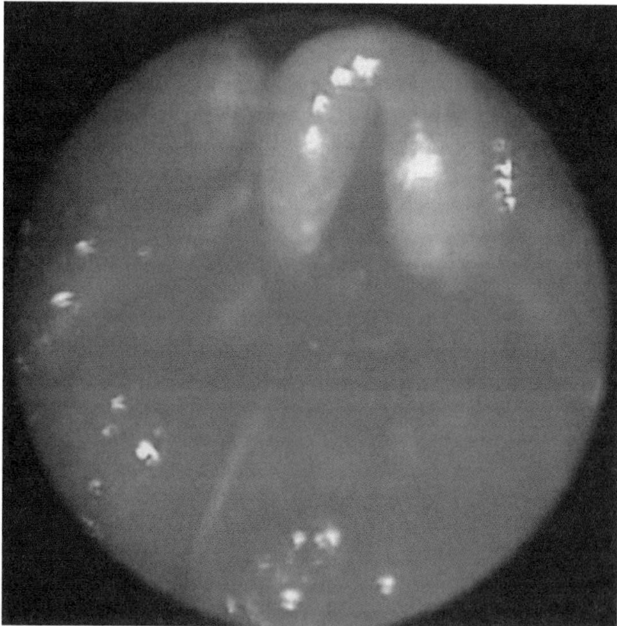

Figure 11-4. Endoscopic view of the airway of a patient with supraglottitis.

Steroids are also often used, but there is currently no conclusive evidence that they provide a benefit.[7] Intubation is usually necessary for 24 to 48 hours. When the supraglottic structures normalize in appearance and a cuff leak develops around the endotracheal tube, extubation can be performed.

Bacterial Tracheitis

Bacterial tracheitis is an infection of the pediatric airway characterized by signs of acute upper airway obstruction caused by narrowing of the airway secondary to purulent debris, which can form pseudomembranes within the trachea. The most common bacteria responsible for tracheitis include *Staphylococcus aureus*, *Haemophilus influenzae*,[8] and *Moraxella catarrhalis*.[9]

Patients normally present with stridor and cough, a symptom complex similar to that of viral croup. Bacterial tracheitis can be either a primary infection or a secondary superinfection after a viral illness, such as croup.[9] High fever and leukocytosis help differentiate bacterial tracheitis from croup. In addition, lateral neck radiographs demonstrate thickened tracheal membranes in approximately 80% of cases.[9]

The diagnosis is confirmed on endoscopy by the presence of thick, purulent secretions. Specimens for tracheal and blood cultures are obtained. At the time of evaluation, therapeutic bronchoscopy is often needed to remove debris and crusting. Endotracheal intubation is usually necessary to support the airway, with reported intubation rates higher than 80%.[10] Treatment consists of appropriate antibiotic therapy and therapeutic bronchoscopy, as necessary.

Retropharyngeal and Parapharyngeal Infections

Deep neck space infections can manifest with symptoms of upper airway obstruction. The pathogen most commonly identified in infections of the retropharyngeal and parapharyngeal spaces is *Staphylococcus aureus*, but Streptococcal species and anaerobic bacteria have also been identified.[11,12]

Patients with retropharyngeal and parapharyngeal infections commonly present with fever, sore throat, odynophagia, limited neck motility and, occasionally, torticollis. Seven percent of patients in one study presented with difficulty breathing.[11] Physical examination may demonstrate pharyngeal erythema, bulging of the pharyngeal soft tissue at the site of the infection (posteriorly for retropharyngeal infections and laterally for parapharyngeal infections), and cervical lymphadenopathy, induration, and erythema, which is usually more pronounced on the affected side.

A lateral neck radiograph may show thickening of the retropharyngeal soft tissue with an infection in this space; however, computed tomography (CT) of the neck with contrast is the radiographic study of choice to

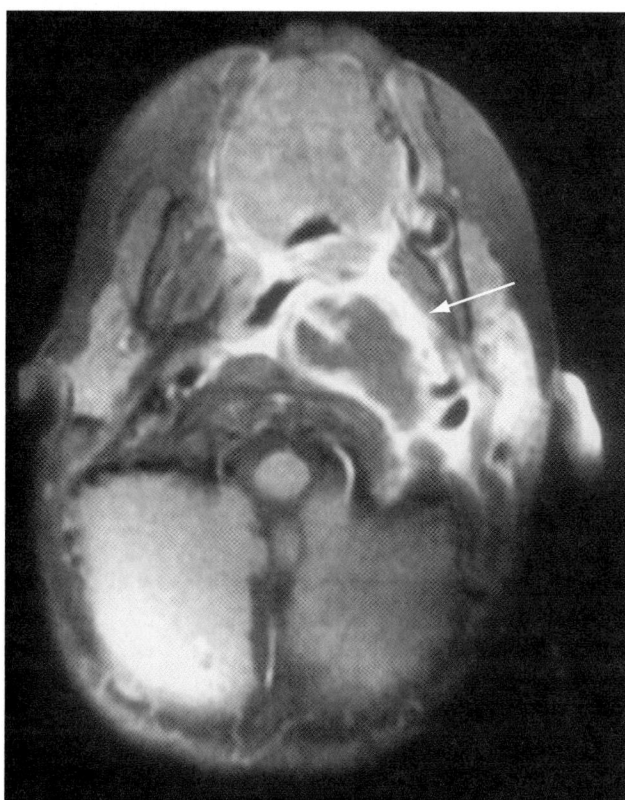

Figure 11-5. Axial CT scan of the head of a child with retropharyngeal abscess *(white arrow)* that compromises the airway.

evaluate these infections (Fig. 11-5). In particular, a study by Wetmore and colleagues[12] has demonstrated a 92% correlation between the presence of a rim-enhancing lesion on a contrast-enhanced CT with the presence of an abscess at the time of surgical intervention.

Patients with retropharyngeal and parapharyngeal infections should be treated with broad-spectrum antibiotics. If there is compromise of the airway, intubation may be necessary. One study[11] has documented that 3% of patients with deep neck space infections require such airway support. Some abscesses can be needle-aspirated. Surgical drainage through an external cervical (for parapharyngeal abscess) or intraoral (for retropharyngeal abscess) approach may be necessary if an abscess fails to resolve with antibiotics and/or needle aspiration.

Tuberculosis

The incidence of laryngeal tuberculosis has risen in recent years secondary to the increasing number of immunocompromised patients and of multidrug-resistant organisms. Patients with laryngeal tuberculosis typically present with hoarseness, cough, odynophagia, dysphagia, and nonspecific symptoms such as weight loss, fevers, and fatigue. Laryngeal tuberculosis may develop in the absence of pulmonary symptoms or a history of pulmonary tuberculosis.[13]

The diagnosis of laryngeal tuberculosis is based on a combination of findings—positive purified protein derivative (PPD) skin testing, characteristic findings on chest radiography, including apical infiltrates and cavitary lesions, and positive sputum samples. Cultures of *Mycobacterium tuberculosis*, a fastidious organism, are difficult to obtain but are necessary to confirm diagnosis and test drug sensitivities. Tissue biopsies and histologic evaluation demonstrate caseating granulomas and acid-fast organisms.

The primary treatment is a multiple chemotherapeutic regimen, including isoniazid, rifampin, and ethambutol. The increasing incidence of drug-resistant *M. tuberculosis* dictates the use of a number of drugs and the need for close monitoring to ensure patient compliance. Patients with severe airway obstruction require tracheostomy.

Fungal Infections

Laryngeal fungal infections are rare in immunocompetent patients. Fungi that may involve the larynx include *Histoplasma capsulatum*, *Blastomyces dermatitidis*, and *Candida albicans*. Symptoms are progressive and include hoarseness, dyspnea, dysphagia, and pain. The diagnosis is confirmed with culture or biopsy, with special stains for fungal elements. The mainstay of treatment is antifungal medications, such as amphotericin B, itraconazole, and ketoconazole, and airway support.

Disorders with Inflammatory Causes

Spasmodic Croup

Spasmodic croup is a noninfectious form of laryngeal inflammation with an unclear cause, although possible triggers include gastroesophageal reflux and allergy. Spasmodic croup affects children 1 to 3 years old and presents with the sudden onset of a barking cough, stridor, and mild dyspnea in the middle of the night. In contrast to children with laryngotracheobronchitis, patients with spasmodic croup do not present with a viral prodrome and fevers. These episodes can be isolated or recur over two or three nights. The airway obstruction from spasmodic croup is usually mild and can be successfully treated on an outpatient basis with humidification and reassurance. Occasionally, a short course of corticosteroids is necessary.

Foreign Bodies

The ingestion or aspiration of a foreign body can present with stridor, depending on its location. Foreign bodies of the glottis and subglottis can present in a manner similar to that of croup, with the sudden onset of inspiratory stridor and dyspnea. Foreign bodies of the tracheal and bronchial airways can present with the sudden onset of cough and persistent wheezing. Finally, foreign bodies of the cervical esophagus can compress the posterior glottis and cause airway obstruction.

The diagnosis of a radiopaque foreign body is easily made with a lateral neck or chest radiograph. However, radiolucent foreign bodies are more difficult to detect. A barium swallow may identify a radiolucent object in the esophagus, but this study is often avoided because the barium may complicate endoscopic removal. A lateral neck radiograph may show subglottic edema similar to that of croup if there is a radiolucent subglottic foreign body. Chest radiography including inspiratory, expiratory, and lateral decubitus views may demonstrate atelectasis, infiltrates, or air trapping in cases of radiolucent objects in the tracheal and bronchial airways. Rigid endoscopy is usually used for the removal of foreign bodies of the upper aerodigestive tract.

Adenotonsillar Hypertrophy

Children with adenotonsillar hypertrophy usually present with chronic airway obstruction and, most notably, obstructive symptoms at night. Symptoms include loud snoring, irregular breathing, nocturnal choking and coughing, restless sleep with frequent awakenings, and daytime hypersomnolence. In severe cases, patients may have failure to thrive or develop congestive heart failure from cor pulmonale. Viral or bacterial upper respiratory infections can precipitate acute airway obstruction or exacerbate existing obstructive symptoms. Patients with craniofacial anomalies, Down syndrome, or central nervous system (CNS) or neuromuscular abnormalities, particularly those that cause hypotonia, are at increased risk of airway obstruction, even with less clinically impressive hypertrophy.

Examination of the tonsils reveals their size and may also demonstrate signs of infection, including erythema and exudates. The inferior poles of the tonsils must be carefully examined, because hypertrophy in this area may not be as readily evident on intraoral examination. Tonsillar size does not always correlate with the severity of symptoms[14]; however, in most cases, the diagnosis is clinically obvious. Multichannel polysomnography, the gold standard in the diagnosis of obstructive sleep apnea, can document the severity of the obstruction in ambiguous cases.

The treatment of acute airway obstruction from adenotonsillar hypertrophy is airway stabilization, with a nasopharyngeal airway or endotracheal intubation. Antibiotics and corticosteroids will treat an underlying infection and reduce the size of the lymphoid tissue.[14] In severe cases unresponsive to medical management, urgent adenotonsillectomy is necessary to relieve the airway obstruction.[15]

Wegener's Granulomatosis

Wegener's granulomatosis is a multisystem inflammatory disorder characterized by a necrotizing granulomatous vasculitis of the vessels of the respiratory tract, kidneys, and other organs. Wegener's has an affinity for the ciliated respiratory epithelium of the upper respiratory tract, particularly the nasal cavity and paranasal sinuses. Not surprisingly, 75% of patients diagnosed with Wegener's granulomatosis display head and neck manifestations,[16] including chronic sinusitis, nasal crusting and obstruction, and mucosal lesions of the nasopharynx.

Laryngeal involvement is present in up to 23% of patients with Wegener's granulomatosis [17] and typically manifests as subglottic stenosis. However, almost 50% of pediatric and adolescent patients who present with Wegener's granulomatosis will develop laryngeal disease.[16] The most common signs and symptoms are dyspnea and hoarseness, although biphasic stridor may develop.

Diagnosis is based on the characteristic pathologic features of necrotizing granulomatous vasculitis in the absence of an underlying infectious cause. In addition, the serologic test for c-ANCA (cytoplasmic pattern antinuclear cytoplasmic antibody) is positive in 90% of patients with active Wegener's granulomatosis.[18] Treatment requires corticosteroids and possibly cyclophosphamide or methotrexate.[18] If laryngeal stenosis severely compromises the airway, surgical dilation or tracheostomy may be necessary.

Sarcoidosis

Sarcoidosis is a chronic granulomatous disease of unknown cause. It usually presents in young adults and is more common in women and African Americans. The most common sites of involvement are the lymph nodes, lungs, spleen, and liver. Although many patients with sarcoidosis are asymptomatic, those patients with symptoms typically complain of respiratory symptoms, including cough and shortness of breath or generalized symptoms, including fever and fatigue.

The larynx is involved in 1% to 5% of patients with sarcoidosis.[19] Sarcoidosis usually involves the supraglottic structures, especially the epiglottis, which may be pale and edematous. The vocal cords are usually not involved.

The diagnosis of sarcoidosis requires histologic documentation of noncaseating granulomas. The diagnosis is also supported by chest radiographs demonstrating bilateral hilar adenopathy and laboratory test results including elevated levels of serum angiotensin-converting enzyme, C-reactive protein, erythrocyte sedimentation rate, and serum and urine calcium. The mainstay of treatment for sarcoidosis is long-term oral corticosteroids or possibly intralesional steroid injections.[19]

Juvenile Rheumatoid Arthritis

Juvenile rheumatoid arthritis (JRA) affects children 16 years of age and younger and is characterized by the persistence of objective inflammatory findings in one or more joints for at least 6 weeks in the absence of other causes of joint inflammation. There are five subtypes of JRA, differentiated based on the systemic symptoms of the disease (e.g., high spiking fevers, rash, lymphadenopathy, hepatosplenomegaly, malaise, and weight loss) and the number of joints involved in the first 6 months of the disease. The cause of JRA is believed to be immune-mediated; however, no autoantibody specific for JRA has been identified.

The airway manifestations of JRA include cricoarytenoid joint arthritis, which can precipitate airway obstruction, and bronchitis obliterans, which can cause marked pulmonary impairment. The diagnosis of these two conditions requires endoscopic examination. The overall diagnosis of JRA is based on the clinical presentation and the exclusion of other sources of joint inflammation. Treatment is medical and may include the use of aspirin, nonsteroidal anti-inflammatory drugs (NSAIDs), gold salts, methotrexate, sulfasalazine, and corticosteroids and physical and occupational therapy.

Laryngeal Trauma

Laryngeal trauma can be the result of blunt or penetrating neck injuries, thermal injuries, caustic ingestions, intubation injuries, high tracheostomy,[20] previous endolaryngeal surgery, and iatrogenic injury to the nerves innervating the larynx, which can result in a unilateral or bilateral vocal cord paralysis usually after thyroid, cardiac, or tracheoesophageal surgery.

In particular, acquired laryngeal stenosis secondary to intubation has been extensively studied. If the pressure of the endotracheal tube exceeds the tracheal mucosal capillary pressure, erosion and ulceration will occur.[21] In the pediatric larynx, the subglottis, which is the narrowest portion of the pediatric upper airway, is particularly susceptible to this type of injury. Other factors contributing to postintubation stenosis include prolonged intubation, superimposed bacterial infections,[22] and possibly gastroesophageal reflux.[23]

These lesions can be difficult to manage and may lead to significant long-term morbidity. It is important to recognize these possible problems and their sequelae and make every effort to prevent them. Surgical technique around the larynx must be meticulous to prevent endolaryngeal scarring or injury to the nerves innervating the larynx. Intubations should be performed with appropriately sized endotracheal tubes that are well secured. Tracheostomies should be performed in children who will require long-term airway support.

Recurrent Respiratory Papillomata

Recurrent respiratory papillomata (RRP) is characterized by multiple and recurrent squamous papillomata that most commonly affect the larynx. The human papillomavirus subtypes 6 and 11 cause juvenile RRP. These viruses, which also reside in the female genital tract, are most likely transmitted to infants during childbirth. However, cases of RRP have been reported after delivery by cesarean section.[24]

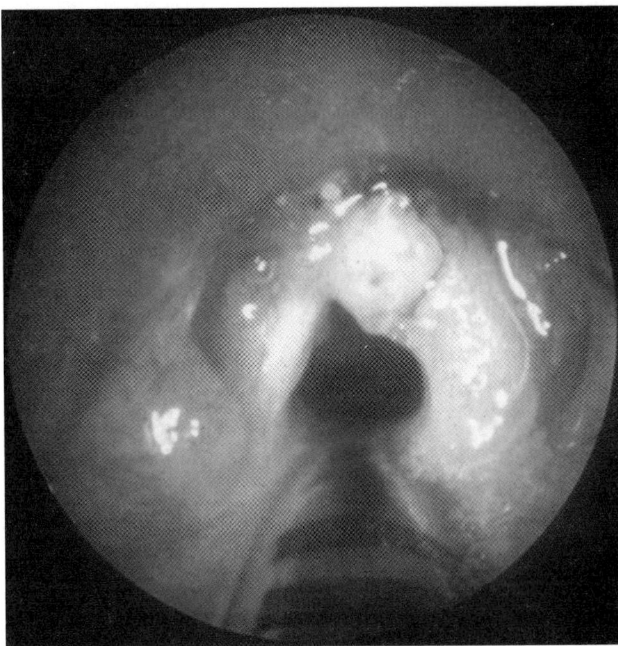

Figure 11-6. Endoscopic view of the airway of a patient with laryngeal papillomas on right vocal cord.

Children with RRP present with hoarseness, dyspnea, and stridor. The lesions typically affect the supraglottic larynx (Fig. 11-6), but careful examination of the entire upper airway is necessary to identify all lesions. The diagnosis is based on histologic evaluation of the lesions. In rare cases, dysplasia and malignant transformation are identified. Given the proliferative and recurrent nature of this disease, treatment usually requires frequent excisions of the lesions. The carbon dioxide (CO_2) laser and surgical microdébrider have both been advocated for the removal of papilloma. Care must be exercised to avoid surgically induced scarring and stenosis of larynx. Other therapies that have been used include photodynamic therapy, systemic interferon therapy,[25] methotrexate,[26] and intralesional cidofovir.[27] The long list of treatment options attests to the difficulty of controlling this disease. Tracheostomy is associated with an increased incidence of tracheal papillomatosis,[28] presumably from direct seeding, and should be avoided if testing is possible. Total remission of the disease occasionally occurs, especially as the patient approaches puberty.

Congenital Laryngeal Abnormalities

Subglottic hemangiomas usually become clinically evident in the first 6 months of a child's life and present with stridor and a crouplike cough. Only 50% of patients with subglottic hemangiomas have associated cutaneous hemangiomas, so a high index of suspicion must be maintained in the absence of visible skin lesions. The diagnosis may be suspected on lateral neck radiographs,

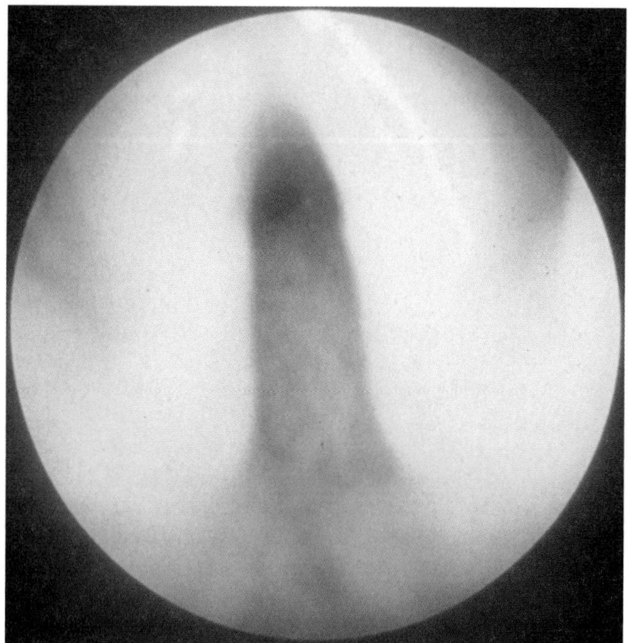

Figure 11-7. Endoscopic view of the airway of a patient with a subglottic hemangioma.

but it should be confirmed endoscopically (Fig. 11-7). Treatment options include local or systemic corticosteroids, laser excision, open surgical excision, and tracheostomy.[29]

Congenital bilateral vocal cord paralysis is most often the result of an Arnold-Chiari malformation. Patients usually present with respiratory distress, stridor, and a normal cry or voice. Diagnosis is made by flexible fiberoptic evaluation of vocal cord mobility. Treatment options include observation or tracheostomy, depending on the severity of the obstruction.

Laryngeal atresia presents immediately after birth with severe respiratory distress and inability to ventilate the patient. Immediate tracheostomy is the only treatment option.

Anaphylaxis

Anaphylaxis is triggered by antigen-specific immunoglobulin E (IgE) antibody activation of mast cells, with subsequently release of potent inflammatory mediators. Signs and symptoms develop rapidly and include itching of the eyes, throat tightness, urticaria, tachycardia, bronchospasm, and airway-compromising edema. Treatment of anaphylaxis consists of establishing an airway and preventing circulatory collapse with intravenous fluids and subcutaneous epinephrine. Corticosteroids and antihistamines also help reverse the effects of the released inflammatory mediators.

Foods, medications, or insect stings can precipitate an anaphylactic reaction. It is important to identify the offending agent so that future episodes can be avoided.

Hereditary Angioedema

Hereditary angioedema is an autosomal dominant deficiency or dysfunction of C1 esterase inhibitor that leads to recurrent episodes of mucocutaneous edema. The edema is usually localized to the face, oral cavity, oropharynx, or larynx. It is nonpitting and not usually associated with urticaria, erythema, or pain. Local trauma usually triggers the edema. Diagnosis is confirmed with complement activation tests. Treatment includes establishing an airway, if necessary, and supportive measures, including subcutaneous epinephrine.

DIAGNOSTIC EVALUATION

Ventilation Assessment

The evaluation of a child with an airway obstruction includes the assessment of the child's ventilation status. In comparison with adults, children have a higher metabolic rate, which leads to increased oxygen consumption and carbon dioxide production. This higher metabolic rate results in a smaller respiratory reserve for children. Clinically, a child can decompensate rapidly with increasing airway obstruction or fatigue from working harder to overcome an obstruction.

Noninvasive methods of monitoring ventilation include pulse oximetry and transcutaneous carbon dioxide monitoring.[30] Determination of arterial blood gas levels can also be used to assess ventilation. However, the results of arterial blood gas testing may not accurately reflect the child's true ventilation status if testing is done while the child is vigorously crying and struggling. An indwelling arterial line overcomes this sampling problem.

Radiologic Evaluation

Radiographic studies of the airway provide significant information for the evaluation of acute upper airway obstruction. In particular, lateral and anteroposterior neck radiographs are valuable to document the patency of the airway lumen, presence of mass lesions, or foreign bodies.[31] These are best recorded using the high-kilovoltage technique to enhance the tracheal air column and deemphasize the cervical spine. To provide the most accurate information, these films should be obtained with the neck in extension and during inspiration. Chest radiographs may demonstrate tracheal or bronchial pathology, intrinsic lung pathology, and distal sequelae of more proximal lesions, such as air trapping or atelectasis in the lungs from airway foreign bodies.

Endoscopic Evaluation

In selected patients, visualization of the airway can be performed with flexible or rigid instrumentation.

Flexible nasopharyngolaryngoscopy (NPL) enables a dynamic assessment of the airway to the level of the larynx and is the preferred method of diagnosing a vocal cord paralysis. This procedure is usually performed at the bedside or in the office, without sedation. A nasal vasoconstrictor and topical anesthetic can be applied to make the procedure more comfortable for the patient. As a precautionary note, flexible NPL should not be performed on children with suspected epiglottitis, because it may precipitate a complete airway obstruction.

A complete endoscopic evaluation of the subglottis and lower airways is best performed under general anesthesia. By using only an inhalational anesthetic, the dynamic movement of the airways can be assessed with a flexible bronchoscope as the patient breathes spontaneously. Rigid bronchoscopy, which offers superior optics and the ability to ventilate the patient, should also be performed.[32] A complete endoscopic evaluation is essential, because studies have demonstrated that multiple airway lesions may be found in one patient.[33,34]

MANAGEMENT OF ACUTE AIRWAY OBSTRUCTION

Nonsurgical Interventions

Observation

If the airway is stable, the patient may be admitted to an intensive care unit or other high-surveillance unit for observation and continuous monitoring. These units must have personnel available to secure the airway, if necessary.

Oxygen and Humidification

Supplemental oxygen can be administered by nasal cannula, face tent, or face mask to facilitate oxygenation. Humidification of inspired oxygen or air is believed to soothe inflamed mucosa and liquify secretions to aid expectoration.[4] Humidified oxygen is recommended for the treatment of LTB even though studies have not demonstrated a significant benefit.

Medical Therapy

Racemic Epinephrine

The efficacy of nebulized racemic epinephrine in the treatment of patients with LTB has been well documented.[35] Its action is mediated through α-adrenergic–mediated vasoconstriction of the airway mucosa and the subsequent reduction of edema.[5] Its effects last approximately 30 to 60 minutes. In the past, concern for a rebound effect and worsening of airway obstruction after the use of racemic epinephrine has led to the recommendation that children who have been given racemic epinephrine be admitted to the hospital for observation. However, research has shown that rebound rarely happens; it is probably safe to discharge patients from the emergency department if they are stable 3 hours after the administration of the racemic epinephrine.[4,5,35]

Corticosteroids

The anti-inflammatory effects of corticosteroids have been proven to reduce airway edema in patients with LTB,[1] postintubation edema,[36] and Epstein-Barr virus–mediated adenotonsillar hypertrophy.[37] In particular, a meta-analysis of studies evaluating the treatment of LTB has demonstrated that high-dose steroids result in significant clinical improvement at 12 and 24 hours and an 80% reduction in the incidence of intubation.[1]

Dexamethasone is the most commonly used corticosteroid for the treatment of airway obstruction because of its rapid absorption, long half-life, and high anti-inflammatory potency.[38] The usual dosage of dexamethasone for upper airway obstruction from edema is 0.6 to 1.5 mg/kg/day. Methylprednisolone can also be used, at a dosage of 5 to 7 mg/kg/day.[36]

Antibiotics

Most upper respiratory tract infections are uncomplicated viral infections that do not require antibiotics. However, bacterial infections, which may be primary or the result of a superinfection after a viral illness, necessitate antibiotic therapy. In comparison with patients with a purely viral infection, patients with bacterial infections often have a prolonged illness, with more severe signs and symptoms. Bacterial infections of the upper airway that require intravenous antibiotics include acute supraglottitis, bacterial tracheitis, and retropharyngeal and parapharyngeal abscesses.

Streptococcus pneumoniae, Haemophilus influenzae, Moraxella catarrhalis, and *Staphylococcus aureus* are common bacteria that can cause infections precipitating acute airway obstruction. Traditionally, ampicillin was the preferred antibiotic for the treatment of upper airway infections. The increasing incidence of bacterial resistance to antibiotics now dictates the use of more potent antibiotics. For example, patients with *H. influenzae* supraglottitis should be treated with higher generation cephalosporins, such as cefuroxime, cefotaxime, or ceftriaxone or ampicillin-sulbactam. Patients with *S. aureus*-mediated bacterial tracheitis should receive an intravenous antibiotic regimen effective against penicillinase-producing organisms.

Heliox

Heliox is a helium-oxygen mixture used for the management of airway obstruction. Helium, which has a lower density than that of the nitrogen it replaces, reduces the turbulence of this gas mixture. This decreased turbulence enables a more effective flow of oxygen past partially obstructing lesions of the larynx, trachea, and bronchi.

Heliox can be used to maintain oxygenation and potentially avoid intubation in selected patients with transient airway obstruction, or it can be used to maintain oxygenation until definitive airway control has been obtained.[39]

Nasopharyngeal and Oropharyngeal Airways

Nasopharyngeal (NP) and oropharyngeal (OP) airways help overcome airway obstruction from soft tissue collapse of the upper airway. An NP airway, inserted through the nares after lubrication, will bypass upper pharyngeal and soft palate collapse. This airway should only be long enough to bypass the soft palate; otherwise, it may stimulate airway-induced gagging. An OP airway, usually made of hard plastic, prevents obstruction from posterior displacement of the tongue. An NP airway is generally better tolerated than an OP airway.

Endotracheal Intubation

Endotracheal intubation has replaced tracheostomy as the treatment of choice for securing the airway in patients with acute airway compromise, particularly in cases of acute supraglottitis.[6] This paradigm shift is the result of technologic advances and the recognition that pediatric tracheostomies bring their own problems.

Endotracheal intubation can be performed orally or nasally by direct visualization with a laryngoscope, fiberoptic guidance with a flexible bronchoscope, lighted stylet for transcutaneous illumination, laryngeal mask or, rarely, blind attempts. Oral intubation is the most common method of endotracheal intubation, but is contraindicated in children with cervical spinal injuries that require neck immobilization. Endotracheal intubation of any means should be avoided in children who have suffered neck trauma with disruption of the larynx or trachea. Patients with laryngotracheal disruption typically present with subcutaneous emphysema and respiratory distress. They are best managed with emergency tracheostomy and immediate or staged repair of the injury.

Intubated children should remain in the intensive care unit or other high-surveillance unit for close monitoring. These children require sedation and arm restraints to decrease the likelihood of accidental self-extubation.

Transtracheal Ventilation

Transtracheal ventilation requires a large-bore (16-gauge) angiocatheter placed through the cricothyroid membrane. Oxygen is delivered after appropriate connective tubing has been attached to the angiocatheter. This technique can provide additional time in the management of acute airway obstruction; however, it is not a substitute for a more stable airway, such as an endotracheal tube or tracheostomy. In small children, transtracheal ventilation is inherently more difficult to perform because of the softness of the airway cartilages and mobility of the trachea.

Surgical Interventions

If the physician is unable to stabilize a child with an airway obstruction by nonsurgical intervention, surgical intervention, such as endoscopy, cricothyrotomy, or tracheostomy, must be carried out.

Endoscopy

A pediatric bronchoscope can establish an airway, permit ventilation, and facilitate endoscopic evaluation of the airway. The pathologic condition responsible for the obstruction can often be diagnosed with the bronchoscope. In some cases, the obstruction can be relieved through the bronchoscope and the child can then be intubated. Otherwise, a tracheostomy can be performed while the patient is being ventilated through the bronchoscope.

Cricothyrotomy

Cricothyrotomy involves making an incision through the cricothyroid membrane and inserting an endotracheal or tracheostomy tube to permit ventilation. This procedure enables rapid access to the airway in patients with complete airway obstruction that cannot be bypassed with less invasive interventions. Cricothyrotomy is for emergencies only and should be replaced by endotracheal intubation or a formal tracheostomy in a timely manner. If a cricothyrotomy is maintained for a prolonged period, perichondritis of the cricoid cartilage and subsequent subglottic stenosis may develop, leading to chronic airway obstruction and its associated morbidity.

Tracheostomy

Tracheostomy involves making an incision into the trachea a safe distance below the cricoid cartilage and inserting a tracheostomy tube to secure the airway. A tracheostomy is a more preferable type of airway than that obtained with a cricothyrotomy. Emergency tracheostomy can be performed quickly; however, it is associated with a higher incidence of complications including bleeding, especially from the thyroid gland, infection, subcutaneous emphysema, and pneumothorax. These complications must be recognized promptly and managed appropriately.

SUMMARY

Infectious and inflammatory disorders of the pediatric airway can compromise the airway and lead to respiratory distress. Their diagnosis and appropriate management can be lifesaving.

MAJOR POINTS

The general appearance of a patient quickly provides a significant amount of information about his or her respiratory status. Children in respiratory distress may present with tachypnea and signs of air hunger, including restlessness, anxiety, and diaphoresis.

Laryngotracheobronchitis (croup) is a viral upper respiratory tract infection that typically presents in children between 6 months and 3 years of age with a characteristic barking cough, inspiratory stridor, and hoarseness.

The incidence of supraglottitis (epiglottitis), an acute bacterial infection typically caused by *Haemophilus influenzae* type b (HIB), greatly decreased after the development and distribution of the HIB vaccine.

Foreign bodies of the upper aerodigestive tract can present with signs and symptoms that mimic those of other infectious and inflammatory disorders of the airway. A high index of suspicion, appropriate radiologic studies, and endoscopy are necessary for accurate diagnosis and treatment.

Clinically, a child can decompensate rapidly with increasing airway obstruction or fatigue from increased work of breathing necessary to overcome the obstruction.

Endotracheal intubation has replaced tracheostomy as the treatment of choice for securing the airway in patients with acute airway compromise, particularly in cases of acute supraglottitis.

If the physician is unable to stabilize a child with an airway obstruction by nonsurgical intervention, surgical intervention, such as endoscopy, cricothyrotomy, or tracheostomy, must be used.

REFERENCES

1. Kairys SW, Olmstead EM, O'Connor G: Steroid treatment of laryngotracheitis: A meta-analysis of the evidence from randomized trials. Pediatrics 1986;83:683-693.
2. Skolnik N: Croup. J Fam Pract 1993;37:165-170.
3. Baugh R, Gilmore BB: Infectious croup: A critical review. Otolaryngol Head Neck Surg 1986;95:460-466.
4. Stroud RH, Friedman NR: An update on inflammatory disorders of the pediatric airway: Epiglottitis, croup and tracheitis. Am J Otolaryngol 2001;22:268-275.
5. Ewig JM: Croup. Pediatr Annu 2002;31:125-130.
6. Senior BA, Radkowski D, MacArthur C, et al: Changing patterns in pediatric supraglottitis: A multi-institutional review, 1980 to 1992. Laryngoscope 1994;10:1314-1322.
7. Frantz TD, Ragson BM, Quesenberry CP: Acute epiglottitis in adults: Analysis of 129 cases. JAMA 1994;272:1358-1360.
8. Eckel HE, Widemann B, Damm M: Airway endoscopy in the diagnosis and treatment of bacterial tracheitis in children. Int J Pediatr Otorhinolaryngol 1993;27:147-157.
9. Bernstein T, Brilli R, Jacobs B: Is bacterial tracheitis changing? A 14-month experience in a pediatric intensive care unit. Clin Infect Dis 1998;27:458-462.
10. Liston SL, Gehrz RC, Siegel LG, Tilelli J: Bacterial tracheitis. Am J Dis Child 1983;137:764-767.
11. Ungkanont K, Yellon RF, Weissman JL, et al: Head and neck space infections in infants and children. Otolaryngol Head Neck Surg 1995;112:375-382.
12. Wetmore RF, Mahboubi S, Soyupak SK: Computed tomography in the evaluation of pediatric neck infections. Otolaryngol Head Neck Surg 1998;119:624-627.
13. Nishiike S, Irifune M, Doi K: Laryngeal tuberculosis: A report of 15 cases. Ann Otol Rhinol Laryngol 2002;111:916-918.
14. Potsic WP: Sleep apnea in children. Otolaryngol Clin North Am 1989;222:537-544.
15. Potsic WP, Pasquariello PS, Baranak CC, et al: Relief of upper airway obstruction by adenotonsillectomy. Otolaryngol Head Neck Surg 1986;94:476-480.
16. Lebovics RS, Hoffman GS, Leavitt RY: The management of subglottic stenosis in patients with Wegener's granulomatosis. Laryngoscope 1992;102:1341-1345.
17. Langford CA, Sneller MC, Hallahan CW, et al: Clinical features and therapeutic management of subglottic stenosis in patients with Wegener's granulomatosis. Arthritis Rheum 1996;39:1754-1760.
18. Duna GF, Galperin C, Hoffman GS: Wegener's granulomatosis. Rheum Dis Clin North Am 1995;21:949-986.
19. Krespi YP, Mitrani M, Husain S, Meltzer CJ: Treatment of laryngeal sarcoidosis with intralesional steroid injection. Ann Otol Rhino Laryngol 1987;96:713-715.
20. Jackson C: High tracheotomy and other errors as the chief causes of chronic laryngeal stenosis. Surg Gynecol Obstet 1921;32:392-398.
21. Gould SJ, Howard S: The histopathology of the larynx in the neonate following endotracheal intubation. J Pathol 1985;146:301-311.
22. Sasaki CT, Horiuchi M, Koss N: Tracheostomy-related subglottic stenosis: Bacteriologic pathogenesis. Laryngoscope 1979;89:857-865.
23. Koufman JA: The otolaryngologic manifestations of gastroesophageal reflux disease (GERD): A clinical investigation of 225 patients using ambulatory 24-hour pH monitoring and an experimental investigation of the role of acid and pepsin in the development of laryngeal injury. Laryngoscope 1991;101(Suppl 53):1-78.
24. Shah K, Kashima H: Rarity of cesarean delivery in cases of juvenile onset respiratory papillomatosis. Obstet Gynecol 1986;68:795-799.
25. Leventhal BG, Kashima HK, Mounts P, et al: Long-term response of recurrent respiratory papillomatosis to treatment with lymphoblastoid interferon alfa-N1. Papilloma Study Group. N Engl J Med 1991;325:613-617.
26. Avidano MA, Singleton GT: Adjuvant drug strategies in the treatment of recurrent respiratory papillomatosis. Otolaryngol Head Neck Surg 1995;112:197-202.

27. Snoeck R, Wellens W, Desloovere C, et al: Treatment of severe laryngeal papillomatosis with intralesional injections of cidofovir [(S)-1-(3-hydroxy-2-phosphonylmethoxypropyl)cytosine]. J Med Virol 1998;54:219-225.

28. Weiss MD, Kashima HK: Tracheal involvement in laryngeal papillomatosis. Laryngoscope 1983;93:45-48.

29. Sie KCY, McGill T, Healy GB: Subglottic hemangioma: Ten years' experience with the carbon dioxide laser. Ann Otol Rhinol Laryngol 1994;103:167-172.

30. Franconi S, Burger R, Maurer H, et al: Transcutaneous carbon dioxide pressure for monitoring patients with severe croup. J Pediatr 1990;117:701-705.

31. Walner DL, Ouanounous S, Donnelly LF, et al: Utility of radiographs in the evaluation of pediatric upper airway obstruction. Ann Otol Rhinol Laryngol 1999;108: 378-383.

32. Handler SD: Direct laryngoscopy in children: Rigid and flexible fiberoptic. Ear Nose Throat J 1995;74:100-106.

33. Friedman EM, Williams H, Healy GB, et al: Pediatric endoscopy: A review of 616 cases. Ann Otol Rhinol Laryngol 1984;93:517-519.

34. Altman KW, Wetmore RF, Marsh RR: Congenital airway abnormalities requiring tracheostomy: A profile of 56 patients and their diagnoses over a 9-year period. Int J Pediatr Otorhinolaryngol 1997;41:199-206.

35. Brown JC: The management of croup. Br Med Bull 2002;61:189-202.

36. Hawkins DB, Crockett DM, Shum TK: Corticosteroids in airway management. Otolaryngol Head Neck Surg 1983;91:593-596.

37. Snyderman NL, Stool SE: Management of airway obstruction in children with infectious mononucleosis. Otolaryngol Head Neck Surg 1982;90:168-170.

38. Schimmer BP, Parker KL: Adrenocorticotropic hormone, adrenocortical steroids and their synthetic analogs: Inhibitors of the synthesis and actions of adrenocortical hormone. In Harman JG, Limbird LE (eds): Goodman and Gilman's The Pharmacological Basis of Therapeutics, 9th ed. New York, McGraw Hill, 1996, pp 1459-1485.

39. Orr JB: Helium-oxygen gas mixtures in the management of patients with airway obstruction. Ear Nose Throat J 1988;67:866-869.

Foreign Bodies of the Upper Aerodigestive Tract and Caustic Ingestion

DANIEL S. SAMADI, MD

FOREIGN BODIES

Any attempt at removal of a foreign body which does not succeed will make a bad situation worse. The child is usually apprehensive and the parents are aggravated. The physician, therefore, should be wary of falling into the trap of trying to do a removal without adequate instruments or good control of the patient.

Foreign Bodies of the Upper Aerodigestive Tract

Children are inclined to explore their environment through their oral cavity, so ingestion or aspiration of foreign bodies is of particular concern in this age group. Some of the contributing factors in ingestion and aspiration of foreign objects include male gender, immature coordination of swallowing and laryngeal sphincter control, and lack of molars before the age of 4 years for fine chewing. Other risk factors include neurologic disorders, inadequate parental supervision, and an abusive environment. Repeated episodes, multiple foreign bodies, and unusual presentation, such as a very young age, should raise the suspicion of child abuse.

Suffocation from foreign body ingestion and aspiration is the third leading cause of accidental death in children younger than 1 year and the fourth leading cause in children between 1 and 6 years. In the United States, over the last 35 years, there has been a dramatic downturn in the number of childhood deaths from asphyxiation secondary to aspiration of a foreign object. Retained esophageal foreign bodies are now much more common than airway aspirations, and procedures for removal of esophageal foreign objects currently outnumber those for aspirated foreign bodies. Long-standing airway foreign bodies are still associated with considerable morbidity, and early diagnosis remains the key to successful and uncomplicated management of these accidents.

History and Physical Examination

Esophageal Foreign Bodies

More than 75% of esophageal foreign bodies are found in children aged 18 to 48 months, and the most commonly ingested foreign bodies are coins, followed by food particles and bones. The remaining small proportion of offending objects includes buttons, plastic items, marbles, crayons, batteries, screws, and pins. Although ingestions are often asymptomatic and self-resolving, more than two thirds of children with esophageal foreign bodies are brought to medical attention within the first 24 hours after the event. Most foreign body ingestions and aspirations are not witnessed by parents or other caretakers.

Symptoms and signs of ingested foreign bodies are often vague but may include vomiting, dysphagia, ptyalism, gagging, poor feeding, and irritability. Larger ingested foreign bodies may manifest with airway symptoms such as wheezing, stridor, cough, and recurrent aspiration of secretions (Box 12-1).

Box 12-1 Signs and Symptoms of Foreign Body Ingestion

Emesis
Dysphagia
Ptyalism
Gagging
Poor feeding
Irritability
Wheezing
Stridor
Cough
Recurrent aspiration

Most ingested foreign bodies are retained at the level of the cricopharyngeus muscle (upper esophageal sphincter), about 15% at the level of the aortic arch at the midesophagus, and the rest at the level of the lower esophageal sphincter. Quarters are most commonly seen at the level of the cricopharyngeus, whereas smaller coins are seen more distally.

Unrecognized or prolonged esophageal foreign bodies may lead to devastating complications. These may include but are not limited to esophageal diverticulum, mediastinitis, bronchoesophageal fistula, aortoesophageal fistula, and death.

Airway Foreign Bodies

Foreign bodies may be the cause of various acute and chronic diseases of the lung and should be considered in the differential diagnosis of any child with recurrent pneumonia. Children younger than 5 years of age account for more than 80% of the cases of foreign body aspirations. Boys are affected more frequently than girls, by a ratio of about 2:1. The increased incidence of foreign body aspiration in children is most likely secondary to a lack of posterior dentition and the immaturity of neuromuscular mechanisms for swallowing and airway protection (Box 12-2).

Box 12-2 Contributing Factors in Ingestion and Aspiration of Foreign Bodies

Male gender
Immature swallow and laryngeal coordination
Lack of molars before age 4 years
Neurologic disorders
Inadequate parental or caretaker supervision
Abusive environment

In the last 20 years, in the pediatric population, the incidence of foreign body aspiration with subsequent asphyxiation has demonstrated a progressive decline, and this trend has most likely contributed to more prevention measures, improved public awareness, and the introduction of the Heimlich maneuver. Coughing, gagging, and throat clearing are reflexes that protect the airway and indicate partial obstruction. Delivering the Heimlich maneuver to a child with complete airway obstruction may be lifesaving, but can be life-threatening to a child with partial airway obstruction. Probing the hypopharynx with a finger may also force a loose foreign body tightly into the larynx, thereby transforming a partial obstruction into a complete one.

Aspiration of a foreign object usually causes significant coughing, choking, gagging, and wheezing immediately after the event. However, in many cases, the diagnosis is delayed, because most aspirations are not witnessed. The mucosa of the larynx, trachea, and bronchi rapidly adapt to the presence of a foreign object, resulting in a decrease or absence of symptoms, further hindering the clinician's suspicion of a foreign object as the possible underlying cause of distress. The practice of treating asthmatic or croupy children with antibiotics or steroids may also obscure signs and symptoms that would normally be expected with a retained foreign object. Late manifestations may include emphysema, atelectasis, pneumonia, and eventually pulmonary abscess.

The most serious sequela of foreign body aspiration is complete obstruction of the airway. In this situation, the foreign body becomes lodged in the larynx or trachea, leaving minimal room for air exchange. Complete airway obstruction may be recognized in the conscious child as sudden respiratory distress, followed by an inability to speak or cough. Recognition of complete airway obstruction is critical to the success of first aid efforts. Globular objects, such as hot dogs, candies, nuts, and grapes, are the most frequent offenders, whereas rubber balloons, balls, marbles, and other toys are the most common among nonfood objects. Vegetable matter, such as nuts, carrot pieces, beans, sunflower seeds, and watermelon seeds, are uniformly the most common foreign bodies found in the pediatric airway. Nuts with oil on the surface tend to stimulate a robust inflammatory mucosal response. Dried beans may also be associated with greater morbidity because of their ability to swell when exposed to secretions in the airway. Metal foreign bodies in the airway have diminished in incidence, whereas the incidence of plastic foreign bodies in the airway has increased. Because plastic matter is nonirritating and radiolucent, it may remain in the tracheobronchial tree for a prolonged period.

Most foreign bodies pass through the larynx and trachea and become lodged in the distal airway. Larger objects, or those with irregular and sharp edges, may become lodged at the laryngeal inlet. In most cases, the foreign body finds

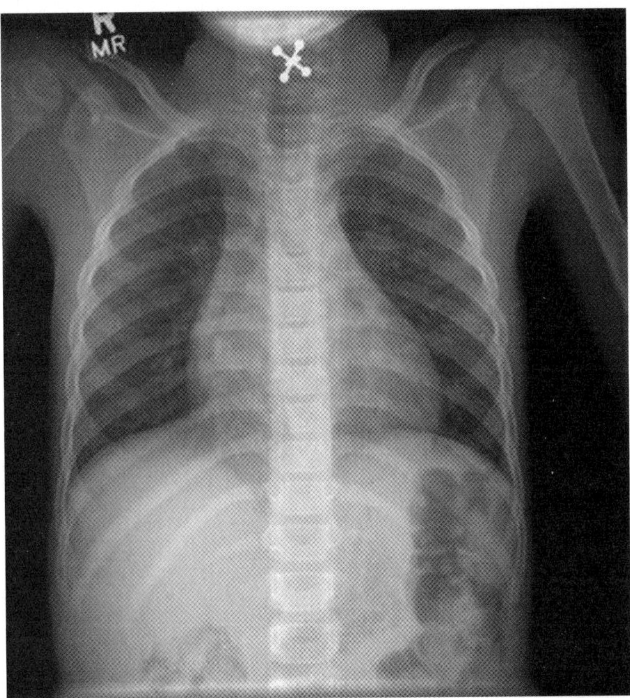

Figure 12-1. Anteroposterior chest radiograph of a child revealing a foreign object ("jack") in the upper esophagus.

its way into the right mainstem bronchus. The tendency for the right mainstem bronchus to be involved is explained by its larger diameter, smaller angle of divergence from the tracheal axis, greater airflow through the right lung, and position of the carina to the left of the midline.

Imaging

Esophageal Foreign Bodies

All patients suspected of harboring esophageal or pharyngeal foreign bodies should undergo anteroposterior and lateral neck radiography and posteroanterior and lateral chest radiography (Figs. 12-1 and 12-2). Although radiolucent objects may not be seen on a neck or chest radiograph, other signs, such as periesophageal inflammation or hyperinflation of the hypopharynx and esophagus, may be seen. Chest radiographs may demonstrate complications such as mediastinitis, pneumothorax, or aspiration pneumonia.

When plain films are normal or equivocal in a symptomatic patient, additional diagnostic procedures may be considered. Barium esophagography may suggest a radiolucent foreign body by demonstrating persistent filling defects, but such studies may pose the risk of aspiration of contrast material. The residual contrast material may also obscure the foreign body at a later endoscopy.

Computed tomography and magnetic resonance imaging are excellent at showing periesophageal soft tissue inflammation and abscess formation, but may require general anesthesia for young children.

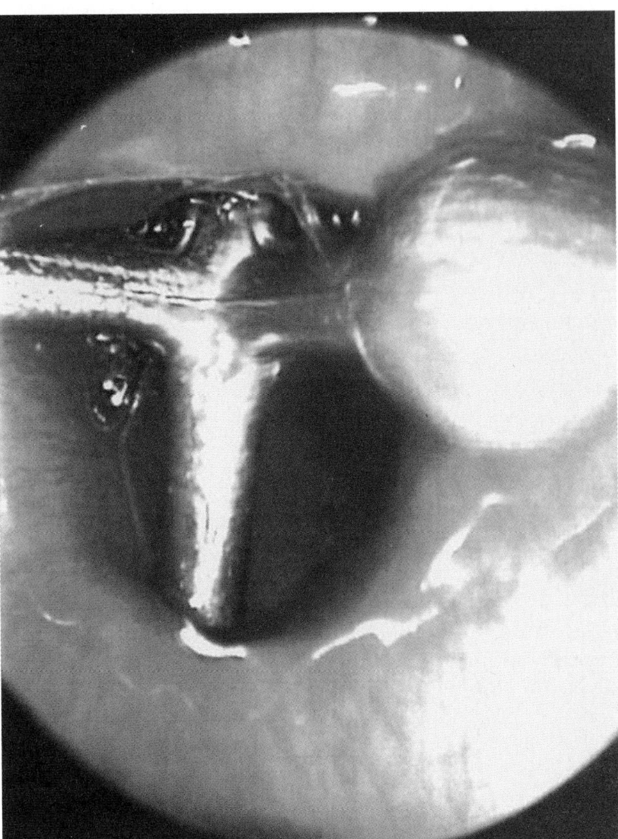

Figure 12-2. Endoscopic view of the airway of a patient with a "jack" in the esophagus at the level of the cricopharyngeal muscle.

Airway Foreign Bodies

Radiographic examination for airway foreign bodies consists of anteroposterior and lateral views of the neck and posteroanterior and lateral radiographs of the chest (Fig. 12-3). Small children may undergo lateral chest

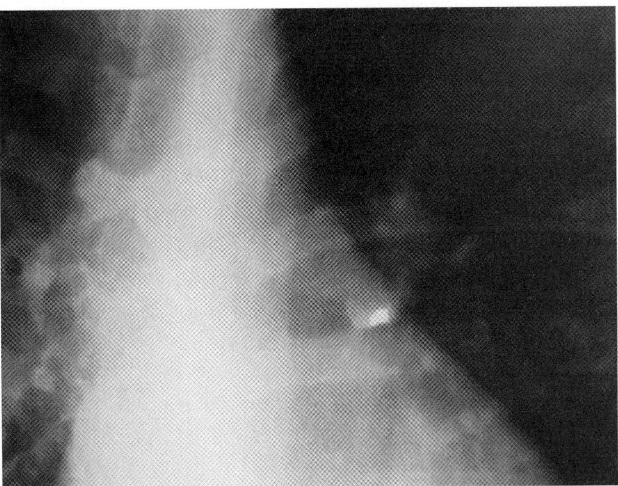

Figure 12-3. Magnified view of an anteroposterior radiograph of the chest showing a tooth in the left mainstem bronchus. Note the filling in the tooth.

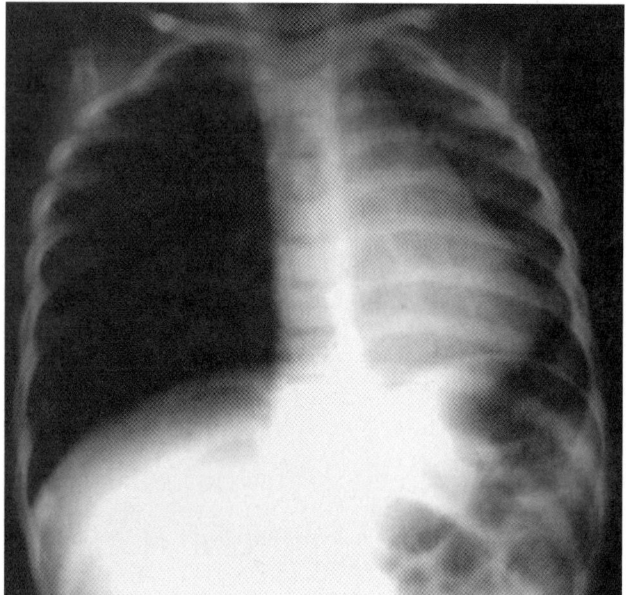

Figure 12-4. Hyperinflation of the right lung as a result of a foreign body in the right mainstem bronchus causing a ball valve effect. The air is trapped distal to the foreign object.

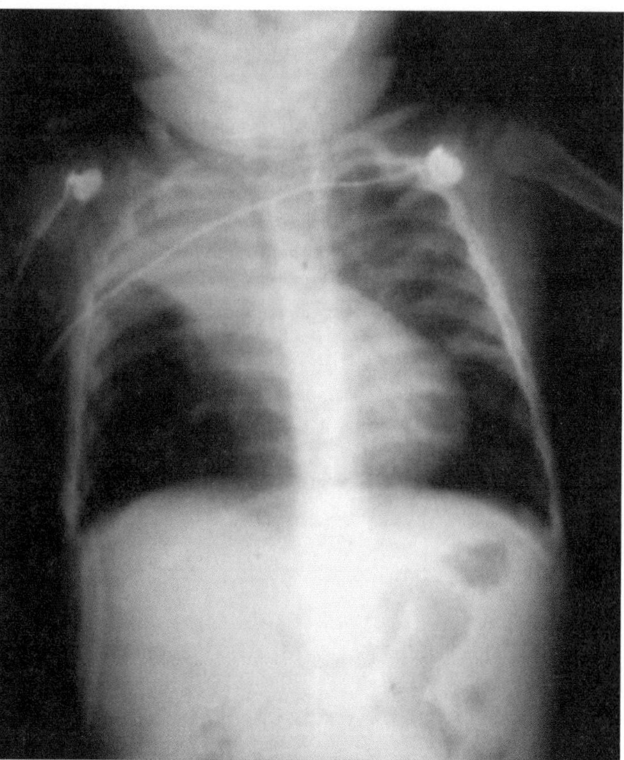

Figure 12-5. Anteroposterior chest radiograph demonstrating consolidation in the right upper lobe distal to a foreign body in the right upper lobe bronchus.

radiography with their arms behind their back and the head extended to visualize the entire airway from the mouth to the carina. Inspiratory and expiratory radiographs of the chest are best for demonstrating unilateral air trapping. Because these views may be difficult to obtain in children, lateral decubitus radiographs are obtained to use the patient's body weight to promote expiratory excursion. Videofluoroscopy offers the additional advantage of multiple views without prolonged radiographic exposure.

Air trapping (obstructive emphysema) is commonly associated with acute aspiration of bronchial foreign bodies. In such cases, air can move past the foreign body on inhalation but not on expiration. The result is hyperinflation of the obstructed lung and mediastinal shift to the opposite side (Fig. 12-4). The opposite side may undergo compensatory atelectasis. Evidence of a consolidation from pneumonia may also be seen (Fig. 12-5).

Neck and chest radiographs are considered an essential part of the evaluation for stridor and airway obstruction, and are obtained when foreign body aspiration is suspected. They are frequently diagnostic in cases of laryngeal foreign bodies, but normal films cannot be used to discount an object in the trachea.

Therefore, in the management of tracheobronchial foreign bodies, history and physical examination, and not radiography, determine the indication for bronchoscopy. Bronchoscopy is considered the definitive diagnostic and therapeutic intervention in the management of tracheobronchial foreign bodies.

Management

Esophageal Foreign Bodies

Coins are the most common foreign bodies ingested by children. Most ingested coins pass spontaneously through the body without any complications. Coins in the distal esophagus have the greatest likelihood of spontaneous passage, and these patients should be followed with subsequent radiographs until the coin has passed into the stomach or beyond. Coins in the proximal esophagus, however, commonly require surgical extraction.

Disk and button batteries may be hazardous if ingested. Problems related to ingestion may include direct caustic injury, absorption of toxins, pressure necrosis, and tissue necrosis from electrical discharge (Figs. 12-6 and 12-7). All batteries lodged in the esophagus must be regarded as emergencies and treated accordingly, and most authors have recommended the use of rigid endoscopy for extraction.

Traditionally, otolaryngologists have advocated rigid endoscopy, with its advantages of better visualization, airway management, and control of foreign body manipulation. However, rigid endoscopy carries with it the risk of general anesthesia and possible esophageal perforation. Flexible endoscopy may be used for the removal of coins and other blunt or smooth esophageal foreign bodies. The final decision in choosing the technique

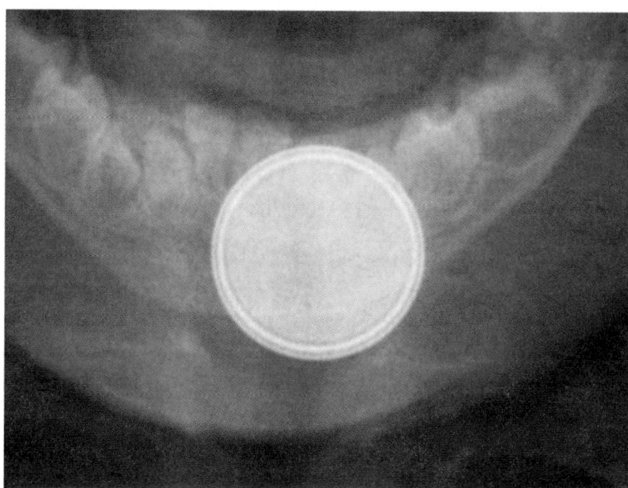

Figure 12-6. Anteroposterior neck radiograph illustrating a disk battery in the upper esophagus. The rim around the edge of the battery serves to distinguish it from a coin, which is a more common esophageal foreign body.

depends on the expertise of the physician involved and availability of the technology.

Airway Foreign Bodies

The treatment of choice for foreign bodies in the upper respiratory tract is prompt diagnosis, followed by endoscopic removal, under conditions of maximum safety and minimum trauma. Unless actual or potential airway obstruction is present, an airway foreign body does not constitute an acute emergency. The endoscopic removal should be scheduled when trained personnel are available, proper instruments have been checked, and techniques have been tested. The situation should be completely and thoughtfully be assessed prior to attempted removal of the foreign body.

Endoscopy needs to be considered as a form of diagnostic and therapeutic techniques. If the findings on history and physical examination are suspicious, endoscopic examination may be indicated to diagnose and possibly provide relief of symptoms. Chest physiotherapy and the use of bronchodilators should be strongly discouraged.

Successful extraction of the foreign body in a child requires the availability of pediatric instrumentation, a skillful anesthesiologist, and a surgeon who has expertise in the pediatric airway. Proper laryngoscopes, bronchoscopes, optical forceps, and telescopes are a few common instruments essential for a foreign body extraction (Fig. 12-8). Trial on a duplicate object on a mannequin board may be important. The use of a team approach, in which an experienced anesthesiologist, scrub technician, circulating nurse, and endoscopist are available, cannot be overemphasized. The procedure should not begin until all members of the team are prepared and the role of each member has been clearly delineated.

External Auditory Canal and Nasal Foreign Bodies

External Ear

Children frequently place small beads, paper, peanuts, or other foreign objects into the ear canal (Fig. 12-9). If the child does not complain, a foreign body may go undetected for weeks or longer. Symptoms of external auditory canal foreign bodies vary depending on the nature and size of the foreign body and how long it has been present. A completely obstructing object may

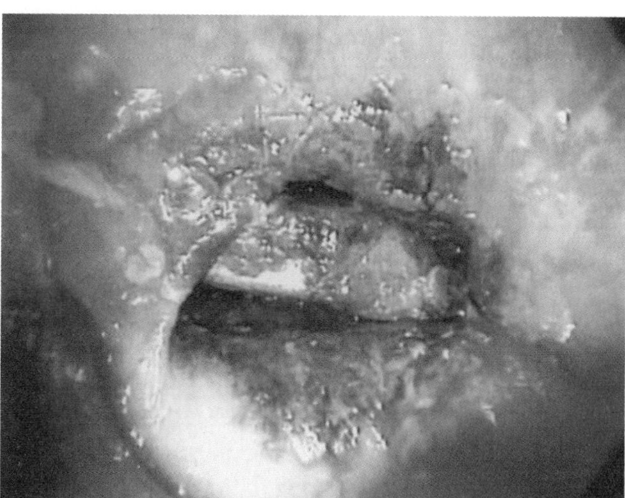

Figure 12-7. Endoscopic view of a disk battery lodged in the upper esophagus for several hours. Note the burns from both caustic and electrical injuries.

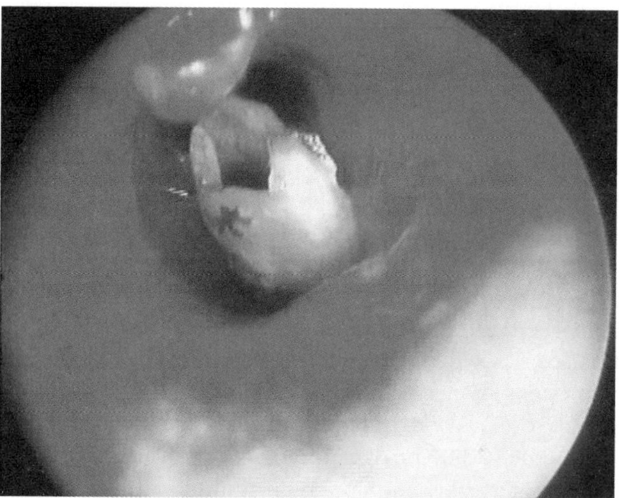

Figure 12-8. Seed lodged in right upper lobe bronchus.

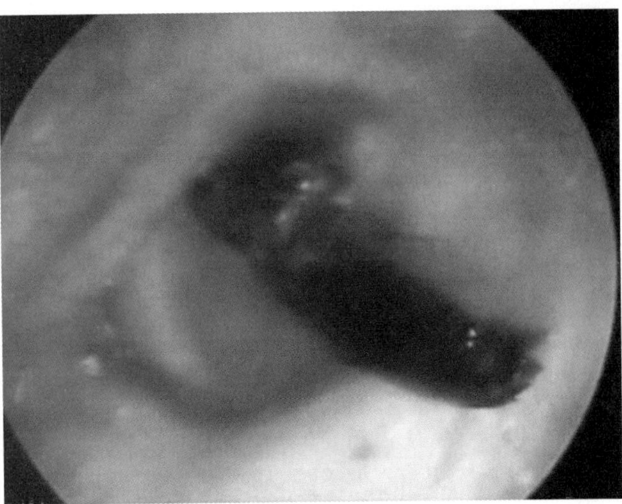

Figure 12-9. Foreign object (insect) in external auditory canal.

cause fullness, hearing loss, and otalgia. A sharp object may cause bleeding. A particularly dangerous foreign body is the lithium battery, because it can be extremely caustic and can cause extensive damage to the external auditory canal, tympanic membrane, and middle ear. These batteries must be removed immediately. Furthermore, the use of irrigation to remove the battery should be strictly discouraged.

Removal of an external auditory canal foreign body may be technically challenging and painful for the child. This problem may be compounded if an unskilled person has unsuccessfully attempted to remove the object, thereby causing local trauma and edema to the ear canal. Additionally, identification of one foreign body does not rule out the presence of others, and it is wise to examine both ears carefully.

The removal of an external auditory canal foreign body requires fine otologic equipment and cooperation from the child. Inappropriate movement may cause further injury to the tympanic membrane or ossicular chain. Restraining the child may be necessary. At times, it may be necessary to remove the foreign body using an operating microscope or under general anesthesia if the child cannot be adequately restrained.

Nose

Objects commonly placed in the nasal cavity by children include beads, toy parts, paper wads, and food. Nasal foreign bodies, unlike those found in the external auditory canal, are rarely noted on examination unless they are suspected. They are most commonly discovered as a result of persistent rhinitis of unknown cause. The presence of a nasal foreign body may interrupt normal mucociliary clearance within the dynamic surface of the nasal mucosa.

Noninert objects may case irritation or even caustic burns. Examples include seeds and beans, which swell on moistening by nasal secretions and become increasingly impacted over time. Plastic and other inert materials may be tolerated for long periods, during which exuberant granulation tissue grows to obscure the foreign body. Button batteries may cause severe chemical burns. If left unnoticed, subsequent septal perforation and eventual saddle nose deformity may occur. Button batteries may cause significant pain and distress in the child, and symptoms of nasal pain should elevate the level of suspicion of a foreign body, even if the incident has not been witnessed.

Common signs and symptoms of nasal foreign bodies include unilateral nasal obstruction, crusting, epistaxis, rhinorrhea, halitosis, and sinusitis. Unless foreign bodies are present in both nasal cavities, signs and symptoms of nasal obstruction, crusting, and rhinorrhea are usually unilateral. Identification of one foreign body does not rule out the presence of others, and it is prudent to examine both sides of the nose fully. Bilateral symptoms may also be seen with acute or chronic adenoiditis. Otitis media is a rare sequela of a nasal foreign body and is usually unilateral in nature. A potential complication of a nasal foreign body is aspiration, and some of the foreign bodies removed from the pediatric aerodigestive tract began as a nasal foreign body.

Topical or systemic antibiotics may be necessary to alleviate the symptoms, but inflammation and infection of the nasal cavity will resolve completely only after the foreign object has been removed. Most foreign bodies are removed by pediatricians and emergency department personnel. Successful removal requires visualization and appropriate instrumentation. Decongestion of the nose may be helpful in reducing mucosal swelling and increasing exposure. An otoscope may be used to perform anterior rhinoscopy. Instruments used to remove the foreign body may include a right-angle hook, cerumen curette, or alligator forceps. The first attempt at removing the foreign body in an awake child is the least difficult one, because most children become more alarmed after the initial manipulation. Restraining the child may be necessary at times. Foreign bodies that are not amenable to removal in the office necessitate extraction under general anesthesia.

Summary

Foreign bodies of the upper aerodigestive tract need to be approached with diligence and careful planning. Proper instrumentation, technical expertise, and a vigilant approach in each situation are warranted to maximize the outcome. The pediatric anesthesiologist plays a crucial role in airway management, especially in urgent circumstances. The overall approach is successful removal of the foreign body while minimizing further injury and morbidity.

MAJOR POINTS

Ingestion of foreign bodies is common in the pediatric population.
Risk factors include male gender, immature swallowing coordination, lack of molars, neurologic disorders, and inadequate parental or caretaker supervision.
There has been a dramatic decrease in childhood deaths from asphyxiation in the United States in the last 35 years.
Retained esophageal foreign bodies are much more common than airway aspirations.
The most common esophageal foreign bodies are coins, followed by food particles and bones.
Most foreign body ingestions and aspirations are not witnessed by parents or caretakers.
Most esophageal foreign bodies are retained at the level of the upper esophageal sphincter.
Disk batteries must be treated as an emergency and immediate extraction is warranted.
Performing the Heimlich maneuver on a child with complete airway obstruction may be lifesaving, whereas it can be life-threatening to a child with partial airway obstruction.
Particles of vegetable matter are the most common foreign bodies found in the pediatric airway.
Most airway bodies dislodge to the right mainstem bronchus.
Plain neck radiographs are essential for the evaluation of suspected foreign body ingestion or aspiration.
Pediatric rigid endoscopic instruments, a skillful anesthesiologist, and a surgeon with expertise in the pediatric airway are required for a successful foreign body extraction.

CAUSTIC INGESTION

The most common cause of an acquired esophageal stricture is a burn from a caustic ingestion. Every effort should be made to prevent accidental ingestion of caustic substances. When ingestion has occurred, accurate assessment of the injury and prompt treatment may help reduce some of the severe sequelae that lead to significant morbidity and mortality.

Most caustic ingestions are accidental. It has been estimated that there are 26,000 caustic ingestions/year in the United States. Children in the first decade of life constitute the largest group affected, with an especially high incidence in the first 3 years of life. Adults attempting suicide form another group, with women outnumbering men. In all reported cases, the most frequent material causing burns was an alkaline substance. It should be emphasized that even small amounts of caustic products can cause severe damage to the esophagus and that once a substance has touched a child's tongue, the natural reflex leads to swallowing.

The Poison Prevention Packing Act of 1970 and the Federal Hazardous Substances Act of 1972, overseen by the U.S. Consumer Product Safety Commission, require child-resistant packaging for substances such as sodium hydroxide or potassium hydroxide in the dry form or in solutions stronger than 2% concentration. The words "Keep out of the reach of children," "Danger," or "Poison" must be placed on the label, depending on the item. On every label, suitable handling and antidote procedures must be listed.

Types of Corrosives

Acids

Most acids are soluble in water. Common acids are hydrochloric (HCl), sulfuric (H_2SO_4), and nitric (HNO_3) acids. Commonly ingested acidic substances are toilet bowl cleaners, swimming pool cleaners, and rust removers. Phenol, an acidic compound, is very caustic. Bleach is usually available in a low concentration and an almost neutral pH. Ingestion of household bleach usually does not result in an esophageal burn.

Alkalis

Alkalis are bases that dissolve in water. Common alkali-containing substances are lyes, ammonia, hair-relaxing agents, nonphosphate detergents, dishwasher soaps, and disk batteries.

Lyes are alkaline agents that contain sodium hydroxide (NaOH), potassium hydroxide (KOH), or calcium hydroxide ($Ca(OH)_2$). Lyes are used in farm cleaning products, soap making, and drainpipe cleaners. Ammonia does not usually cause esophageal injury; however, there is a potential for pharyngeal or laryngeal edema, with subsequent upper airway obstruction.

Hair strengtheners or *hair-relaxing agents* may contain a product with a pH as high as 13. Although the ingestion of these products, mostly from nonchildproof containers, is becoming more prevalent, serious injuries or sequelae are rare (Table 12-1).

Table 12-1 Types of Corrosives

Acids	Bases
Toilet bowl cleaners	Lyes
Swimming pool cleaners	Ammonia
Rust removers	Hair-relaxing agents
Bleach	Dishwasher soaps
	Disk batteries

Table 12-2 Characterictistics of Lesions Caused by Acids and Bases

Feature	Acid Lesion	Base Lesion
Type of necrosis	Coagulation	Liquefaction
Penetration	Superficial	Deep
Prognosis	Good	Unfavorable

Pathology

Acids cause a coagulation necrosis, which eventually forms an eschar. This eschar tends to keep the corrosive from penetrating into deeper layers of tissue. Alkalis, on the other hand, produce liquefaction necrosis, with an edematous loosening of the tissue that allows diffusion of the corrosive into deeper layers. Lesions caused by acids are thus more superficial and have a more favorable prognosis than the deeper alkali lesions (Table 12-2).

From the pathologic standpoint, three stages are seen—acute, intermediate, and late. These stages correspond clinically to the following: (1) immediate pain and discomfort on swallowing, gradually easing over the first 2 weeks; (2) a relatively asymptomatic period lasting for 1 week or longer; and (3) a period of increasing difficulty in swallowing, leading to a complete inability to swallow as a stricture develops.

Management

Management of the patient with a caustic ingestion is based on the timing of presentation, degree of the burn, and pathologic stage of the esophageal burn.

Most patients present during the acute stage. The severity of signs and symptoms at this stage may vary from normal to severe with complications. The initial tasks are to assess the vital signs accurately, obtain the history of the ingestion, assess the severity of signs and symptoms, and decide on and prepare for endoscopic assessment of the degree of the esophageal burn.

It is important to reduce the time of contact with the concentrated substance. Irrigating the contact sites, as well as having the child drink milk or water, may dilute the concentration of the caustic agent. Vomiting can increase the degree of esophageal injury and should be avoided. In the emergency department, it is important to find out what type of substance was ingested or suspected to have been ingested. Information about the composition and concentration of the substance can then be obtained from the nearest poison control center. An attempt should also be made to estimate how much of the substance was ingested.

Examination of the patient may reveal burns of the lips, chin, or hands as a result of manipulation of the substance or following regurgitation. Patients may be in severe pain and unable to swallow their own saliva. There may be burns in the mouth, which do not necessarily correlate with burns in the esophagus; thus, it should not be assumed that if there are no burns in the mouth, then esophageal burns are not present, and vice versa.

Other signs of upper airway edema, stridor, hoarseness, and cough should be dealt with immediately. Mediastinitis from a rupture of the esophagus may cause severe chest pain, especially on respiration. The abdomen should be examined for signs of pain and rigidity, signifying perforation with peritonitis. Lateral and anteroposterior chest radiographs are essential in all cases as a baseline and to detect evidence of mediastinitis or aspiration pneumonia.

If complications such as acute airway compromise, mediastinitis, peritonitis, or esophageal perforation are suspected, immediate otolaryngologic and general surgical consultation should be obtained. Once these complications have been excluded, the aim of management is to prevent stricture formation in the esophagus by reducing the amount of granulation tissue, activity of fibroblasts, or both. It is difficult to know whether to treat all cases of children with a history of caustic ingestion or only those with symptoms, and it is also difficult to predict which children have suffered burns, so all symptomatic patients should be treated until esophagoscopy has confirmed the diagnosis. Most children who are asymptomatic may have no burn or a first-degree burn. In most of these cases, a stricture should not develop. Some physicians opt for no treatment in these children.

Analgesics may be necessary. Antibiotics may reduce the bacterial and granulation tissue load and lead to enhanced epithelialization. The patient should remain on intravenous hydration or, if able to swallow, be allowed to attempt a clear liquid diet. Food particles trapped on necrotic tissue may enhance granulation tissue formation. Aggressive antireflux treatment with H_2-receptor blockers or proton pump inhibitors should be started immediately.

The use, dosage, and length of treatment of corticosteroids therapy remain controversial. The most commonly accepted form of steroid treatment is early administration within the first 8 hours of injury. Most authors have noted that early steroid therapy inhibits the inflammatory response and granulation tissue formation, with a subsequent decrease in stricture formation in children with moderate to severe esophageal burns. A combination of antibiotic and steroid therapy has been found to be most effective in reducing stricture formation. Since the extent of esophageal injury cannot be determined until esophagoscopy has been performed, some physicians opt to treat all cases with steroids initially, stopping them if no burn is found during esophagoscopy. If steroids are continued, a 6-week taper may be required.

Esophagoscopy

There is poor correlation between oral or pharyngeal ulceration and esophageal injury. Direct visualization is the only accurate method to diagnose esophageal burns. Most authors have agreed that it is safe to observe asymptomatic patients without the need for endoscopy; however, for patients who have two or more signs of oral burns, such as dysphagia, pain, vomiting, drooling, or stridor, esophagoscopy is warranted.

The suggested timing for endoscopy ranges from 24 to 72 hours following the ingestion. If esophagoscopy is performed within the first 24 hours of injury, a lesion may be overlooked. If esophagoscopy is performed beyond 72 hours after the event, there may be an increased risk of esophageal perforation, because the esophageal wall is weakest during that period. Although controversy exists about the use of a rigid versus flexible esophagoscope for the examination, most experts have advocated performing rigid esophagoscopy of symptomatic patients 24 to 72 hours after ingestion. The esophagoscope should not be advanced beyond the first area of a severe burn, because this increases the danger of perforation.

If no burn seen is on endoscopy, all medications are stopped and an esophagogram is obtained prior to discharge. A second esophagogram is repeated in 6 to 8 weeks. If the results are normal and the patient is asymptomatic, no follow-up is necessary.

With a mild to moderate burn, the combination of antibiotics and corticosteroid therapy should be continued for 3 to 6 weeks and gradually tapered over that time. The child is maintained on intravenous fluids and a clear liquid diet, and may be advanced to a soft diet after a few days. An esophagogram is obtained 6 to 8 weeks after injury and the patient is seen for follow-up evaluation every 3 months for 1 year. If dysphagia or an esophagogram shows evidence of early stricture formation, dilation may be necessary.

Patients with severe esophageal burns are treated initially in a similar manner to those with less severe burns. As soon as the extent of the burn has been discovered by esophagoscopy, steroids are discontinued. Steroids increase the risk of esophageal perforation by interfering with wound healing at the site of injury. In patients with severe burns, the goal is to keep a tube or stent in place to prevent stricture, or to perform repeated dilations until scar formation is mature. At times, the esophagus may need to be rested with a gastrostomy or jejunostomy tube. Placement of a nasogastric tube or passing a string through the esophagus has been advocated by some to maintain the esophageal lumen. If a stricture develops, dilation may be necessary; this may be accomplished with the use of balloon dilation under radiographic visualization, prograde dilation, or retrograde dilation.

There is an estimated 1000-fold increase in the likelihood of development of esophageal carcinoma following a caustic ingestion. Some authors have advocated esophagectomy with various choices of reconstruction because of the high risk of development of squamous cell carcinoma. Additionally, if dilation fails, esophageal replacement may be the only alternative. Colonic interposition, gastric pull-up, and microvascular free jejunum transfer have all been used for esophageal reconstruction. Every effort should be made to maintain esophageal function for as long as possible.

Summary

Pediatric caustic ingestion remains a significant clinical problem in the United States and may lead to significant morbidity and mortality. When ingestion has occurred, accurate assessment of the injury and prompt treatment may help reduce some of the severe complications. Every effort should be made to prevent accidental ingestion of caustic substances. Parental and caretaker education and other outreach programs may help in reducing these accidents.

MAJOR POINTS

- Prevention is the best means for avoidance of caustic ingestion.
- Acids cause coagulation necrosis and eschar formation, preventing further penetration into deeper layers of tissue.
- Alkalis produce liquefaction necrosis and tissue disintegration, allowing further diffusion of the corrosives into deeper layers.
- Irrigation of the contact site will dilute the concentration of the caustic agent.
- Information about the pH and concentration of the substance should be obtained from the nearest poison control center.
- Most children present with no burns or first-degree burns.
- The aim of all management in caustic ingestion is to prevent stricture formation in the esophagus.
- The use of corticosteroid therapy remains controversial.
- If endoscopy is indicated, most authors have suggested timing of the examination within 24 to 72 hours following ingestion.
- Primary management of caustic ingestion is medical therapy, with surgical intervention indicated for severe strictures and other complications.
- There is an estimated 1000-fold increase in the likelihood of development of esophageal carcinoma following a caustic ingestion.

SUGGESTED READING

Foreign Bodies

Arjmand EM, Muntz HR Stratmann SL: Insurance status as a risk factor for foreign body ingestion or aspiration. Int J Pediatr Otorhinolaryngol 1997;42:25-29.

Black RE, Johnson DG, Matlak ME: Bronchoscopic removal of aspirated foreign bodies in children. J Pediatr Surg 1994;29:682-684.

Esclamado RM, Richardson MA: Laryngotracheal foreign bodies in children: A comparison with bronchial foreign bodies. Am J Dis Child 1987;141:259-262.

Heimlich HJ: A life-saving maneuver to prevent food choking. JAMA 1975;234:398-401.

Reilly JS: Prevention of aspiration in infants and young children: Federal regulations. Ann Otol Rhinol Laryngol 1990;99:273-276.

Reilly JS, Walter MA: Consumer product aspiration and ingestion in children: Analysis of emergency room reports to the National Electronic Injury Surveillance System. Ann Otol Rhinol Laryngol 1992;101:739-741.

Reilly JS, Walter MA, Beste D, et al: Size/shape of aerodigestive foreign bodies in children: A multi-institutional study. Am J Otolaryngol 1995;16:190-193.

Rimell FL, Thome A Jr, Stool S, et al: Characteristics of objects that cause choking in children. JAMA 1995;274:1763-1766.

Stool SE, McConnel CS Jr: Foreign bodies in pediatric otolaryngology: Some diagnostic and therapeutic pointers. Clin Pediatr (Phila) 1973;12:113-116.

Svensson G: Foreign bodies in the tracheobronchial tree: Special references to experiences in 97 children. Int J Pediatr Otorhinolaryngol 1985;8:243-251.

Caustic Ingestion

Alford BR, Harris HH: Chemical burns of the mouth, pharynx, and esophagus. Ann Otol Rhinol Laryngol 1959;68:122-128.

Christesen HBT: Prediction of complications following caustic ingestion in adults. Clin Otolaryngol 1995;20:272-278.

Christesen HBT: Prediction of complications following unintentional caustic ingestion in children. Is endoscopy always necessary? Acta Paediatr 1995;84:1177-1182.

Crain EF, Gershel JC, Mezey AP: Caustic ingestions. Am J Dis Child 1984;138:863-865.

Haller JA, Bachman K: The comparative effect of current therapy on experimental caustic burns of the esophagus. Pediatrics 1964;34:236-245.

Holinger PH, Johnston KC: Caustic strictures of the esophagus. Illinois Med J 1950;98:246-248.

Krey H: On the treatment of corrosive lesions in the esophagus: An experimental study. Acta Otolaryngol Suppl (Stockh) 1952;102:1-45.

Lovejoy FH Jr: Corrosive injury of the esophagus in children. N Engl J Med 1990;323:668-670.

Moore WR: Caustic ingestions. Pathophysiology, diagnosis and treatment. Clin Pediatr (Phila) 1986;25:192-196.

Ritter FN, Newman MH, Newman DE: A clinical and experimental study of corrosive burns of the stomach. Ann Otol Rhinol Laryngol 1968;67:830-836.

Spain DM, Molomut N, Haber A: The effect of cortisone on the formation of granulation tissue in mice. Am J Pathol 1950;268:710-715.

Tucker JA, Turtz ML, Silberman HD, et al: Tucker retrograde esophageal dilation. Ann Otol Rhinol Laryngol (Suppl) 1974;83:1-35.

Wjiburg FA, Beukers MM, Bartelsman JF, et al: Nasogastric intubation as sole treatment of caustic esophageal lesion. Ann Otol Rhinol Laryngol 1985;94:337-341.

Yarington CT Jr, Heatley CA: Steroids, antibiotics, and early esophagoscopy in caustic esophageal trauma. N Y State J Med 1963;63:2960-2963.

Zargar SA, Kochhar R, Nagi B, et al: Ingestion of corrosive acids. Gastroenterology 1989;97:702-707.

Management of Chronic Upper Airway Obstruction

KAREN B. ZUR, MD
IAN N. JACOBS, MD

Documentation of conditions leading to chronic airway obstruction dates back thousands of years. The paradigm of care throughout the centuries has focused on prompt management and identification of the safest methods to secure the airway. Chronic airway obstruction refers to any condition (e.g., infectious, inflammatory, tumor, congenital, acquired) that blocks the airway anywhere along the laryngotracheal complex (e.g., supraglottis, glottis, subglottis, trachea).

Historically, airway obstruction was related to infectious agents such as diphtheria, tuberculosis, syphilis, croup, and typhoid. Children requiring an artificial airway in such conditions underwent high tracheotomies, leading to the development of subglottic stenosis. With the introduction of toxoids and vaccinations, the rates of inflammatory and infectious conditions requiring an artificial airway have significantly decreased. Consequently, subglottic stenosis secondary to this cause has dramatically decreased.

In the mid to late 1960s, prolonged intubation and mechanical ventilation were introduced to manage pulmonary and airway compromise. As a result of increased survival rates of premature infants with the advent of prolonged intubation for management of hyaline membrane disease, bronchopulmonary dysplasia (BPD), and other neonatal pulmonary conditions, the rates of subglottic stenosis in this population have increased.

The surgically created artificial airway (tracheostomy or tracheotomy) was introduced thousands of years ago. The earliest known references have been linked to ancient Egyptian tablets, circa 3600 BC (Fig. 13-1), and to Hindu writing, circa 2500 BC.[1,2] In regard to more modern medical history, its use gained popularity in the early 1800s. Perhaps one of the most famous references to the link between upper airway obstruction and the tracheostomy tube was in 1799, when George Washington suffered from an acute airway obstruction secondary to a peritonsillar abscess or acute epiglottitis. This led to his death. One of his surgeons recommended a tracheostomy, but this issue was vetoed by his two other physicians, claiming lack of experience and benefit.[3,4] In 1808, Caron performed the first successful tracheostomy in a child.[5] In those days, most indications for placement of a tracheostomy tube were for the treatment of diphtheria. Chevalier Jackson popularized the concept of using a tracheostomy tube for airway obstruction in the early 1900s. His 1909 publication about the technique for and experience with tracheostomy is still the standard. Early in his studies, Jackson

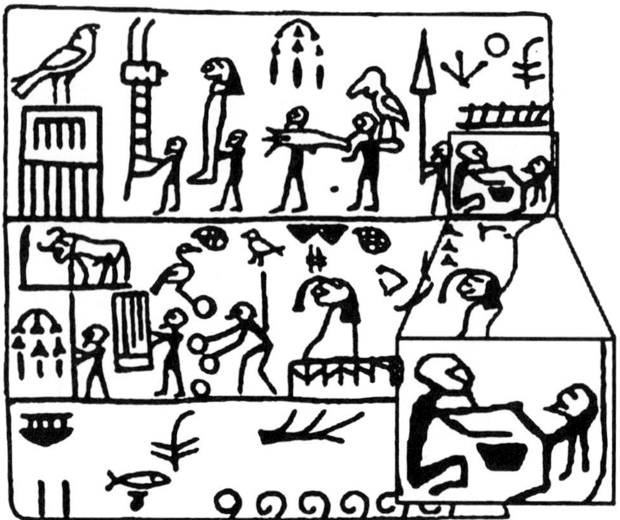

Figure 13-1. Possibly the earliest reference to the creation of a tracheostomy is found in Egyptian tablets. This illustration is thought to depict either a human sacrifice, which was uncommon in Egyptian culture, or fenestration of the trachea. (From Pahor AL: Medicine and Surgery in Ancient Egypt. Available at http://www.touregypt.net/featurestories/humansac.htm. Reprinted by permission of InterCity Oz.)

recognized that patients with chronic airway stenosis do not outgrow the obstruction; however, he believed that the surgical manipulation of the laryngotracheal complex might inhibit future growth of the larynx.[6] This was later refuted in modern practice.[5,7]

PRESENTATION

The presentation of chronic airway obstruction is variable and dependent on the degree of airway compromise and age of the patient. A young infant with airway obstruction may present with noisy breathing during sleep, stridor, retractions, weak cry, feeding difficulty, failure to thrive, and/or cyanosis. On the other hand, an older child with a similar level of pathology may experience various degrees of these symptoms or only dyspnea on exertion. In the hospitalized infant or child, failure to extubate may manifest as stridor, desaturations, cyanosis, respiratory distress, and retractions; these may indicate an acquired or congenital stenosis. Often, a congenital airway compromise may be exacerbated by the injury or inflammation of an indwelling endotracheal tube.

Finally, chronic cough and recurrent croup may also be seen and, in these cases, asthma, tracheomalacia, and gastroesophageal reflux disease (GERD) must be excluded. The diagnosis is often elusive and a child may be treated for a period of time with nebulizers, with no improvement or even worsening of symptoms in cases of tracheomalacia. The theory behind this phenomenon is that smooth muscle relaxation is exacerbated by calcium channel blockers, leading to worsening malacia.

The hallmark of airway compromise is stridor. In a patient with mild to moderate stridor, the clinician can tailor the workup of physiologic narrowing based on the quality and timing of the stridor. The loudness is important, because a sudden loss of the stridorous sound, in the appropriate clinical setting, may mark an impending respiratory failure caused by progressive airway obstruction. Inspiratory stridor is indicative of collapse at the level of the supraglottic larynx because of the flaccid nature of the cartilage in this level; with significant collapse and the Bernoulli effect, the physiologic narrowing that normally occurs during inspiration is exacerbated and manifests as high-pitched inspiratory stridor. Expiratory stridor suggests a more distal pathology affecting the intrathoracic trachea and mainstem bronchi. This finding is because of the physiologic narrowing of these segments during expiration; it is exacerbated with stenosis or tracheomalacia. Finally, biphasic stridor is consistent with a fixed obstruction at a level supported by more rigid cartilage, as in the glottic and subglottic regions, because airflow through these regions is affected during inspiration and expiration.

Infants and children who have undergone a tracheostomy because of chronic lung disease may fail a capping or decannulation trial because of subglottic stenosis, glottic stenosis, or tracheomalacia related to the initial intubation, placement of a high tracheostomy tube (see later, "Tracheotomy"), or softening of the tracheal wall at the level of the tracheal stoma (suprastomal collapse).

Older children may not experience stridor as a manifestation of airway obstruction. Manifestation of airway obstruction may include recurrent croup, chronic cough, dyspnea on exertion, dysphagia, and hoarseness. Dysphagia may result from difficulty breathing while feeding in the younger patient with a high larynx (the larynx descends with age, allowing improved ability to eat and breathe simultaneously). A patient with subglottic stenosis may or may not experience hoarseness. This depends on the degree of obstruction in the subglottis, altering the airflow through the vocal folds and leading to dysphonia (abnormal voice), and on the involvement of the glottis or supraglottis by the scar tissue.

EVALUATION

Obtaining an accurate history is paramount to the prompt diagnosis. Often, children with subglottic stenosis are unsuccessfully treated for prolonged periods for asthma or protracted croup. Information about the onset of symptoms, history of airway manipulation or intubation, history of caustic or foreign body ingestion, feeding difficulties, changes in voice, and birth and perinatal data should be obtained. Response to prior therapy should be ascertained as well.

Physical Examination

A complete visual examination and head and neck examination must be performed on each patient. The clinician should note any signs of distress, such as retractions, nasal flaring, stridor, and cyanosis, that might indicate an impending respiratory failure requiring emergent care. At the onset of the airway evaluation, the acuity and stability of the airway must be established. Distinguishing stridor from stertor (upper airway noise caused by nasal or pharyngeal obstruction) may be difficult for the untrained clinician. If symptoms do not usually occur at rest or during sleep, it is important to try to simulate conditions that exacerbate the symptoms, maintaining the patient's safety at all times. For example, in a child with exercise-induced dyspnea, an exercise stress test (treadmill) may be necessary. The head and neck examination should note any unusual findings, such as craniofacial anomalies, midface hypoplasia, nasal stenosis, and hemangiomas. Intraoral and neck masses should be excluded, as well as causes of extrinsic airway compression or obstruction. Flexible nasopharyngoscopy should be performed to evaluate the base of the tongue, supraglottis, and glottic larynx. The clinician should note supraglottic collapse, vocal fold motion impairments, and pooling of secretions. The latter two are often associated with swallowing difficulty, and appropriate referrals and evaluations should be pursued.

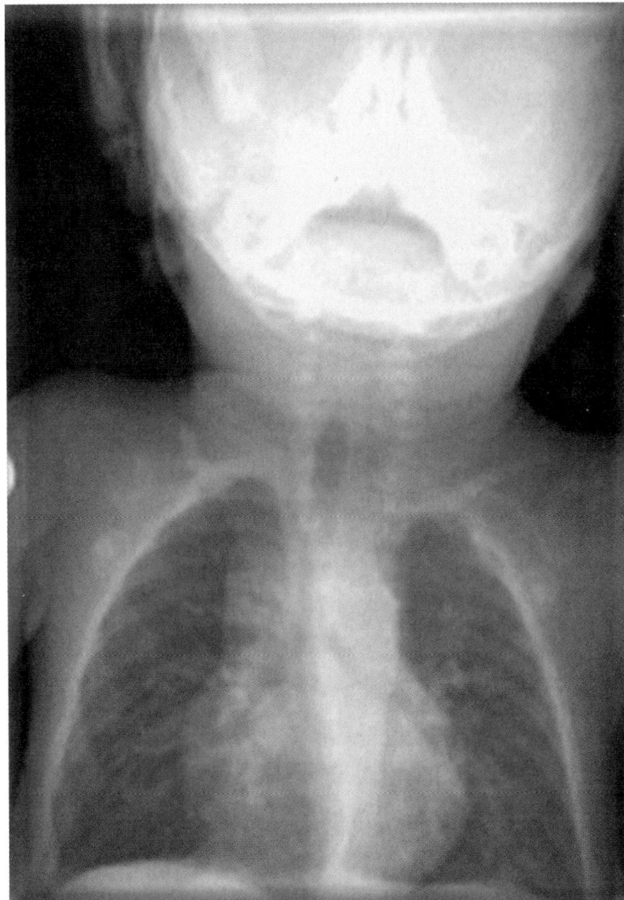

Figure 13-2. Shown is a posteroanterior neck radiograph of a normal subglottis in an infant with laryngomalacia. The radiograph was done to exclude other airway lesions.

Radiographic Evaluation

The routine use of plain radiographs to diagnose subglottic stenosis is often unnecessary. On the other hand, airway radiographs can be used to provide supplemental information prior to or following endoscopy (the gold standard). For example, anteroposterior and lateral neck radiographs may be used in cases of mild laryngomalacia (diagnosed in the office) to exclude synchronous airway lesions; however, in more significant cases of laryngomalacia, and in almost all other pathologic conditions, a radiograph should not replace an airway endoscopy (Fig. 13-2). Chest radiographs (anteroposterior and lateral) should be obtained to evaluate the pulmonary status, especially in patients with a known history of problems such as bronchopulmonary dysplasia, hyaline membrane disease, and aspiration pneumonias. Patients with a known history of recurrent pneumonias should undergo computed tomography (CT) scanning of the chest to determine whether chronic parenchymal damage has occurred.

Airway fluoroscopy, depending on the skills and resources of the institution, may be useful to diagnose dynamic problems of the airway, such as tracheomalacia. In addition, barium swallow is an excellent screening tool if vascular rings or compression are suspected (Fig. 13-3). Magnetic resonance angiography (MRA) may be used to delineate the vascular anatomy in the chest. Vascular rings may be well visualized on MRA (Fig. 13-4).

During endoscopy, extrinsic vascular compression (e.g., innominate compression, vascular sling, or rings) leading to tracheomalacia may be noted, and an MRA or CT with contrast might be considered to evaluate for feasibility of repair (Fig. 13-5). Planning is done in consultation with the cardiothoracic service.

A newer tool that supplements this evaluation is the cine magnetic resonance imaging (cine MRI). Cine MRI has the benefit of providing a high-resolution image of the airway without the risk of ionizing radiation that was inherent in earlier studies, such as airway fluoroscopy.[8] The main advantage of cine MRI is its ability to obtain a good sagittal view of the entire airway, from nasal passages to trachea, while assessing concurrent dynamic processes and pathologies. It allows an instant evaluation of the entire airway so that diffuse collapse versus discrete levels of obstruction can be isolated, and an association between the two types

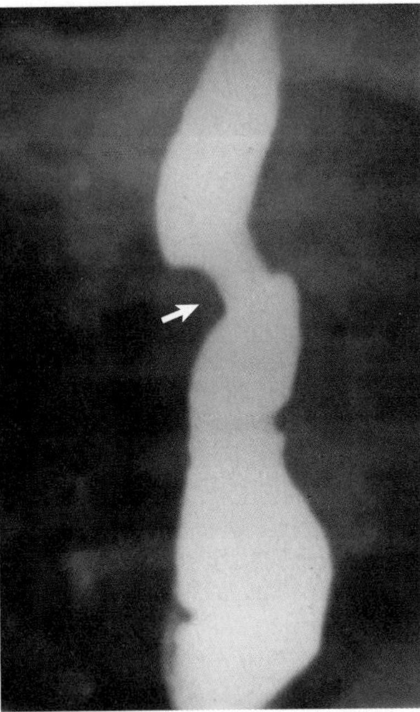

Figure 13-3. Barium swallow, revealing a vascular ring. Note the external esophageal compression (*arrow*).

of obstructions can also be made. One limitation of the use of cine MRI involves missing short bursts of obstruction because of short periods of respiration during sleep.[8] A team of interventional radiologists and anesthesiologists may be needed at cine MRI evaluations. At home, to visualize obstructions as they occur most accurately, no artificial airway is placed unless necessary; at that point, an experienced clinician should be available to manage the airway.

Endoscopic Evaluation

The gold standard of the airway evaluation is rigid endoscopy under general anesthesia. A combination of flexible laryngoscopy and bronchoscopy under light sedation, as well as rigid microlaryngoscopy, rigid bronchoscopy, and esophagoscopy, provide a comprehensive, multidisciplinary, aerodigestive evaluation critical to proper diagnosis and treatment. During endoscopy, photodocumentation is used to follow the progression of stenosis, improvement in stenosis, and/or operative results. The aim of the endoscopy is to identify specific sites of obstruction, degree of lumen compromise, length of narrowing, and any associated lesions and pathologic processes.

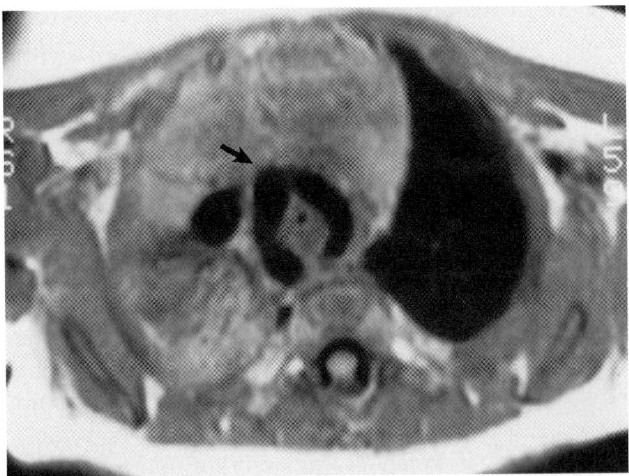

Figure 13-4. Magnetic resonance angiogram of a vascular ring (*arrow*).

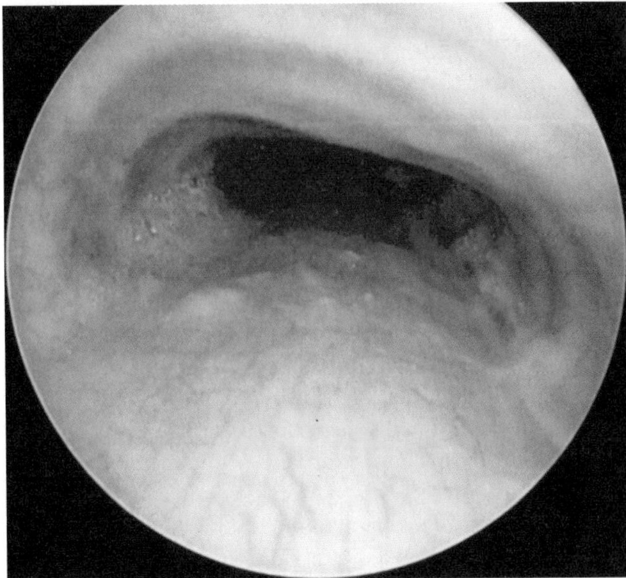

Figure 13-5. Extrinsic tracheal compression caused by innominate artery compression. (Courtesy of Mike J. Rutter, MD, Cincinnati Children's Hospital Medical Center.)

Laryngoscopy

Flexible laryngoscopy provides a dynamic assessment of the larynx and pharynx. After decongestion with topical oxymetazoline, the flexible laryngoscope (Fig. 13-6) is passed through the nares into the posterior pharynx. The nasopharynx, pharynx, and larynx can be visualized with the flexible scope. Dynamic conditions such as laryngomalacia, supraglottic stenosis, or pharyngolaryngomalacia may be seen best with the flexible laryngoscope.

Rigid laryngoscopy is accomplished with the metal laryngoscope, which is placed in the vallecula and used for exposure of the larynx. Several types of laryngoscopes are used, such as the Lindholme, Benjamin, and Dedo laryngoscopes (Fig. 13-7). After the laryngoscope exposes the larynx, magnified views of endolaryngeal structures are obtained with the Storz-Hopkins telescopic rod or operating microscope (Fig. 13-8). The base of the tongue, supraglottis (epiglottis, arytenoids, interarytenoid region), and vocal folds are viewed to exclude obstructing masses or discrete lesions. Masses, cysts, tumors, and granulomas should be sought out and excluded.

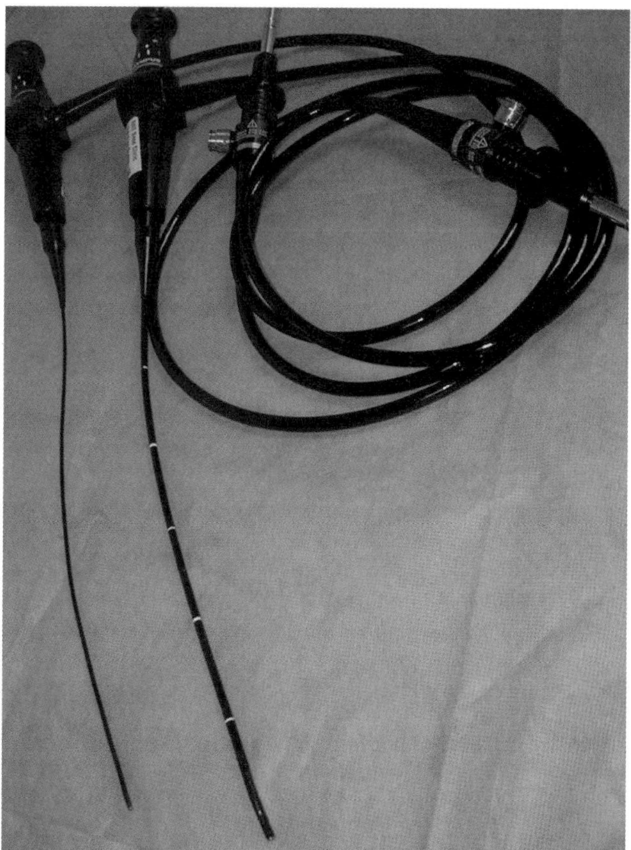

Figure 13-6. Flexible laryngoscopes measuring 2.2 mm *(left)* and 3.7 mm *(right)* in diameter are used to view the larynx following intranasal passage.

Bronchoscopy

Bronchoscopy is performed to evaluate the caliber and shape of the immediate subglottis, cervical trachea, carina, and mainstem bronchi. The same flexible laryngoscope used for flexible laryngoscopy may be passed into the subglottis and trachea after topical anesthesia of the vocal cords. Often, flexible bronchoscopy is performed to evaluate the dynamic nature of the larynx and trachea. Conditions such as tracheobronchomalacia are best visualized with the flexible bronchoscope when the patient is breathing spontaneously.

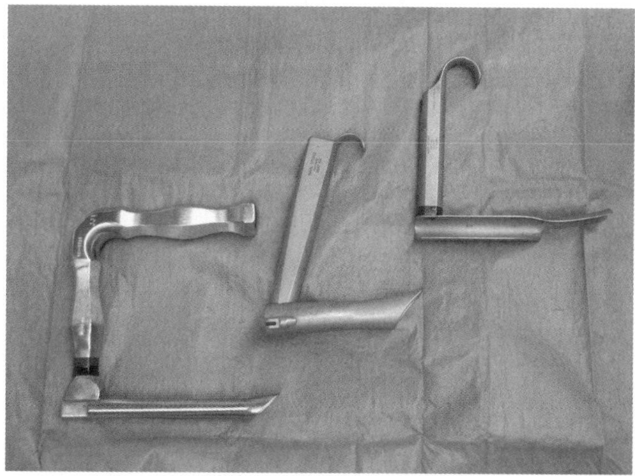

Figure 13-7. Selection of operating laryngoscopes. *Left to right*, The Dedo, Lindholme, and Benjamin laryngoscopes.

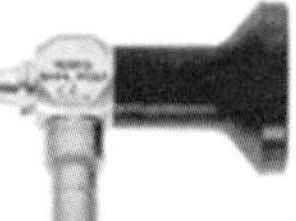

Figure 13-8. The Storz-Hopkins rod is a telescope used to magnify the view of the larynx, subglottis, and trachea. It can be used alone or inside a hollow, rigid ventilating bronchoscope.

The rigid, open tube, ventilating bronchoscope stents the airway open by lifting the trachea anteriorly during the procedure, while providing an excellent magnified view of the lesion via the telescope. Because of the technique used for rigid endoscopic evaluations, dynamic lesions such as tracheomalacia may be missed. Therefore, the internal telescope may be used alone for evaluation of the tracheal airway.

Esophagoscopy

Esophagoscopy with biopsy is an important component of the airway evaluation to exclude the possibility that significant reflux and/or eosinophilic esophagitis have affected the airway. There is a strong association between these two processes and airway inflammation and edema.[9] In addition, congenital problems such as esophageal atresia, hiatal hernia, and foreign bodies need to be excluded. Plain films and barium esophograms are useful for delineating basic anatomy. Flexible esophagoscopy with air insufflation provides the best visualization of the esophageal, gastric, and duodenal mucosa (Fig. 13-9A). Biopsies may be taken at these sites to evaluate for esophagitis or eosinophilic esophagitis (EE). Mild EE is diagnosed in cases in which 5 to 10 eosinophils per high-power field (hpf) are found, moderate EE with 10 to 20 eosinophils/hpf, and severe EE with more than 20 eosinophils/hpf (see Fig. 13-9B).

Sizing the Airway With the Endotracheal Tube Leak Test

The endotracheal tube (ETT) leak test is helpful to size the airway. It provides the surgeon and anesthesiologist a standardized way to communicate about the degree of obstruction and provides information about the appropriately sized ETT to be used in case of an emergency or other surgical procedure. To size the airway, following the endoscopic evaluation, an ETT is inserted into the airway and the anesthesiologist is asked to check for an air leak. Normally, an appropriately sized tube should leak at less

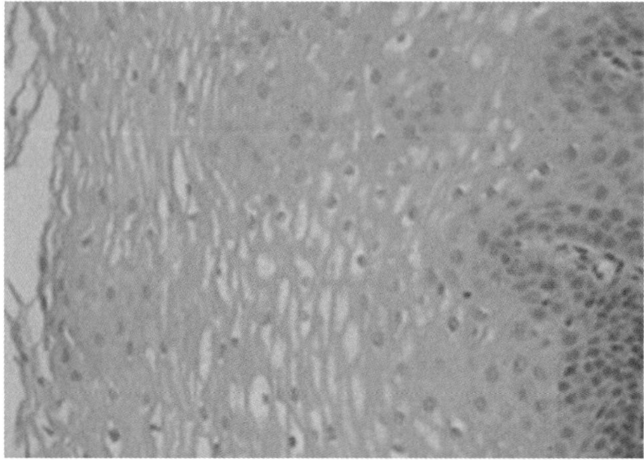

A

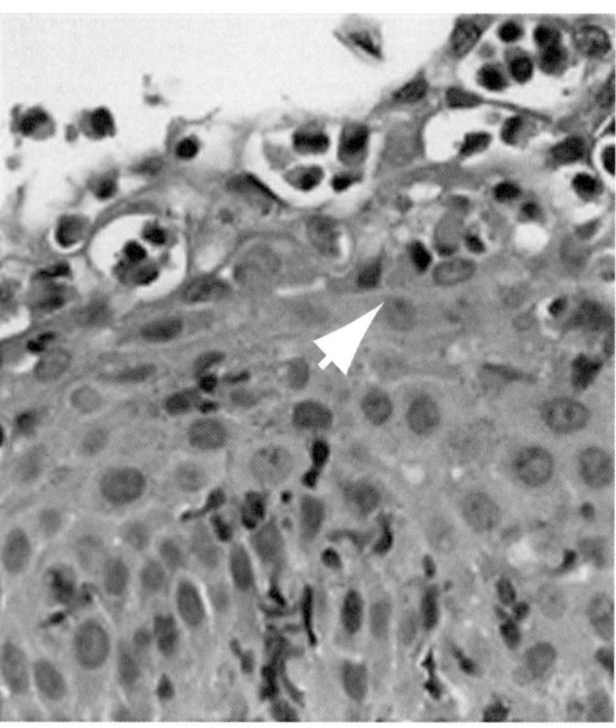

B

Figure 13-9. Eosinophilic esophagitis may be associated with laryngitis, cough, and failed airway reconstruction. This micrograph shows a normal esophageal biopsy specimen (**A**) and a classic eosinophilic specimen (**B**). Note the eosinophils scattered throughout the specimen *(arrowhead)*. (Courtesy of the Gastroenterology Division, Cincinnati Children's Hospital Medical Center.)

than 20 to 25 cm H_2O during a Valsalva maneuver. The ETT size that ultimately fits the airway is compared with the expected ETT size based on age (Table 13-1). There are several formulas that may be used to estimate the appropriate ETT. The easiest one to remember is as follows[10]:

$$(\text{Age}/4) + 4$$

The Cotton-Myer classification[11] is a grading system used to standardize how the severity of subglottic lumen obstruction is quantified. Using this technique to determine airway size, the degree of obstruction is graded as follows: grade I, 0% to 50%; grade II, 51% to 70%: grade III, 71% to 99%; and grade IV, no detectable lumen (Fig. 13-10).

Table 13-1 Guidelines for Pediatic Tracheal Tube Size

Child's Age	Expected Internal Diameter (mm)
Premature	
1000 g	2.5
1000-1500 g	3.0
1500-2500 g	3.5
Normal newborns	3.5-4.0
6-12 mo	4.0-4.5
1-2 yr	4.5
4 yr	5.0
6 yr	5.5
8 yr	6.0
10 yr	6.5
Older than 12 yr	
Female	7.0-8.5
Male	8.0-10.0

Modified from Jacobs IN, Pettignano MM, Pettignano R: Airway management. In Czervinske MP, Barnhart SL (eds): Perinatal and Pediatric Respiratory Care, 2nd ed. St. Louis, WB Saunders, 2003, p 209.

The final issue to consider is the stage of stenosis. Often, early active inflammation will manifest with edema, granulation, and a friable laryngeal and subglottic mucosa. The "active" larynx, or the acutely inflamed larynx, must be documented and treated prior to consideration of reconstruction. If this is seen, the patient should be evaluated for contributing factors such as GERD and eosinophilic esophagitis. When the stenosis comes into a mature scar, the larynx is then amenable to operative intervention.

Pulmonary Evaluation

Collaboration with the pulmonologist provides the otolaryngologist with another dimension in regard to airway evaluation and management. Most of the patient population presenting for treatment of chronic airway obstruction have a history of immature lung development because of prematurity or are actively presenting with pulmonary compromise requiring better toilet, medical management or ventilatory support with or without continuous positive airway pressure (CPAP) or bilevel positive airway pressure (BiPAP). With the assistance of the pulmonologist, a comprehensive approach to the care of the patient will ensure better early and late care. Furthermore, appropriate tests can be carried out and interpreted (e.g., chest CT, pulmonary function tests, bronchoalveolar washout, sleep studies) in a timely and comprehensive manner.

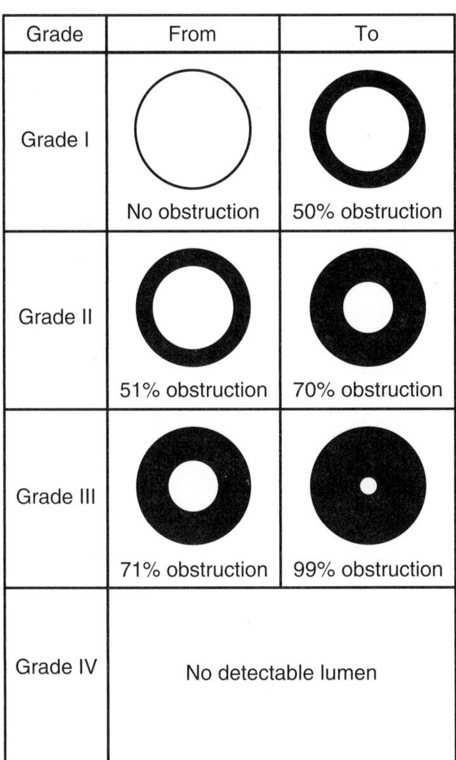

Figure 13-10. The Myer-Cotton classification for subglottic stenosis. (From Myer CM 3rd, Hartley BE: Pediatric laryngotracheal surgery. Laryngoscope 2000;110:1875-1883.)

Gastroenterologic Evaluation

Gastroesophageal Reflux Disease

Gastroesophageal reflux disease can adversely affect the airway prior to and following reconstruction.[10] It is not unusual to encounter clinical or subclinical GERD in patients with chronic upper airway obstruction. In the nontracheotomized population, chronic retractions and increased respiratory efforts create a negative pressure that is sufficient to predispose the young child to reflux, emesis, and potential aspiration.

It is well known that 67% of infants older than 4 months are expected to have esophageal reflux.[12] More than of 85% of neonates can have reflux.[13] Pathologic reflux is a condition that leads to feeding abnormalities, failure to thrive, aspiration or respiratory complications, esophagitis, and/or esophageal strictures. In patients with a compromised airway, the effluent can irritate the supraglottic, glottic, and/or subglottic mucosa, exacerbating the obstruction and may lead to a pneumonitis or, in severe cases, to aspiration pneumonia.

A gold standard for the evaluation of pediatric GERD has not been established. There are several tools that have been extensively used to evaluate the gastroesophageal tract for evidence of reflux or esophagitis. A visual inspection of the tract and biopsies will reveal macroscopic and microscopic mucosal changes that should be managed medically. In addition to an esophagogastroduodenoscopy (EGD), 24-hour reflux monitoring has been advocated.[14-16] In studies of adults, pH probe monitoring for 24 hours has been used and normal and abnormal values established. For example, an intraluminal pH less than 4 for 15 seconds is considered a reflux episode, and a reflux index score of 5% is abnormal (i.e., pH 4 for 5% of the time). Unfortunately, no such values have been established for the pediatric population, which limits its value.

The issue of pH probe monitoring as a contributor to extraesophageal disease (e.g., laryngitis) is controversial. Double- and triple-probe monitors have been developed in an attempt to define the level of reflux. More controversy has developed because of false-positive and false-negative results, as well as biases in reporting of the data. The newer probes allow measurement of proximal esophageal and hypopharyngeal reflux events. False-positive results may be seen, according to some authorities, because of the presence of the probe, which can promote reflux. Proximal false-negative results have also been reported by pH studies and postcricoid mucosal biopsies.[17] Again, all these published studies are controversial, and data for the pediatric population are limited.

Another method of evaluating reflux is the impedance probe (IMP). Because nonacid reflux disease (bile) may be aspirated and lead to pneumonitis, as well as airway inflammation, knowledge of any reflux episode could be informative. The multichannel IMP was developed to detect impedance changes along the digestive tract. The onset of a retrograde bolus reflux event is defined as a decrease in impedance in the distal intraluminal impedance measurement (IMP channels that proceed to the more proximal channels.) The end of a reflux episode, as defined by IMP evaluation, is a return of the impedance value to at least 50% of the initial value.

IMP studies have been performed in infants and children, but with limited reports in the literature.[18] Some are flawed by lack of control data in normal patients. IMP studies can be performed on patients who are on acid suppression therapy, because the goal of the study is to measure any bolus (nonair) reflux episode that is missed on pH probe monitoring. Thus, IMP studies can be viewed as a complement to endoscopy and pH probe and manometry studies in the complex patient. More research needs to be done in the pediatric population with regard to this potentially revolutionary tool.

Eosinophilic Esophagitis

Eosinophilic esophagitis (EE), an allergic condition of the esophagus, may be diagnosed on EGD biopsies. Microscopic analysis focuses on the number of eosinophils/hpf (see Fig. 13-9). EE is graded as mild, moderate, or severe (more than 24 eosinophils/hpf). Clinically, EE may lead to laryngeal edema and result in poor healing after airway reconstruction. Because it is often related to food allergies, allergy testing (patch testing) is essential. Treatment includes elimination of certain foods, antihistamines, and oral fluticasone. Repeat EGD with biopsies is necessary to show resolution of EE prior to laryngotracheal reconstruction.

Dysphagia

The evaluation of dysphagia in patients with chronic airway obstruction is of paramount importance. There are several reasons for this: (1) nutrition is often compromised in patients with high caloric expenditure because of airway obstruction; (2) patients with a compromised airway often are premature or had sustained injury to the upper aerodigestive tract; (3) patients who are tracheostomy-dependent often have an altered laryngeal elevation mechanism that may disrupt swallowing; and (4) patients with dysphagia are at risk of aspiration because of poor ability to manage their secretions and pooling.

For the otolaryngologist about to perform an airway reconstruction, knowledge of the swallowing status of the child is important for two reasons, to ensure adequate nutrition and establish safety of swallowing and risk of postreconstruction aspiration. Assessing the risk of aspiration is vital, because certain procedures that have been designed to improve the airway can increase the chances of aspiration (e.g., arytenoidectomy, transverse cordotomy, posterior cricoid graft). There are several factors that might contribute to a risk of aspiration—delayed swallowing mechanism development; anatomic (e.g., laryngotracheal or tracheoesophageal clefts), physiologic (e.g., lack of coordination), neurologic (e.g., vocal fold paralysis, cortical or brainstem pathology), and behavioral and postsurgical factors (some of the airway procedures disrupt the muscles that suspend the larynx and help in the swallowing coordination); and poor hypopharyngeal sensation, occasionally because of severe reflux disease.

The swallowing evaluation should be multidisciplinary and involve a trained speech-language pathologist, gastroenterologist, pulmonologist, nutritionist, and feeding team. A detailed history about feeding, choking with liquids or solids, weight loss or failure to thrive, and drooling provide the clinician with an idea about the severity of potential problems. Aversion to feeds is also elicited. Information about a history of Nissen fundoplication and G-tube feeding should be sought. All these help determine whether aspiration is related to oral intake, gastroesophageal content reflux, or aspiration of saliva.

There are a few tools that can be used to assess the risk of aspiration and evaluate the swallowing mechanism: the video swallow study (VSS), the modified barium swallow study (MBSS), and videofluoroscopy. The VSS helps define the anatomy and physiology of swallowing while observing the patient swallow barium-laden liquids, purées, and solids under fluoroscopy. Poor oral, pharyngeal, and esophageal phases of the swallow can be observed. Compensatory mechanisms that the patient adapts or compensation as taught by the speech pathologist can be visualized; these include head positioning, thickening the feeds, and use of a bottle or nipple. The VSS and MBSS can demonstrate frank aspiration, penetration, or barium residues in the hypopharynx. The disadvantages of fluoroscopy include the risk of radiation exposure and the need to use barium. The procedure is operator-dependent and, more important, requires the patient to be an oral feeder. Those patients who have not developed oral feeding skills cannot undergo this examination.

A more recent addition to the armamentarium of the evaluation of swallowing in the pediatric population is the functional endoscopic evaluation of swallowing (FEES). This procedure is an endoscopic, flexible nasolaryngoscopic examination performed concomitantly with a speech pathologist who feeds the patient with dyed solids, semisolids, and liquids while the hypopharynx and larynx are visualized. Particular attention is paid to the presence or absence of coating of the vallecula, pooling of secretions, penetration or aspiration of the food matter between the vocal folds, and vocal fold motion. The advantages of FEES are the evaluation of concurrent orolaryngeal and speech mechanisms, ability to evaluate nasal, velopharyngeal, and laryngeal structure and function, ability to tolerate various food textures, compensatory mechanisms, and addition of sensory testing. The disadvantages are the need to place a nasopharyngeal scope in a potentially uncooperative child, potential discomfort, inability to visualize the oral and esophageal phases of swallowing, and momentary inability to visualize the hypopharynx during the actual swallow.

CHRONIC AIRWAY CONDITIONS

Acquired Subglottic Stenosis

A small percentage of premature infants who are intubated and ventilated may develop subglottic and/or laryngeal stenosis (Fig. 13-11). The exact cause of laryngeal stenosis is unknown at this time. The severity of stenosis is graded using the Cotton-Myer grading system with the endotracheal tube leak test. Laryngeal stenosis may involve the vocal cords, with reduced vocal cord abduction seen on rigid laryngoscopy under spontaneous ventilation. Palpation of the arytenoids may reveal fixation if the stenosis extends from the subglottis to the interarytenoid area, mimicking bilateral vocal fold paralysis. The scar may be limited to the interarytenoid region and then classified as posterior glottic stenosis.

Treatment depends on severity. Mild cases may be managed conservatively or treated endoscopically with the laser. More severe cases require open laryngotracheal reconstruction (LTR) once the GI, pulmonary, and swallowing systems have been cleared.

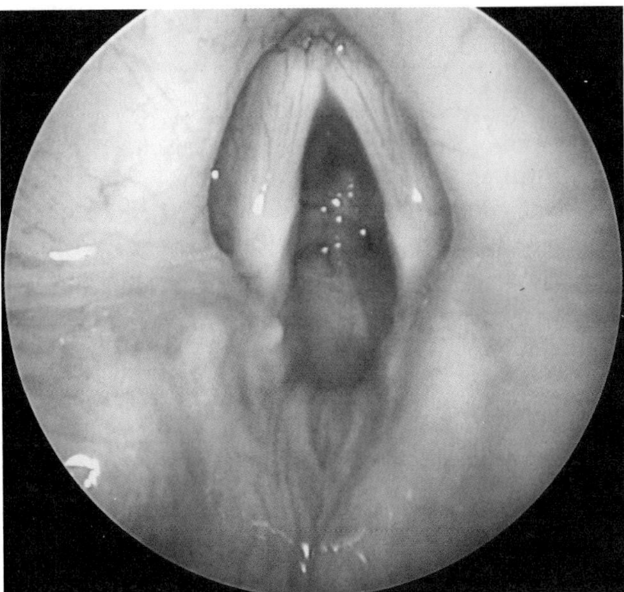

Figure 13-11. Acquired subglottic stenosis. Cotton-Myer grade III subglottic stenosis. Note the normal-appearing vocal folds in white. The subglottis is almost completely obstructed but, because of a pinhole airway, is labeled as a grade III as opposed to a grade IV, or complete, subglottic stenosis.

Congenital Subglottic Stenosis

Congenital subglottic stenosis is a rare condition, with an elliptic narrowing of the subglottic airway from failure of the cartilage to recanalize (Fig. 13-12). The vocal cords are usually mobile. Severity may vary and mild cases may be managed without tracheotomy. More severe cases may require tracheotomy or LTR.

Tracheal Stenosis

Tracheal stenosis may be congenital or acquired. Acquired tracheal stenosis may be related to endotracheal tube or cuff erosion injuries. An overinflated endotracheal cuff may cause pressure necrosis of the tracheal mucosa, which leads to a tracheal narrowing.

This may require tracheal resection and primary anastomosis. Long-segment congenital tracheal stenosis may be challenging to manage. The patient may have multiple complete tracheal rings (Fig. 13-13). Depending on the severity, treatment may consist of observation,[19] tracheal resection, or primary anastomosis or slide tracheoplasty.[20]

Subglottic Hemangiomas

Congenital cavernous hemangiomas have a predilection for the subglottic region of the larynx, as well as other head and neck sites (Fig. 13-14). The patient may present with crouplike symptoms and biphasic stridor. Treatment, which depends on severity and clinical experience, may include observation, corticosteroids, laser, tracheotomy, interferon, or open resection. Often, a mild subglottic stenosis is associated with subglottic hemangiomas, and a laryngotracheoplasty with a thyroid alar graft might be needed for the symptomatic child who requires resection of the lesion.

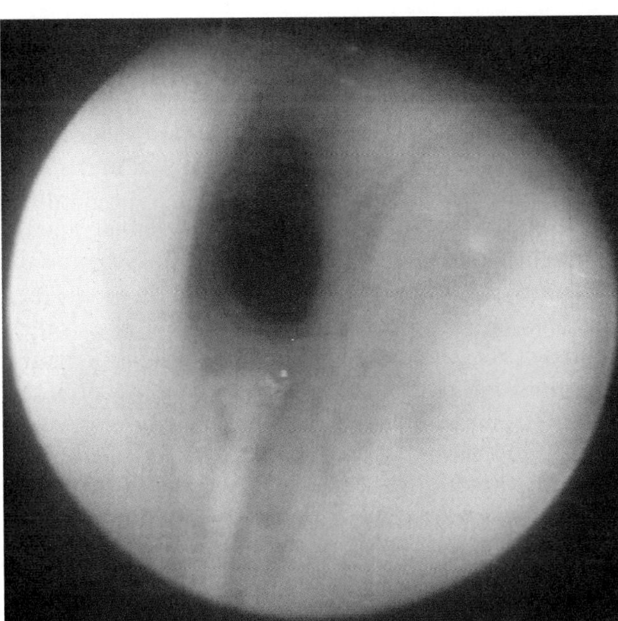

Figure 13-12. Congenital subglottic stenosis. Note the elliptic nature of the cricoid cartilage.

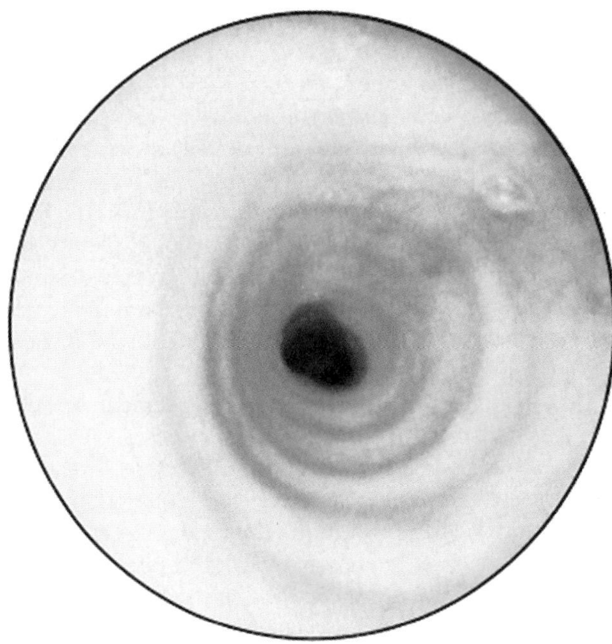

Figure 13-13. Tracheal stenosis caused by complete tracheal rings. (From Handler SD, Myer CM 3rd: Atlas of Ear, Nose and Throat Disorders in Children. Hamilton, Ontario, BC Decker, 1998.)

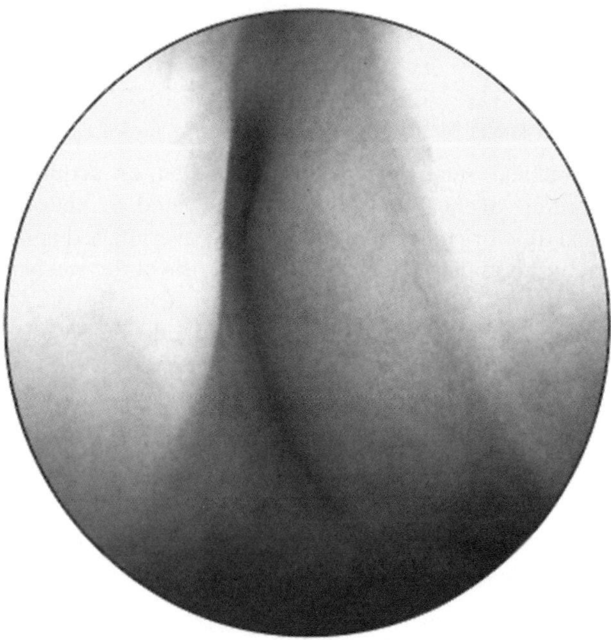

Figure 13-14. Subglottic hemangioma. Note the fullness on the undersurface of the right vocal fold, representing the hemangioma. (From Handler SD, Myer CM 3rd: Atlas of Ear, Nose and Throat Disorders in Children. Hamilton, Ontario, BC Decker, 1998.)

Recurrent Respiratory Papillomatosis

Recurrent respiratory papillomatosis (RRP) is the most common benign laryngeal neoplasm in children and the most common cause of pediatric hoarseness. Human papillomavirus (HPV), most commonly subtypes 6 and 11, has been implicated as the cause of RRP. Type 11 appears to be more virulent and is associated with more airway obstruction, pulmonary spread, and need for a tracheostomy.[21]

RRP most commonly involves the larynx; the other common extralaryngeal sites are the oral cavity, trachea, and bronchi. The classic clinical presentation is that of chronic hoarseness, stridor, and respiratory distress. Additional symptoms such as chronic cough, paroxysms of choking, recurrent pneumonia, failure to thrive, shortness of breath, and dysphagia may be mistaken for conditions such as asthma, croup, allergy, bronchitis, and vocal fold nodules.

The treatment of RRP is surgical débridement without permanent damage to underlying structures such as the vocal folds. Children who develop RRP before 3 years of age typically have frequent recurrences, requiring multiple surgical débridement procedures during the first few years of life.[21] The most commonly used techniques involve carbon dioxide laser, pulsed dye laser, cold instrumentation, and a microdébrider. In certain relentless situations or with distal spread to the lungs, adjuvant therapy with cidofovir, interferon alfa, and other experimental chemotherapeutic regimens have shown variable responses.

MANAGEMENT

Surgical Intervention

Once the severity of the airway obstruction has been ascertained, and after feeding, swallowing, pulmonary, GI, and voice concerns have been addressed, a decision can be made regarding the direction of management of chronic airway obstruction. In cases of very mild obstruction, with no overt symptoms or complications, it is possible to closely observe the child. Regular endoscopies to assess structural progression versus resolution of the obstruction are important. During the period of observation, it is important to exclude underlying reflux and esophagitis and to ensure optimal pulmonary status. In cases with more significant symptoms or obstruction, and following proper evaluation (see earlier), an appropriate intervention is chosen.

Tracheotomy

The indications for tracheotomy include severe upper obstruction, long-term ventilation, and pulmonary toilet. A tracheostomy tube is a plastic or metallic hollow tube that is surgically placed into the trachea to bypass the obstruction (Fig. 13-15A).

Tracheotomy may be required immediately in cases of acute airway obstruction in which traditional intubation with an endotracheal tube is not possible because of severe subglottic stenosis or difficult anatomy precluding oral or nasal intubation, such as trauma, or in patients with congenital airway problems such as laryngeal atresia.

In infants and small children, unlike in adults, emergency tracheostomy is rarely indicated or performed. Every attempt is made to establish an artificial airway by intubation or ventilation with a bronchoscope. Close cooperation with a trained anesthesiologist is vital. A horizontal skin incision is created at the level of the cricoid cartilage, superficial tissue and the strap musculature are retracted, and the laryngotracheal complex is exposed in the midline. A vertical incision is created through the third tracheal ring and retention sutures are placed laterally on the trachea in case the tube has become dislodged postoperatively. This allows anterior traction on the trachea in case of emergency (see Fig. 13-15B). The skin is then sutured to the tracheal edges and the tracheostomy tube is inserted. To confirm that the length and width of the chosen tracheostomy tube are appropriate for the child's airway, endoscopy is performed following the procedure. An ultrathin flexible scope is passed through the tracheostomy tube to be certain that the position of the tube is above the carina. Tracheostomy ties are placed and secured around the child's neck. A postoperative chest radiograph may be obtained to exclude a pneumothorax, although with meticulous midline technique, this complication is rare. The choice of the type of

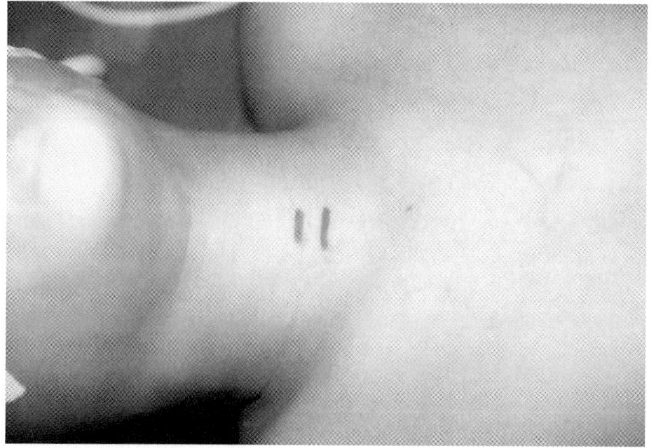
A

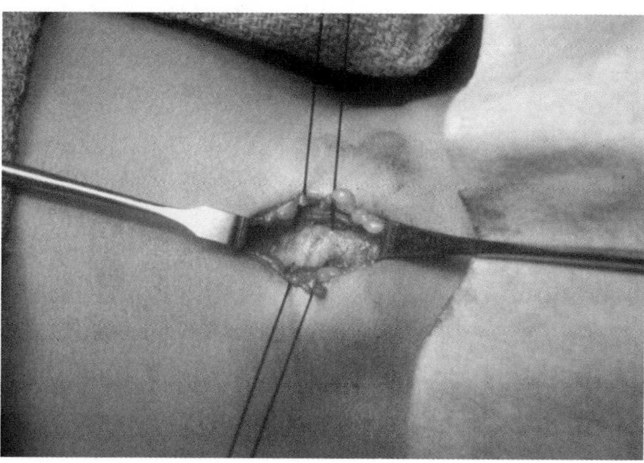
B

Figure 13-15. Tracheostomy placement. **A**, Infant in a hyperextended position for a tracheostomy. **B**, Two stay sutures placed lateral to the midline of the tracheal incision, prior to entering the airway.

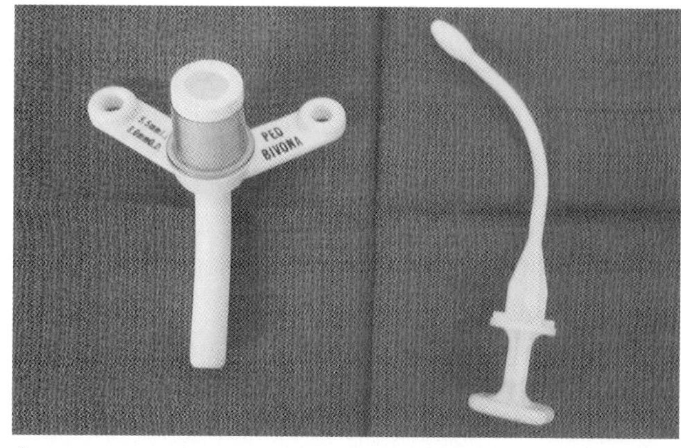

A

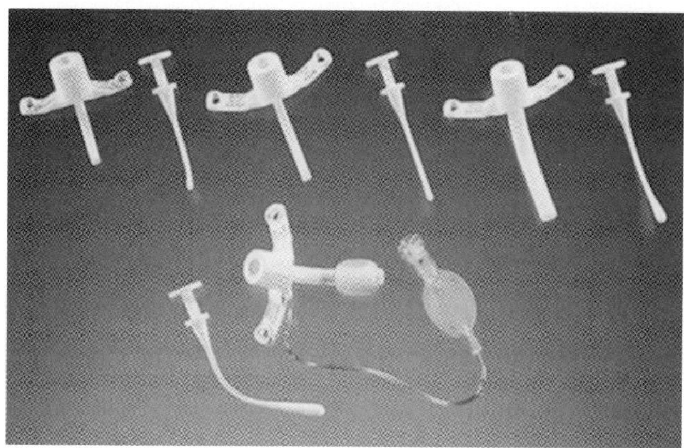
B

Figure 13-16. Bivona (**A**) and Shiley (**B**) tracheostomy tubes.

tracheostomy tube used is institution-dependent. The most common tubes used today are the Bivona and Shiley tubes (Fig. 13-16 and Table 13-2).

The greatest risk associated with an indwelling tracheostomy is death secondary to tube obstruction or an accidental dislodgment. Mortality related to the presence of a tracheostomy tube has been reported to approximate 0.5%.[22] It is therefore incumbent on the clinician to educate the family and caretakers regarding proper care at home. Specific tracheostomy care protocols have been developed and are used by many hospitals and medical centers. Caretakers should be well trained in all aspects of tracheostomy tube care, including routine tracheostomy tube changes, emergency problems, and normal stomal care. A standard set of equipment must always be available for emergency tracheostomy tube changes (Table 13-3). Having tracheostomy tubes one half-size smaller and similarly sized endotracheal tubes is necessary to avoid disaster. In addition, portable oxygen, suction, and resuscitation equipment must always be near the patient. The family must always travel with this equipment. Portable pulse oximetry monitors are helpful, especially during sleep.[23]

The surgical risks of a tracheotomy include bleeding, infection, pneumothorax, and loss of the airway. Bleeding is most likely because of and may be associated with a coagulation defect related to liver disease, coagulopathy, and other medical conditions; these should be controlled, if possible, prior to elective tracheostomy placement. Hemorrhage because of thyroid bleeds or vascular injuries are less common with proper surgical technique. Bleeding may also be seen in the tracheostomy-dependent child because of granulation (inflammatory tissue) at the tracheostomy site.

Postoperative chest radiography is performed to check for the presence of pneumothorax, pneumomediastinum, or subcutaneous emphysema, reported to occur in 3% to 9% of cases.[24] These occur because of intraoperative pleura injury low in the neck or because of a tension pneumothorax, seen in patients in whom the wound had been sutured tightly, allowing no air egress out of the neck. The latter problem is usually seen in ventilated patients. The treatment in most cases is expectant, with placement of a chest tube for larger pleural injuries.

Table 13-2 Commonly Used Tracheostomy Tubes and their Equivalent Dimensions

Brand	Inner Diameter (mm)	Outer Diameter (mm)	Length (mm)
Shiley			
3.0 neonatal (00NT)	3.0	4.5	30
3.5 neonatal (0NT)	3.5	5.2	32
4.0 neonatal (1NT)	4.0	5.9	34
3.0 pediatric (00PT)	3.0	4.5	39
3.5 pediatric (0PT)	3.5	5.2	40
4.0 pediatric (1PT)	4.0	5.9	41
4.5 pediatric (2PT)	4.5	6.0	42
5.0 pediatric (3PT)	5.0	7.1	44
5.5 pediatric (4PT)	5.5	7.7	46
Bivona			
2.5 neonatal	2.5	4.0	30
3.0 neonatal	3.0	4.7	32
3.5 neonatal	3.5	5.3	34
4.0 neonatal	4.0	6.0	36
2.5 pediatric	2.5	4.0	38
3.0 pediatric	3.0	4.7	39
3.5 pediatric	3.5	5.3	40
4.0 pediatric	4.0	6.0	41
4.5 pediatric	4.5	6.7	42
5.0 pediatric	5.0	7.3	44
5.5 pediatric	5.5	8.0	46
Portex			
3.0	3.0	5.0	36
3.5	3.5	5.8	40
4.0	4.0	6.5	44
4.5	4.5	7.1	48
5.0	5.0	7.7	50
5.5	5.5	8.3	52

Table 13-3 Equipment Needed for Tracheotomy Care and Tracheostomy Tube Changes

Tracheotomy Care	Tracheostomy Tube Change
Tracheostomy tube and obturator	Tracheostomy tube and obturator
One size smaller tracheostomy tube	One size smaller tracheostomy tube
Pipe cleaners	Blanket roll
Sterile water	Lubricant
Container for sterile water	Tracheotomy tie, collar
Gauze	Scissors
Portable suction machine	Stethoscope
Flexible suction catheter	Resuscitation bag with mask
Humidity valves (nose)	Oxygen supply
Tracheostomy gauze dressing	Clean wet and dry gauze
Oxygen	
Tracheostomy collar	

In our experience with proper midline surgical techniques, this complication is exceedingly rare.

Less common operative complications include injury to the esophagus and recurrent laryngeal nerve(s); both lie adjacent to the trachea. These complications should be rare with meticulous surgical technique. Sudden relief of obstruction and rapid CO_2 clearance may lead to pulmonary edema and respiratory arrest, respectively. Mechanical ventilation is necessary to manage these situations.

The most consistently fatal and feared postoperative complication, as noted earlier, is tube obstruction by dried blood or dried secretions. Proper suctioning protocols and humidification are mandatory. Tube dislodgment into a false tract and accidental decannulation can lead to death as well. The appearance of subcutaneous air in a ventilated patient should alert the family or the clinician to tube dislodgment. Unexplained cyanosis, desaturations, sudden audible phonation in a tracheotomized child who cannot usually be heard, retractions, and irritability should alarm the caregiver about tube obstruction of any cause.

Less common complications include hemorrhage from the tracheostomy stoma related to infection, granulation, and, rarely, tube erosion through the tracheal wall into the innominate artery. The latter manifests with unmistakable massive hemorrhage and must be managed emergently with digital pressure, cuffed endotracheal tube placement, and surgery or angiography with embolization. Innominate artery injury is less common with the use of the softer nonmetal tracheostomy tubes. More minor bleeding because of infection or granulation tissue can be managed with antibiotics, humidification, and excision of the granulation.

Ventilated patients with an endotracheal tube or tracheostomy tube may develop subcutaneous emphysema, pneumomediastinum, or pneumothorax because of overzealous positive pressure ventilation. Subcutaneous emphysema can be managed expectantly with placement of a cuffed tube, whereas a pneumothorax requires placement of a chest tube.

Moreover, tracheostomy tube placement may result in structural alteration in the trachea and subglottis. Placement of a high tracheostomy tube through the cricothyroid membrane, in absolute emergency situations, may result in subglottic stenosis. Suprastomal collapse, softening of the anterior tracheal wall at the upper stoma because of the presence of the tracheostomy tube, may occur in various degrees of severity. Severe collapse can lead to proximal suprastomal obstruction, necessitating surgical reconstruction prior to extubation or maintenance of a safe airway above the tracheostomy stoma in cases of accidental decannulation.

Finally, when the tracheostomy is no longer medically necessary, the child will undergo a decannulation process to remove the tube. This will require a preliminary airway evaluation, including a microlaryngoscopy and bronchoscopy (MLB), to make sure that the airway is adequate, followed by repair of the suprastomal collapse and granulation. In 50% to 90% of cases, a persistent tracheocutaneous fistula (TCF) will result.[24,25] This is managed by surgical excision of the tract from the skin to the trachea and skin closure.

Endoscopic Approaches to Repair of Glottic and Subglottic Stenosis

There are certain conditions that are amenable to endoscopic, minimally invasive approaches of repair. The technique involves suspension microlaryngoscopy, in which a laryngoscope with a wide orifice is inserted transorally and suspended in the vallecula (Fig. 13-17). A microscope with a focal length deep enough to magnify the structures of the larynx and/or trachea (400 mm) is then used by the surgeon. The technique of repair is with or without a laser. Discussion of the merits of various lasers (CO_2, KTP) versus cold steel is beyond the scope of this chapter. Conditions leading to chronic airway obstruction that are potentially amenable to endoscopic management include base of tongue cysts and masses, glossoptosis (base of tongue collapse), RRP, laryngomalacia, arytenoid prolapse, arytenoid subluxation leading to posterior glottic stenosis, small posterior glottic scar or web, bilateral vocal fold paralysis, small subglottic web, subglottic cysts, and tracheal hemangiomas.

Anterior Cricoid Split

Neonates who have been intubated for a prolonged period who fail extubation because of minimal subglottic stenosis and who meet strict eligibility criteria[19] (Box 13-1) may benefit from a cricoid split to augment the airway. The reason for the strict criteria is that if

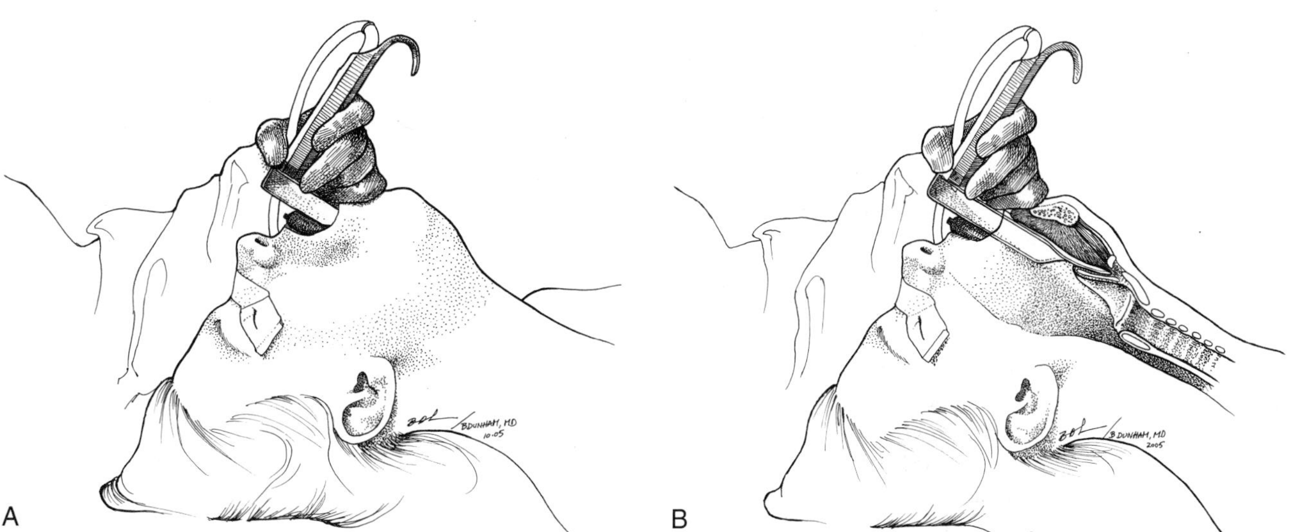

Figure 13-17. Laryngoscope suspended in the vallecula. **A**, Head positioning of the patient in the operating room. **B**, Actual placement of the laryngoscope in the vallecula to expose the larynx fully. (Courtesy of Dr. Brian Dunham.)

Box 13-1 Criteria for Performing Anterior Cricoid Split

Extubation failure on at least two occasions secondary to laryngeal pathology
Weight >1500 g
No assisted ventilation for 10 days prior to evaluation
Supplemental oxygen requirement <35%
No congestive heart failure for 1 mo prior to evaluation
No acute upper or lower respiratory tract infection at time of evaluation
No antihypertensive medications for 10 days prior to evaluation

successful, the cricoid split will lead to extubation and no need for further ventilatory support.

The cricoid split is a surgical alternative to placement of a tracheostomy tube, expanding the cricoid framework without a graft. The procedure involves a horizontal skin incision at the level of the cricoid, with elevation of subplatysmal skin flaps and exposure of the laryngotracheal complex by retracting the strap muscles laterally. The anterior cricoid is then incised. Occasionally, if the stenosis involved a posterior subglottic component, a posterior cricoid split may be useful as well. The patient remains intubated for approximately 10 days to allow fibrosis to occur between the split ends of the cricoid, thus expanding the airway. The patient is then re-evaluated endoscopically prior to extubation.

Augmentation Procedures: Laryngotracheal Reconstruction

Expansion procedures to aid in tracheostomy tube removal in the child with glottic or subglottic stenosis include placement of anterior, posterior, or combined grafts to augment the cricoid and/or tracheal airway. The management of laryngotracheal stenosis in children includes several approaches that have already been discussed—a tracheostomy tube and wait- and- see policy for the milder forms of narrowing; endoscopic maneuvers for moderate cases; anterior cricoid cartilage split for the management of evolving subglottic stenosis in the neonate; and open surgical procedures using grafts of various types, with or without intraluminal stents, for severe cases.[5]

Laryngotracheal reconstruction (or laryngotracheoplasty; used interchangeably in this chapter) refers to an augmentation or expansion procedure with use of a graft(s). The aim of this surgical method is to reestablish airway continuity without the need for a tracheostomy tube. For this reason, the candidate for an LTR should have good pulmonary reserve, requiring no ventilatory support, and be medically stable. The preoperative workup should include the comprehensive evaluation delineated earlier. It is important to note the aspiration risk in such patients. Often, patients at risk for aspiration may not develop aspiration pneumonia because of a high-grade subglottic stenosis, physically impeding the flow of refluxed material and food into the trachea and lung. The decision whether to reconstruct such a patient is not easily made and should be done in collaboration with the family, caretaker, speech-language pathologist, and pulmonologist. It would be counterproductive to augment the airway of an aspirator, which would then increase the risk for recurrent pneumonias and possible need for a tracheostomy tube.

Once the decision has been made regarding the eligibility for reconstruction, the choice of reconstruction includes augmentation or resection. Resection will be described in the next section. Another element that needs to be decided is whether the procedure should be single-staged or double-staged. A single-staged procedure means that at the conclusion of the surgery, the tracheostomy tube will no longer be present, whereas a double-staged procedure means that a tracheostomy tube or similar type of stent will be present at the end of the case (see next section).

The augmentation procedure involves placement of an autogenous cartilage graft between the split cricoid cartilage and/or split tracheal wall. Numerous graft materials have been reported in the literature over the years, but the most commonly used graft is the cartilaginous rib. Other sources of cartilage grafts, reported in both adult and pediatric studies, have included auricular cartilage, hyoid, thyroid ala, septal cartilage, and thyrotracheal autografts.[5,26,27] Regardless of the source of cartilage, studies have shown that autogenous cartilage used in the anterior and posterior pediatric larynx survives, grows, and undergoes neovascularization.[7] Some potential problems related to the use of autogenous grafts of cartilage include partial graft resorption and potential donor site complications (in the case of rib grafts, pneumothorax). Numerous reports of the use of alloplastic materials have been published, but have not been universally accepted or used in large human series as an alternative graft material.[28]

Technique. With the patient under general anesthesia, intubated with a tracheostomy tube or ETT, a horizontal skin incision is made at the level of the cricoid. Subplatysmal flaps are elevated and the soft tissue overlying the laryngotracheal complex retracted laterally. The cricoid cartilage is then split and the airway inspected for synchronous airway lesions. The subglottic scar is excised. Once an adequate subglottic lumen has been created, a decision is made regarding placement of a posterior graft, an anterior graft, or both. This depends on the location of the narrowing. The harvested cartilage graft is then shaped to fit the cricoid defect and placed between the cut cricoid cartilage edges posteriorly, anteriorly, or in both locations.

In a single-stage procedure, the patient is nasotracheally intubated for a predetermined period. Usually, for anterior grafts, it is 3 to 5 days. If more complex reconstruction has been performed, the intubation can last more than of 10 days. Following this period of stenting with an endotracheal tube, the patient is reevaluated endoscopically. If the repair appears intact, the child can be extubated.

There are certain situations that guide the surgeon when performing a double-stage laryngotracheal reconstruction. The benefit of maintaining the tracheostomy tube is ensuring a safe decannulation process, avoiding the need for postoperative sedation while the patient is nasotracheally intubated. Patients who are unlikely to benefit from a single-stage procedure include the following: (1) neurologically compromised children; (2) very young children; (3) patients who required supraglottic reconstruction in addition to LTR; (4) patients with glottic pathology (e.g., vocal fold paralysis, edema); (5) children in whom the tracheostomy stoma is very distal to the level of stenosis with healthy intervening tracheal rings, and (6) tracheomalacia patients. Some tracheostomy-dependent patients may not be candidates for decannulation (need for overnight ventilatory support), but would benefit from proximal airway reconstruction to allow the development of communication and verbal skills.

Resection Procedures: Partial Cricotracheal Resection

Patients with discrete levels of obstruction, grade III or IV subglottic stenosis, often benefit from a graft-free resection procedure. Two resection procedures are used to manage subglottic or tracheal stenosis, partial cricotracheal resection (CTR) or tracheal resection, respectively. This chapter focuses on the more complex CTR.

The CTR procedure involves resection of the anterior cricoid plate, remaining anterior to the cricothyroid joint, resection of the proximal tracheal stenosis, maintaining the first healthy tracheal ring intact, and removal of the posterior cricoid scar in a submucosal plane, below the level of the cricoarytenoid joint. Once the scar has been removed, the trachea is sutured to the posterior cricoid mucosa and anterior thyroid lamina. Chin to chest sutures are placed for 10 days to allow healing of the anastomosis without the potential for head extension and tracheal separation in case of patient agitation. CTR, just like LTR, can be performed in a single- or double-stage procedure, with similar indications for each, as described earlier.

Complications following a CTR could be potentially devastating. Anastomotic dehiscence can lead to partial or complete separation of the trachea from the thyroid cartilage, leading to severe airway compromise and possible death if not identified promptly. Sudden subcutaneous air in the neck or chest, tachypnea, fever, neck cellulitis, stridor, or acute hoarseness should alert the clinician to an occult or complete laryngotracheal separation. Immediate management in the operating room is a necessity. Intubation should not be attempted at the bedside, because false-passage intubation and its complications may be life-threatening.

Wound infection, bleeding, and pneumothorax are minor possible complications and can be managed routinely. Nonjudicious dissection of the trachea during the procedure may lead to unilateral or bilateral vocal fold paralysis because of injury to the recurrent laryngeal nerve(s). This injury must be excluded in any CTR patient with postextubation stridor or dyspnea. Nocturnal or exertional stridor may be a manifestation of arytenoid prolapse, which is commonly seen following CTR.[29] Flexible, awake, and sedated nasopharyngoscopy can reveal this potential complication, related to destabilization of the posterior cricoid support of the arytenoid cartilages. An endoscopic arytenoidectomy might be required to manage this.

Decannulation

Once a patient has been deemed ready for tracheostomy tube removal, decannulation is undertaken. In most situations, an MLB is performed to ensure an adequate airway and to repair stomal problems, which might include placing a "pexy" (or a tether) suture to alleviate a collapsed suprastomal region (Fig. 13-18A) or excision of obstructive suprastomal granulation tissue[30] (Fig. 13-18B). Subsequently, the patient is admitted for a tracheotomy downsizing and capping trial while on continuous pulse oximetry. Capping means placement of a tracheostomy

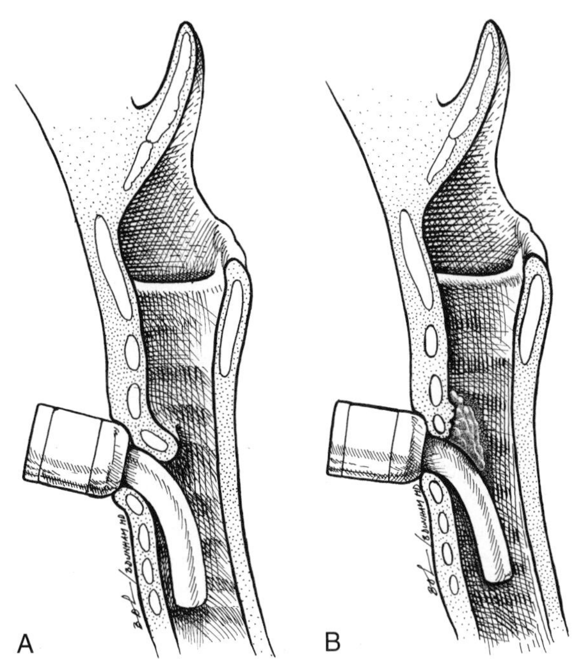

Figure 13-18. **A,** Suprastomal collapse. **B,** Suprastomal granulation. (Courtesy of Dr. Brian Dunham).

tube plug or cap on the anterior limb of the tracheostomy tube to allow the child to breath naturally through the mouth and/or nose. It is essential to watch the child sleeping as well as awake. An overnight observation period is used. If a capping trial is successful, without retraction, stridor, or desaturations, the tracheostomy tube is then removed and the stoma is covered with a bandage. The remaining tracheocutaneous tract or fistula (TCF) will heal in the ensuing several months. If it does not heal completely, surgical closure is undertaken. Care is taken to ensure that there is no recurrence of the airway obstruction, which would prevent complete spontaneous closure of the TCF.

SUMMARY

The management of chronic airway obstruction in the pediatric population is a challenging multidisciplinary effort. With close monitoring and a trained staff, these patients can often resume a healthy, tracheostomy-free lifestyle. Associated medical issues such as lung disease, reflux, and swallowing disorders must be excluded and/or treated prior to venturing into airway reconstruction.

MAJOR POINTS

The presentation of chronic airway obstruction is variable and dependent on the patient's age and severity of the compromise.

Chronic cough and recurrent croup may be manifestations of asthma, gastroesophageal reflux disease, and tracheomalacia, and should be carefully distinguished from upper airway stenosis or compromise.

Stridor is a common presentation of airway compromise in young children. It is important to realize that other manifestations of airway obstruction may include recurrent croup, chronic cough, dyspnea on exertion, dysphagia, and hoarseness.

A thorough history and physical examination are paramount to an accurate diagnosis.

The gold standard of the airway evaluation is rigid endoscopy under general anesthesia.

Esophagoscopy with biopsy is an important component of the airway evaluation to exclude the possibility that significant reflux and/or eosinophilic esophagitis affect the airway.

Once the severity of the airway obstruction has been ascertained, and after feeding, swallowing, pulmonary, GI, and voice concerns have been addressed, a decision can be made regarding the direction of management of chronic airway obstruction.

REFERENCES

1. Pahor AL: Ear, nose and throat in Ancient Egypt. J Laryngol Otol 1992;106:773-779.
2. Graamans K, Pirsig W, Biefel K: The shift in the indications for the tracheotomy between 1940 and 1955: An historical review. J Laryngol Otol 1999;113:624-627.
3. Wallenborn WM: George Washington's terminal illness: A modern medical analysis of the last illness and death of George Washington, 1997. Available at http://gwpapers.virginia.edu/ articles/wallenborn.html.
4. Morens DM: Death of a president. N Engl J Med 1999; 341:1845-1849.
5. Cotton R: The problem of pediatric laryngotracheal stenosis: A clinical and experimental study on the efficacy of autogenous cartilaginous grafts placed between the vertically divided halves of the posterior lamina of the cricoid cartilage. Laryngoscope 1991;101:1-34.
6. Jackson C: Laryngeal stenosis—growth of the larynx as a factor in treatment. Laryngoscope 1932;2:887-898.
7. Pashley N, Jaskunas J, Waldstein G: Laryngotracheoplasty with costochondral grafts—a clinical correlate of graft survival. Laryngoscope 1984;94:1493-1496.
8. Shott SR, Donnelly L: Cine magnetic resonance imaging: Evaluation of persistent airway obstruction after tonsil and adenoidectomy in children with Down syndrome. Laryngoscope 2004;114:1724-1729.
9. Brown P: Medical management of gastroesophageal reflux. Curr Opin Pediatr 2000;12:247-250.
10. McMurray JS, Prescott CA: Tracheostomy in the pediatric patient. In Cotton RT, Myer CI (eds): Practical Pediatric Otolaryngology. Philadelphia, Lippincott-Raven, 1999, pp 575-593.
11. Myer CM 3rd, O'Connor DM, Cotton RT: Proposed grading system for subglottic stenosis based on endotracheal tube sizes. Ann Otol Rhinol Laryngol 1994;103:319-323.
12. Nelson SP, Chen EH, Syniar GM, et al: Prevalence of symptoms of gastroesophageal reflux during infancy. A pediatric practice-based survey. Pediatric Practice Research Group. Arch Pediatr Adolesc Med 1997;151:569-572.
13. Gold BD: Outcomes of pediatric gastroesophageal reflux disease: In the first year of life, in childhood, and in adults. Oh, and should we really leave *Helicobacter pylori* alone? J Pediatr Gastroenterol Nutr 2003;37(Suppl 1):S33-S39.
14. Walner DL, Stern Y, Gerber ME, et al: Gastroesophageal reflux in patients with subglottic stenosis. Arch Otolaryngol Head Neck Surg 1998;124:551-555.
15. Halstead LA: Gastroesophageal reflux: A critical factor in pediatric subglottic stenosis. Otolaryngol Head Neck Surg 1999;120:683-688.
16. Walsh SV, Antonioli DA, Goldman H, et al: Allergic esophagitis in children: A clinicopathological entity. Am J Surg Pathol 1999;23:390-396.
17. Tolia V: Gastroesophageal reflux and supraesophageal complications: Really true or ballyhoo? J Pediatr Gastroenterol Nutr 2002;34:269-273.

18. Skopnik H, Silny J, Heiber O, et al: Gastroesophageal reflux in infants: Evaluation of a new intraluminal impedance technique. J Pediatr Gastroenterol Nutr 1996;23:591-598.

19. Cotton R: Management of subglottic stenosis. Otolaryngol Clin North Am 2000;33:111-130.

20. Rutter MJ, Cotton RT, Azizkhan RG, et al: Slide tracheoplasty for the management of complete tracheal rings. J Pediatr Surg 2003;38:928-934.

21. Wiatrak BJ, Wiatrak DW, Broker TR, et al: Recurrent respiratory papillomatosis: A longitudinal study comparing severity associated with human papilloma viral types 6 and 11 and other risk factors in a large pediatric population. Laryngoscope 2004;114:1-23.

22. Wetmore RF, Marsh RR, Thompson ME, et al: Pediatric tracheostomy: A changing procedure? Ann Otol Rhinol Laryngol 1999;108:695-699.

23. Jacobs I, Pettignano M, Pettignano R: Airway management. In Czervinske MP, Barnhart SL (eds): Perinatal and Pediatric Respiratory Care, 2nd ed. Philadelphia, WB Saunders, 2003, pp 207-232.

24. Wetmore R, Handler S, Potsic W. Pediatric tracheostomy: Experience during the past decade. Ann Otol Rhinol Laryngol 1982;91:628-632.

25. Sautter NB, Krakovitz PR, Solares CA, et al: Closure of persistent tracheocutaneous fistula following "starplasty" tracheostomy in children. Int J Pediatr Otorhinolaryngol 2006; 70:99-105.

26. Zur KB, Urken ML: Vascularized hemitracheal autograft for laryngotracheal reconstruction: A new surgical technique based on the thyroid gland as a vascular carrier. Laryngoscope 2003;113:1494-1498.

27. Caputo V, Consiglio V: The use of patient's own auricular cartilage to repair deficiency of the tracheal wall. J Thorac Cardiovasc Surg 1961;41:594-596.

28. Chan KH, Reilly JS, Hashida Y: A staged laryngotracheal reconstruction using alloplast (Proplast) in the canine model. Int J Pediatr Otorhinolaryngol 1990;18:227-239.

29. Rutter MJ, Link DT, Hartley BE, et al: Arytenoid prolapse as a consequence of cricotracheal resection in children. Ann Otol Rhinol Laryngol 2001;110:210-214.

30. Gray RF, Todd WN, Jacobs I: Tracheostomy decannulation in children: Approaches and techniques. Laryngoscope 1998;108:8-12.

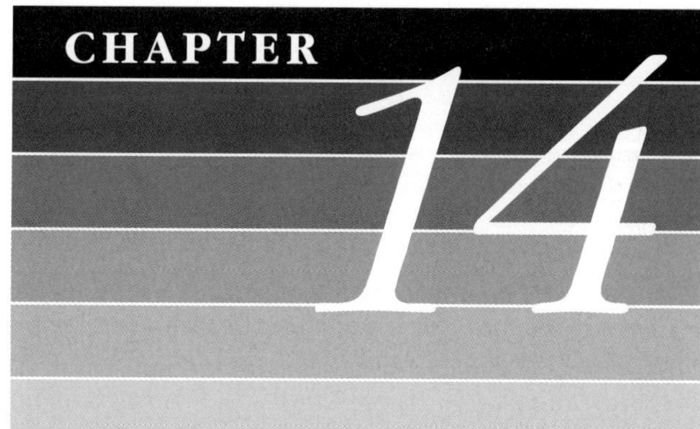

Sleep-Disordered Breathing

RALPH F. WETMORE, MD

Although sleep-disordered breathing (SDB) in children was recognized as long ago as 1976, the report of normative pediatric sleep data by Marcus in 1992 led to a surge of investigation into the effects of nighttime airway obstruction on the quality of life of children who suffer with it.[1,2] The study of sleep medicine, in both children and adults, has blossomed into a separate medical specialty, and medical and surgical treatments have been shown to be effective in relieving symptoms. Although further work needs to be done to understand this disorder fully, a major hurdle has been bridged in that the nature of SDB has been brought to the attention of practicing clinicians.

DEFINITIONS

Patterns of breathing during sleep may be categorized into one of several types. Primary snoring (PS) consists of snoring without a change in sleep architecture, alveolar ventilation, or gas exchange abnormalities. The incidence of PS on a habitual basis ranges from 7% to 10% of children.[3] Most children with PS do not progress to SDB.[4]

Upper airway resistance syndrome (UARS) describes the effect of negative intrathoracic pressure changes on inspiration during sleep. These changes are caused by airway obstruction that may lead to electroencephalographic arousals and major sleep fragmentation, but not to frank apnea. In addition to the repeated transient electroencephalographic arousals, an increase in snoring occurs just prior to the arousal. Changes in the respiratory pattern include an increase in the time of inspiration and a coinciding decrease in the time of expiration, but no change in gas exchange abnormalities.[5] UARS is found most often during rapid eye movement (REM) sleep. It is difficult to document in children because it usually requires direct measurement of intrathoracic pressure in the esophagus, a procedure difficult to perform in most children. In assessing the quality of life in children with SDB, de Serres and associates have shown that UARS is more common than obstructive apnea.[6]

Obstructive apnea (OA) is the absence of any gas exchange that results from complete obstruction of the upper airway during a respiratory effort. During sleep, these obstructive episodes result in electroencephalographic arousals, sleep fragmentation, and gas exchange abnormalities.

During an episode of central apnea, there is an absence of gas exchange that results from an absence of a respiratory effort. Episodes of central apnea are abnormal if they are longer than 20 seconds in duration or associated with one of the following: oxygen desaturation below 90%, bradycardia, or nighttime arousals.[7,8] Mixed apnea episodes contain both obstructive and central elements.

Hypopnea is a partial obstruction during sleep that may result in electroencephalographic arousal, sleep fragmentation, and changes in ventilation and gas exchange. In children, there has been a lack of consensus of what actually constitutes a hypopnea. Catterall and colleagues have described a hypopnea as breath with a 50% reduction in airflow.[9] Gould and co-workers have described it as a 50% reduction in respiratory effort.[10] Guilleminault and associates have reported both a reduction in airflow and associated oxygen desaturation.[11] Block and colleagues have suggested a reduction in airflow and respiratory effort in association with a fall in oxygen saturation.[12] Complete (obstructive apneas) and partial obstructions (hypopneas) intermingled with periods of normal sleep and ventilation are defined as the obstructive sleep apnea syndrome (OSAS).

A respiratory event-related arousal (RERA) is a gradual increase in the end-inspiratory negative intrathoracic pressure of at least 5 cm H_2O during five or more breath cycles, followed by an arousal or awakening.[13] This subtle measure of a significant respiratory disturbance may be more important in children than in adults.

EVALUATION

To use the indices of SDB that describe the severity of obstruction in adults, one must recognize that SDB affects children differently than adults. Children have much briefer episodes of obstruction and more partial obstructions, although the frequency of obstructive events is much more common than in adults. An apnea of 10 seconds may be significant because it may represent several missed breaths in a young child. For example, an apnea of 6 seconds lasting the duration of one and one-half to two breaths may result in significant oxygen desaturation. Because the obstructive events are very short, there may be fewer gas exchange abnormalities (hypoxia, hypercapnea), although repeated arousals during the night may affect sleep architecture.

The apnea index (AI) is a measure of the number of apneas per hour of sleep. In adults, the normal AI ranges between 5 and 10.[14] In children, the normal range (0.1 ± 0.5) reflects the fact that an apnea of almost any duration is abnormal in a child, whereas normal adults may have a low incidence of obstructive events.[2]

The respiratory disturbance index (RDI) is a measure of complete and partial obstructive events, the number of apneas and hypopneas per hour of sleep. A RDI greater than 20 is abnormal in adults, although the RDI in a child should not exceed 5. Because of the significance and number of hypopneas in children, the RDI is probably a better measurement of SDB in children than the AI. To classify a child with UARS, the RDI should not exceed 5.[5] Variability in event reporting (i.e., the definition of an apnea and a hypopnea) among centers has made both clinical and experimental interpretation of sleep studies difficult.[15]

The measurement of oxygen saturation is important in any evaluation of SDB. A decrease of oxygen saturation more than 3% to 5% is thought to be abnormal.[16] Similarly, carbon dioxide exchange abnormalities, such as a peak end-tidal CO_2 greater than 53 mm Hg or an end-tidal CO_2 greater than 45 mm Hg for 60% of the total sleep time (TST), is abnormal.[2] Because of the high number of hypopneas and the short duration of apneas, gas exchange abnormalities are much less frequent in children. Arousals tend to be less frequent in children; along with less gas exchange abnormalities, this decrease in arousals may result in less daytime hypersomnolence.[17]

Pathophysiology

Obstructive apnea can be found in 1% to 3% of children, with an equal male-to-female prevalence.[18] There is a higher incidence of SDB in the African American population.[19] The peak incidence of SDB in children mirrors the peak age for the narrowing effect of lymphoid hyperplasia on the airway—2 to 6 years of age.[7] Snoring remains the most common symptom and most affected children are of normal weight, in contrast to the predilection for obesity in affected adults. Symptoms of SDB frequently appear in those as young as 2 years of age, but a delay in diagnosis is common, averaging 3.3 years in one series.[20]

As in adults, the most common site of obstruction in children with SDB is the pharynx. Isono and associates used endoscopic examinations to demonstrate a narrow pharynx in children with SDB compared with controls.[21] Although a major anatomic cause of airway obstruction in adults is the deposition of fat in the lateral pharyngeal musculature,[22] in children, hyperplastic lymphoid tissue, specifically the tonsils and adenoid, produce a similar obstructive effect on the pharyngeal airway. The severity of symptoms does not appear to be related to the size of the tonsils and adenoid, and apnea may persist following tonsillectomy and adenoidectomy or may reappear years later. This is especially true of children suffering with obesity, whose pattern mirrors the obstruction observed in the adult population.

Disorders that affect the skull base or narrow the nasopharynx predispose the child to SDB and include the following orocranial features described by Guilleminault and colleagues: small chin, steep mandibular plane, retroposition of the mandible, long face, high hard palate, elongated soft palate, and enlarged lingual tonsil.[5] Conditions in the nose that favor the development of SDB include a nasal cavity narrowed by enlarged turbinates or nasoseptal deviation. Similarly, the nasopharynx may be blocked by enlarged adenoid tissue. Laryngeal or tracheobronchial lesions are rarely the site of obstruction in children.

In addition to the anatomic blockage caused by adenotonsillar hypertrophy, obstruction of the airway at night is often the result of dynamic neuromuscular factors that may be subtle in children who are otherwise healthy. SDB in children may be associated with primary hypoventilation (pickwickian syndrome), although the incidence of this condition is much lower in children than adults. Sedative drugs, such as anticonvulsants, may predispose the child to nighttime obstruction. A familial incidence of OA has been reported to occur in 20% to

25% of first-degree relatives of patients with apnea.[23,24] This compares with an incidence of OA in the general pediatric population of up to 1% to 3%.

POPULATIONS AT RISK

The most common cause of SDB in children is the result of lymphoid hyperplasia, as mirrored by a prevalence of nighttime obstruction in both preschool and school-age children when the size of tonsillar and adenoid tissue is greatest compared with the size of the airway. Craniofacial syndromes that contain one or more of the orocranial features outlined by Guilleminault and co-workers as predisposing to SDB have a high incidence of OA.[5] Apert's and Crouzon's syndromes are distinguished by midface hypoplasia, narrow nasopharynx, and altered skull base. In Treacher Collins syndrome, features such as a small chin, steep mandibular plane, and retroposition of the mandible, in association with a long face, all predispose to SDB. Children with Down syndrome have an altered skull base and relative macroglossia, features that lead to nighttime obstruction. Adenotonsillar hypertrophy, often the result of frequent upper respiratory illnesses, is common in Down syndrome children, as is generalized hypotonia, which predisposes to obstruction. In Hunter's and Hurler's syndromes, glycogen storage deposition in the pharyngeal musculature, in association with adenotonsillar hypertrophy, leads to airway obstruction.

Although nasoseptal deviation is uncommon in children, complete or near-total obstruction of one or both nares may cause symptoms of SDB. Other nasal conditions that rarely cause symptoms include nasopharyngeal stenosis or the presence of a large antrochoanal polyp that blocks the nasopharynx. In children younger than 2 years, laryngeal or tracheal conditions such as bilateral vocal cord paralysis, laryngomalacia, tracheomalacia, or mass lesions may cause significant nighttime obstruction.

The presence of allergy alone does not cause SDB; however, swelling of the respiratory mucosa in addition to increased secretions may be have a cumulative effect with other anatomic obstructions. A high prevalence of allergy has been seen in children with habitual (obstructive) snoring.[25] Similarly, viral upper respiratory infections may exacerbate symptoms because of an increase in secretions and the size of the tonsillar and adenoid tissue. Asthma frequently mimics obstructive apnea during sleep. Both apnea and asthma patients may have fits of coughing and difficulty breathing during sleep, and it is important to distinguish which condition is the cause, so that treatment can be effective. Gastroesophageal reflux may also contribute to nighttime obstruction by various mechanisms. Chronic exposure of the pharynx to acid secretions from the stomach may lead to chronic inflammation and swelling of the pharyngeal, and even the nasal mucosa in severe cases. Episodes of gastroesophageal reflux that reach the level of the larynx may cause laryngospasm with resulting apnea or may result in microaspiration or frank aspiration. Episodes of obstruction that result in apnea may also precipitate gastroesophageal reflux as the child generates high intrathoracic pressure in an attempt to overcome the obstruction. Finally, children with neuromuscular disorders such as cerebral palsy and muscular dystrophy are at risk for SDB because their underlying hypotonia is exacerbated during sleep, with a resultant increase in pharyngeal obstruction.[26]

CONSEQUENCES

During normal sleep, changes in respiration include a decrease in minute ventilation and functional residual capacity. REM sleep is marked by irregular breathing, with a variable rate and tidal volume and frequent central apneas. Children have more REM sleep; this is significant because, in one series, 55% of OAs occurred during REM sleep.[27] Children tend to have normal sleep stage distribution and architecture, but there is an increase in the AI, duration of apnea, and degree of desaturation during REM sleep. There is also an increase in the number and severity of obstructive events as the night progresses.[27]

Evidence that SDB may have a negative impact on daytime behavior and school performance remains controversial. A meta-analysis of 17 reports[28] failed to show a causal relationship between SDB and behavior and performance, citing poor sampling, insufficient consideration of confounders, and imprecise use of statistical tools. Conversely, others have shown a higher prevalence of behavior problems in children with mild SDB, including externalizing and hyperactivity-type behaviors.[29] Animal studies have demonstrated neural apoptosis in the cortex and hippocampus in rats subjected to chronic hypoxia.[30]

Although childhood obesity has become more prevalent in the last decade, many children with SDB are often small and skinny, preferring food that does not require chewing. Anosmia that results from nasal obstruction at night may also impair appetite in affected children. The expenditure of calories because of increased work of breathing may have an impact on growth and body habitus. Bar and associates have suggested that SDB may have a negative effect on growth hormone secretion at night.[31] Williams and colleagues have shown a significant improvement in weight following adenotonsillectomy, with 65% of patients having increases of 15% or more.[32] Marcus and co-workers have demonstrated a growth spurt in patients following tonsillectomy and adenoidectomy, and suggested that this is the result of a decrease in calories in the work of breathing.[33]

The presence of SDB has been shown to have adverse effects on the cardiorespiratory system. Obstruction that results from adenotonsillar hypertrophy can cause an increase in mean pulmonary artery pressure, a value that normalizes following tonsillectomy and adenoidectomy.[34] Brown and associates have reported 11 cases of children with cor pulmonale secondary to adenotonsillar hypertrophy; the cardiac symptoms disappeared following surgical intervention.[35] The presumed mechanism of right heart failure begins as decreased minute volume ventilation, secondary to upper airway obstruction leading to pulmonary ventilation-perfusion abnormalities and chronic alveolar hypoventilation. The resulting hypercapnia and hypoxia lead to respiratory acidosis and pulmonary artery constriction, and ultimately increased to right ventricular work and hypertrophy. Eventually, ventricular dilation can occur.[35] Although adults tend to have tachyarrhythmias with SDB, children are more prone to have bradyarrhythmias. Systemic hypertension has been shown to result from SDB.[36]

The effects of long-standing nasal obstruction in young children remain controversial, but elongation of the midface resulting in an adenoid facies has been documented.[37] Similarly, chronic airway obstruction has been shown to lead to malocclusion of the teeth.[38]

SYMPTOMS AND SIGNS

Daytime symptoms of SDB are listed in Box 14-1. Chronic mouth breathing is common, but constant loud breathing is often associated with significant nighttime obstruction. Decreased appetite often occurs because of hyposmia and aversion to food that requires chewing. Abnormal daytime behavior seen with SDB runs the gamut of symptoms, from shyness to hyperactivity and aggressive behavior. Morning headaches are the result of chronic hypoxia and nighttime hypercapnea. Because children have fewer gas exchange abnormalities and often nap during the daytime, they show less symptoms of daytime hypersomnolence. Gozal and associates have shown that only 13% of children with SDB fall asleep in less than 10 minutes during daytime sleep laboratory studies.[39] Also, because children manifest fewer gas exchange abnormalities, pickwickian symptoms such as hypersomnolence are rare. The current trend of obesity in children may make these symptoms more prevalent.

Nighttime symptoms of SDB are listed in Box 14-2. Notable among these are loud snoring, apnea, choking, and gasping. In children with asthma, it may be difficult to distinguish between coughing that is caused by upper airway obstruction and coughing from reactive airway disease. Abnormal sleep positions, including hyperextension of the head, a frequent sign of SDB, and sitting upright or prone with the knees tucked beneath the rest of the torso, are common. Many children with SDB resist going to bed because of unpleasant nighttime symptoms.[40] Enuresis is not uncommon in children with SDB and may be multifactorial. An increase in urine production and salt excretion has been shown in patients with SDB. Affected patients also have more nocturnal micturations. Hormonal effects that may account for enuresis include an increase in atrial natriuretic peptide release, a decrease in activity of the renin-angiotensin-aldosterone system, and an increase in catecholamine levels. Sleep-related confusion and an increase in intra-abdominal pressure during obstructive episodes may contribute to enuresis.[41]

Physical signs of SDB may be varied but often point to the source of obstruction. Because adenotonsillar hypertrophy is the most common cause of SDB, enlarged tonsillar tissue is a common physical finding (Fig. 14-1); however, several studies have failed to show a correlation between the size of the tonsil and adenoid tissue and the severity of SDB.[42] Although the size of the adenoid tissue cannot be determined on direct examination, a lateral

Box 14-1 Daytime Symptoms of Sleep-Disordered Breathing

Chronic mouth breathing
Hyponasal speech
Diminished appetite
Morning headaches
Nasal obstruction
Hyposmia
Abnormal behavior

Box 14-2 Nighttime Symptoms of Sleep-Disordered Breathing

Loud snoring
Choking and gasping
Retractions
Abnormal sleep positions
Night terrors
Abnormal sleep positions
Teeth grinding
Enuresis
Apnea
Coughing
Restless sleep
Rocking
Somnambulism
Sleep talking
Head banging

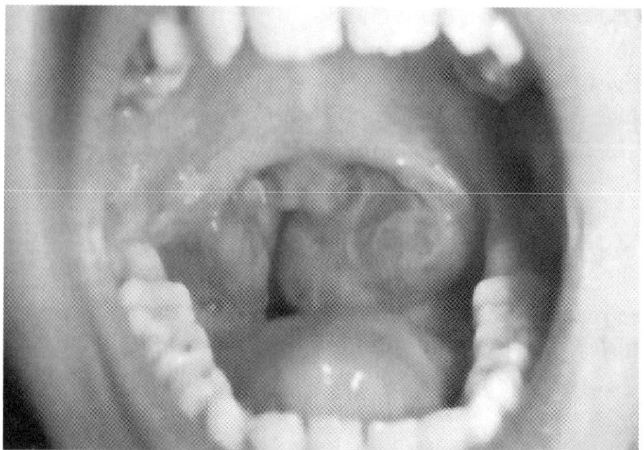

Figure 14-1. Examination of the oropharynx reveals markedly enlarged tonsils.

neck radiograph or fiberoptic examination can be used to make this assessment. Children with long-standing nasal obstruction may develop a particular facies manifested by several characteristics, including a long midface and an open-mouth posturing. Similarly, craniofacial syndromes with maxillary or mandibular hypoplasia predispose affected patients to SDB. In children with cleft palate who have undergone posterior pharyngeal flap surgery to correct velopharyngeal insufficiency, the presence of the flap may cause obstruction of the nasopharynx, with resultant sleep apnea. Although nasal polyps are rare in children not afflicted with cystic fibrosis, the presence of a large antrochoanal polyp in an older child or adolescent may obstruct the nasopharynx. Evidence of a pharyngeal flap or a large antrochoanal polyp may be seen on examination of the pharynx. Nasopharyngeal stenosis, a rare complication following adenotonsillar surgery, may also result in SDB (Fig. 14-2). Children affected by neuromuscular disorders that cause hypotonia, especially during sleep, are usually easily recognized. Signs of right heart failure may be seen rarely on physical examination.

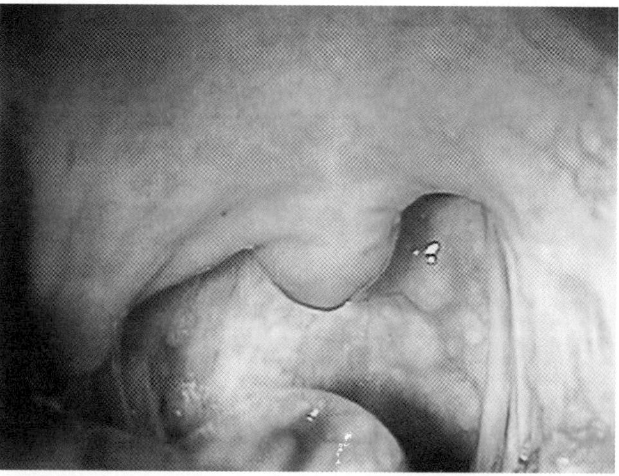

Figure 14-2. Nasopharyngeal stenosis, a rare complication of tonsil and adenoid surgery, may cause sleep-disordered breathing.

DIAGNOSIS

A history elicited from the family and physical examination of the affected child remain as the major source of clinical information used in the decision to perform surgery in many patients with SDB. Much controversy, however, exists about to the accuracy of information obtained on history and physical examination. Several studies have demonstrated a poor correlation between an elicited history and polysomnography.[43-45] The problem with many of these studies is that variable criteria for apneic and hypopneic episodes have been used to determine the presence of sleep-disordered breathing, and the issue of UARS as a cause of symptoms remains unaddressed.

Until rather recently, the lack of pediatric sleep centers has left few alternatives to history and physical examination in the diagnosis of SDB. Inexpensive screening tools such as pulse oximetry and videotapes or audio tapes are helpful in diagnosis when symptoms are severe, but may not be accurate in the evaluation of children with mild symptoms. In addition, polysomnography has been assumed to be the gold standard in the evaluation of SDB, but outcomes data are lacking in patients with neurocognitive disorders. Children with mild symptoms of SDB and neurocognitive disorders may have a normal polysomnogram but benefit from tonsil and adenoid surgery. Conversely, the value of tonsil and adenoid surgery in children with mild forms of SDB (UARS, primary snoring) and neurocognitive disorders has not been well substantiated (Box 14-3).[28]

Because obtaining a polysomnogram from every child with suspected SDB is not feasible or practical, and because polysomnography may not represent the gold standard in diagnosing neurocognitive symptoms in patients with airway obstruction, clinical judgment should still be used to determine candidates for surgery or further investigation of SDB.[46] Symptoms that may predict a negative polysomnogram include a lack of

Box 14-3 Favored Indications for Polysomnography

- Children younger than 2 years of age
- Patients with a craniofacial disorder
- Patients with persistent symptoms following surgical treatment
- Parental request
- A sleep disorder or unclear clinical picture

Table 14-1 Polysomnography: Measured Parameters

Oral and Nasal Airflow	Chest Wall Movements
Electrocardiography	Pulse oximetry
Electroencephalography (EEG)	Electromyography (pharyngeal musculature)
Electro-oculography	pH probe

consistent snoring and daytime mouth breathing. On the contrary, symptoms that may predict an abnormal polysomnogram include observed apneic spells, constant snoring, and restless sleep.[13]

By most measures, polysomnography remains the gold standard in the diagnosis of SDB. Table 14-1 lists the parameters that should be measured during sleep, as recommended by the American Thoracic Society.[47] Oral and nasal airflow are measured by thermistors that detect airflow. Chest wall movements can be recorded by respiratory inductive plethysmography, a method that also allows for semiquantitative measurement of airway obstruction. Sleep staging is performed by electroencephalographic analysis, although electro-oculography confirms episodes of REM sleep. Cases in which gastroesophageal reflux is suspected as a cause of nighttime obstruction are an indication for a pH probe, which can be used in conjunction with formal polysomnography. Electromyography of the muscles that dilate the pharynx is helpful in synchronizing episodes of upper airway obstruction.

In patients scheduled for adenotonsillectomy, Weatherly and co-workers have compared polysomnograms and clinical findings of SDB. Three criteria were used to analyze polysomnograms: (1) one OA episode/hour; (2) more than five apneas or hypopneas/hour of sleep; and (3) more than one apnea, hypopnea, or RERA/hour of sleep. The use of a higher criterion (i.e., a more sensitive measure of respiratory disturbance) resulted in a better correlation between the polysomnogram and the clinical diagnosis of SDB.[13]

Polysomnography is expensive and may require an overnight hospital stay to ensure compliance. Because of an alteration in sleep in a different environment (first-night effect), polysomnography may not be representative of the child's chronic nighttime breathing. Because polysomnography is expensive and may be difficult to obtain because of limited testing situations, most authors still recommend using clinical judgment in recommending patients for surgery. The clinical situations listed in Box 14-3 lend themselves to a formal sleep study. Several conditions exist in which the child undergoes normal polysomnography and still may be considered for surgical intervention (i.e., adenotonsillectomy). These include problems eating because of adenotonsillar hypertrophy, persistent daytime mouth breathing that may interfere with orthodontic treatment, and behavioral or neurocognitive disorders that may be the result of UARS.

In an attempt to obtain objective evidence of SDB and without performing polysomnography, several home monitoring techniques have been developed. Asking the parent or caregiver to videotape the sleeping child, especially during episodes of noisy breathing, may provide evidence of apnea or significant airway obstruction.[48] At times, these videotapes may demonstrate frank apnea that may not be appreciated on an audio tape alone. Audio recording of sleep (sleep sonography) is economical and can be performed at home, eliminating concerns about the first-night effect of sleeping in the hospital situation. Although sleep sonography may not be representative of a full night's sleep, Potsic has shown good correlation with polysomnography.[49] A nighttime pulse oximetry recording has good predictive value of SDB if the study is positive. A negative result does not exclude obstructive sleep apnea.[50]

The most economical radiologic study in the evaluation of a child with SDB is the lateral neck radiograph. Although it provides a *static* view of the upper airway, it is excellent for assessing the size of the adenoid and tonsillar tissue and analyzing the upper tracheal and laryngeal airways (Fig. 14-3). Cephalometric radiographic studies of the upper airway provide a similar static view. Videofluoroscopy of the upper airway can provide a

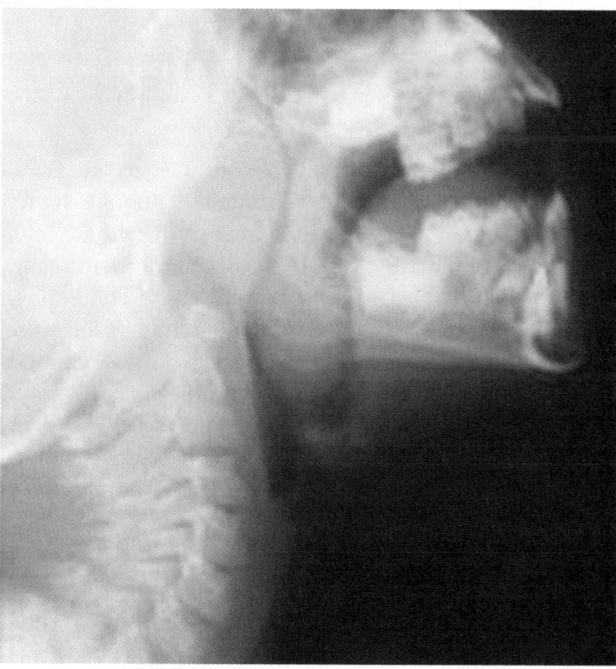

Figure 14-3. Lateral neck radiograph demonstrates enlarged tonsils and adenoids.

dynamic view of the upper airway, but this study is difficult to do in the sleeping patient, especially a child. Cine or spiral computed tomography (CT) may also provide an excellent view of the upper airway but may necessitate sedation in young children. Finally, magnetic resonance imaging (MRI) studies have been shown to be useful in demonstrating fat planes surrounding the pharyngeal musculature in adults. They may show similar planes in obese children and may also document obstruction by hyperplastic lymphoid tissue.

Flexible nasopharyngoscopy and laryngoscopy can be performed in the office setting in awake children. These procedures allow assessment of both nasal cavities, the size of the adenoid and tonsillar tissue, and any pathology of the supraglottic larynx. Both can be performed in infants and children using topical anesthesia with lidocaine and oxymetazoline as a decongestant. In the surgical setting, flexible endoscopy performed under general anesthesia may demonstrate where airway obstruction occurs during normal sleep.

Two quality of life measures of SDB have been described for use in children. As initially described by de Serres and colleagues, the OSD-6 instrument was used to document large improvements in short-term quality of life in patients with SDB before and following adenotonsillectomy.[51] In many cases, however, the documentation of SDB was by history and physical examination alone and not by polysomnography. Sohn and Rosenfeld have validated the OSA-18 instrument with polysomnography and have shown it to be useful for further investigation of SDB.[52]

MANAGEMENT

Nonsurgical Treatment

Weight Loss. The deposition of fat in the muscles planes surrounding the pharynx contributes to the airway obstruction that causes SDB in adults. Although hyperplastic lymphoid tissue causes similar obstruction in children, the accumulation of fat in the same muscle planes may also play a role in obstruction in obese children. An epidemic of obesity in children and adults has led to an increase in SDB in both age groups.[53] Obese children should consult with a nutritional expert skilled in weight loss (Box 14-4) as part of a comprehensive treatment program for SDB that may also include a tonsillectomy, adenoidectomy, and other medical or surgical therapy.

Artificial Airways. Various dental devices have been used in the management of SDB in adults. Most of these act to keep the pharyngeal airway patent, thereby preventing episodes of complete obstruction. Unfortunately, poor compliance prevents most of these devices from being used in children. In selected cases, use of a soft nasal airway during sleep to keep the airway open may be tolerated and prevent the need for more invasive airway intervention, such as a tracheostomy.

Box 14-4 Nonsurgical Treatment of Sleep-Disordered Breathing

Weight loss
Artificial airway
Antibiotic therapy
Treatment of allergies
Treatment of gastroesophageal reflux
Supplemental oxygen
Nasal continuous positive airway pressure (CPAP), bilevel positive airway pressure (BiPAP)

Respiratory Stimulants. Medications that have been shown to decrease the symptoms of SDB in adults, such as medroxyprogesterone, tricyclic antidepressants, or naloxone, have been shown to be ineffective in children. The only exception is the treatment of central apnea in neonates with caffeine or theophylline.

Antibiotic Therapy. A course of antibiotic therapy may produce a decrease in the size of tonsil and adenoid tissue, but the effect is frequently short-lived.[3]

Treatment of Allergies. In general, nasal allergies alone rarely cause SDB. They may be contributory, however, and aggressive treatment may result in less secretions and an improved nasal airway. Typically, allergic therapy includes antihistamines, nasal steroids, and, in selected patients, immunotherapy. The use of steroidal nasal sprays has also been shown to provide some benefit in decreasing the size of the adenoid tissue, thereby improving the nasal airway.[54,55]

Treatment of Gastroesophageal Reflux. Children with gastroesophageal reflux may benefit from aggressive medical management of their reflux. These measures include elevating the head of the bed at night and the use of antacids, histamine receptor antagonists (ranitidine), and proton pump inhibitors (omeprazole). In severe cases, surgical intervention with a fundoplication may be necessary.

Supplemental Oxygen. Use of supplemental oxygen at night administered by mask or nasal prongs may correct episodes of oxygen desaturation. Because this therapy fails to correct abnormalities in ventilation, there is no change in the end-tidal carbon dioxide level or incidence of apneas.[56]

Nasal CPAP/BiPAP. The use of continuous positive airway pressure (CPAP) delivered to the nose by mask has been shown to be effective in children even younger than 2 years of age.[57,58] Continuous positive pressure acts to keep the airway patent during inspiration, countering the effect of negative intrathoracic pressure, which tends to precipitate collapse of the pharyngeal airway. Patients are typically titrated during polysomnography to determine an effective continuous positive pressure that will keep the airway patent. As in adults, compliance remains a problem, with approximately 10% to 20% of patients being unable to tolerate this form of treatment.[57] Therefore, the use of CPAP is reserved for children in whom simpler therapeutic options, such as a tonsillectomy and adenoidectomy, have failed. Side effects of therapy that lead to noncompliance include nasal congestion, rhinorrhea, nasal dryness, and difficulty tolerating the mask or obtaining a satisfactory mask fit. In adults, heated humidification and the use of various masks or pillows have improved compliance and should be considered in the management of children.[59] Development of midface hypoplasia and nasal deformities such as columella necrosis have been reported as complications of CPAP therapy in children.[60,61] Padman and associates have described the use of bilevel positive airway pressure (BiPAP) to maintain airway patency.[62] The advantage of this therapy is that different levels of positive pressure can be delivered during inspiration and expiration, allowing treatment to be tailored to the patient. The equipment required to deliver BiPAP tends to be heavier, noisier, and more expensive, and many centers reserve its use for cases that cannot be managed effectively with CPAP.[62]

Surgical Treatment

Tonsillectomy and Adenoidectomy. Because the major cause of SDB in children is related to lymphoid hyperplasia in the form of adenotonsillar hypertrophy, most cases are relieved by tonsillectomy and adenoidectomy (Box 14-5).[63,64] In addition to relieving symptoms of frank apnea, tonsillectomy and adenoidectomy may be curative for children with habitual snoring or UARS, who also have normal polysomnograms. Quality of life measures, even in the realm of behavioral and emotional disorders, have been used to confirm symptomatic improvement following surgery.[65,66] In most cases, the results of tonsil and adenoid surgery are dramatic, and no follow-up studies are necessary. In cases in which severe SDB was documented prior to surgery, especially in the presence of conditions such as obesity, Down syndrome, or neuromuscular disorders, postoperative polysomnography is necessary to determine whether additional therapy is required.

Box 14-5 Surgical Treatment of Sleep-Disordered Breathing

- Tonsillectomy, adenoidectomy
- Craniofacial procedures
- Nasal surgery
- Pharyngeal surgery
- Tracheostomy

Although adenoidectomy alone may suffice in patients with enlarged adenoid tissue, but small tonsils, and symptoms of habitual snoring or UARS, most experts have recommended performing both a tonsillectomy and adenoidectomy in children with OA. Until a decade ago, techniques for adenoidectomy were limited to the use of a curette or adenotome for removal and packing or chemical cauterization or electrocautery for hemostasis. Tonsillectomy was performed using cold dissection or electrocautery.[67] With cold dissection techniques, bleeding vessels could be ligated or cauterized. Proponents of the cold dissection technique have cited studies that show less postoperative pain compared with electrocautery tonsillectomy.[68] In the last 5 years, the microdébrider has appeared as a tool for both tonsillectomy and adenoidectomy.[69] Lymphoid tissue is shaved down, and hemostasis is then obtained in the surgical bed using electrocautery. With use of the microdébrider, a small layer of lymphoid tissue usually remains in the nasopharynx and tonsillar fossae. For a tonsillectomy, this technique actually results in a subcapsular tonsillectomy because the capsule of the tonsil is not excised. Proponents of this technique have claimed that their patients suffer less postoperative pain because the pharyngeal musculature is not exposed and there is a decreased rate of delayed hemorrhage, although data to support those claims are forthcoming. The harmonic scalpel is another instrument that has been shown to be as effective as electrosurgical techniques in excising the tonsils.[70] Cold ablation (coblation) is an additional method for excising the tonsils, and proponents have cited decreased postoperative pain as an advantage.[71,72] Radiofrequency ablation can be used to reduce the size of the tonsil,[73] but anecdotal reports have suggested that tonsillar regrowth can be an issue in children treated with this technique.

For most children 4 years of age or older, tonsillectomy and adenoidectomy remain a daytime surgical procedure, with patients being observed for several hours following the procedure. Children with comorbidities and those identified by history or polysomnography as having severe obstructive symptoms should remain overnight for observation. Some children may even require monitoring in the intensive care setting. Selected children younger than 4 years may be candidates for discharge the same day if they exhibit no symptoms of airway obstruction postoperatively and seem able to maintain their hydration; however, several studies have demonstrated that children younger than 4 years are at higher risk for complications.[74-76] Ross and associates have recommended a planned admission for all children younger than 36 months undergoing a tonsillectomy.[77] Use of humidification, corticosteroids, antibiotics, and antiemetics in selected cases has improved the early postoperative course in many patients, allowing for same-day discharge.[78]

Craniofacial Procedures. In children with a craniofacial disorder that includes midface or mandibular hypoplasia, correction of the disorder frequently improves the upper airway, with a resultant decrease in SDB. Children with Apert's or Crouzon's syndrome and SDB may show marked improvement following midfacial advancement procedures.[79] Similarly, Treacher Collins patients may benefit from mandibular advancement that allows the tongue to move forward, expanding the pharyngeal airway. In cleft palate children with SDB secondary to a posterior pharyngeal flap to correct velopharyngeal insufficiency, takedown or revision of the flap may lead to the resolution of symptoms.

Nasal Surgery. Although the nasal cavities are rarely the site of obstruction in children, septoplasty or inferior turbinate reduction may result in an improved nasal airway and resolution of symptoms. Children afflicted with cystic fibrosis are prone to develop nasal polyps, a condition that often results in SDB. Nasal polypectomy or endoscopic sinus surgery may improve the nasal airway, although polyps and chronic sinus infection are frequently recurrent.

Pharyngeal Surgery. More complex pharyngeal surgery that may be necessary in a selected group of children with SDB includes either a hyoid advancement or uvulopalatoplasty. In the hyoid advancement procedure, the hyoid is released from its surrounding attachments and advanced anteriorly, drawing the tongue base in the same direction and opening the pharyngeal airway. Although uvulopalatoplasty is undertaken more often in adults, it may provide benefit in selected patients. Excision of the uvula, along with redundant palatal mucosa, increases the size of the pharyngeal inlet.[80]

Tracheostomy. Tracheostomy remains the surgical procedure of last resort in cases of severe SDB. Because their airway is otherwise normal, children with a tracheostomy performed solely for SDB may cap their tube during the daytime and function relatively normally. Treatment of the underlying anatomic abnormality may allow the tracheostomy to be removed at a later time.

SUMMARY

Although not a new disorder, sleep-disordered breathing has become increasingly identified as a condition that affects the overall growth and development of children. Symptoms that were once ignored or minimized are now treated with due regard for their significance, resulting in more efficient sleep at night and improved performance during the daytime. The growth of sleep centers for diagnosis and treatment of SDB and the recognition of sleep disorders by families and primary care practitioners as a serious medical problem have brought sleep medicine to its rightful place among the pediatric specialties that have the greatest impact on the health of our children.

MAJOR POINTS

The incidence of sleep-disordered breathing (defined as nighttime breathing that ranges from UARS to OSAS) falls in the 1% to 3% range.

Although the pathophysiology of SDB in children and adults is similar, normative data show differences between these populations. An apnea of almost any duration is abnormal in a child, and children tend to have briefer and more frequent episodes of apnea and more partial obstructions (hypopneas). An RDI above five events/hour is abnormal in a child, whereas an abnormal value in an adult is more than 20 events/hour.

Groups of pediatric patients at risk for SDB include those with adenotonsillar hypertrophy, craniofacial disorders, Down syndrome, mucopolysaccharidoses, and children with neuromuscular disorders.

Sleep-disordered breathing can affect growth, behavior, and school performance and may have deleterious effects on both the cardiovascular system and development of the face.

In many cases, sleep disorders may be diagnosed by history and physical examination, although polysomnography remains the gold standard for diagnosis. Ancillary diagnostic procedures short of full polysomnography may also provide objective evidence of SDB.

Both medical and surgical treatment may be used in the management of children with OSAS. Children with UARS and normal findings on polysomnography may also benefit from such treatment.

REFERENCES

1. Guilleminault C, Eldridge FL, Simmons FB, et al: Sleep apnea in eight children. Pediatrics 1976;58:23-30.
2. Marcus C, Omlin K, Basinski D, et al: Normal polysomnographic values for children and adolescents. Am Rev Respir Dis 1992;146:1235-1239.
3. Bower CM, Gungor A: Pediatric obstructive sleep apnea syndrome. Otolaryngol Clin North Am 2000;33:49-75.
4. Marcus CL, Hammer A, Loughlin GM: Natural history of primary snoring in children. Pediatr Pulmonol 1998;26:6-11.
5. Guilleminault C, Pelayo R, Leger, D, et al: Recognition of sleep-disordered breathing in children. Pediatrics 1996; 98:871-882.

6. de Serres LM, Derkay C, Astley S, et al: Measuring quality of life in children with obstructive sleep disorders. Arch Otolaryngol Head Neck Surg 2000;126:1423-1429.
7. Marcus CL: Sleep-disordered breathing in children. Am J Respir Crit Care Med 2001;164:16-30.
8. Bower CM, Buckmiller L: What's new in pediatric obstructive sleep apnea? Curr Opin Otolaryngol Head Neck Surg 2001; 9:352-358.
9. Catterall JR, Calverley PM, Shapiro CM, et al: Breathing and oxygenation during sleep are similar in normal men and normal women. Am Rev Resp Dis 1985;132:86-88.
10. Gould GA, Whyte KF, Rhind GB, et al: The sleep hypopnea syndrome. Am Rev Respir Dis 1988;137:895-898.
11. Guilleminault, C, Connolly S, Winkle R, et al: Cyclical variation of the heart rate in sleep apnoea syndrome. Mechanisms, and usefulness of 24 h electrocardiography as a screening tool. Lancet 1984;1:126-131.
12. Block AJ, Boysen PG, Wynne JW, et al: Sleep apnea, hypopnea and oxygen desaturation in normal subjects. A strong male predominance. N Engl J Med 1979;300:513-517.
13. Weatherly RA, Ruzicka DL, Marriott DJ, et al: Polysomnography in children scheduled for adenotonsillectomy. Otolaryngol Head Neck Surg 2004;131:727-731.
14. Guilleminault C, van den Hoed J, Mitler MM: Clinical overview of the sleep apnea syndromes. In Guilleminault C, Dement WC (eds): Sleep Apnea Syndrome. New York, Raven Press, 1990, pp 1-8.
15. Tang JPL, Rosen CL, Larkin EK, et al: Identification of sleep-disordered breathing in children: Variation with event definition. Sleep 2002;25:72-79.
16. American Thoracic Society: Cardiorespiratory sleep studies in children: Establishment of normative data and polysomnographic predictors of morbidity. Am J Respir Crit Care Med 1999;160:1381-1387.
17. McNamara F, Issa FG, Sullivan CE: Arousal pattern following central and obstructive breathing abnormalities in infants and children. J Appl Physiol 1996;81:2651-2657.
18. Gislason T, Benediktsdottir B: Snoring, apneic episodes, and nocturnal hypoxemia among children 6 months to 6 years old. An epidemiologic study of lower limit of prevalence. Chest 1995;107:963-966.
19. Redline S, Tishler PV, Hans MG, et al: Racial differences in sleep-disordered breathing in African-Americans and Caucasians. Am J Respir Crit Care Med 1977;155:186-192.
20. Richards W, Ferdman RM: Prolonged morbidity because of delays in the diagnosis and treatment of obstructive sleep apnea in children. Clin Pediatr 2000;39:103-108.
21. Isono S, Shimada A, Utsugi M, et al: Comparison of static mechanical properties of the passive pharynx between normal children and children with sleep-disordered breathing. Am J Respir Crit Care Med 1998;157:1204-1212.
22. Schellenberg JB, Maislin G, Schwab RJ: Physical findings and the risk for obstructive sleep apnea. The importance of oropharyngeal structures. Am J Resp Crit Care Med 2000;162:740-748.
23. Douglas NJ, Luke M, Mathur R: Is the sleep apnoea/hypopnoea syndrome inherited? Thorax 1993;48:719-721.
24. Redline S, Thishler PV, Tosteson TD, et al: The familial aggregation of obstructive sleep apnea. Am J Respir Crit Care Med 1995;151:682-687.
25. McColley SA, Carroll JL, Curtis S, et al: High prevalence of allergic sensitization in children with habitual snoring and obstructive sleep apnea. Chest 1997;111:170-173.
26. Margardino TM, Tom LW: Surgical management of obstructive sleep apnea in children with cerebral palsy. Laryngoscope 1999;109:1611-1615.
27. Goh DYT, Galster, Marcus CL: Sleep architecture and respiratory disturbances in children with obstructive sleep apnea. Am J Respir Crit Care Med 2000;162:682-686.
28. Ebert CS, Drake AF: The impact of sleep-disordered breathing on cognition and behavior in children: A review and meta-synthesis of the literature. Otolaryngol Head Neck Surg 2004;131:814-826.
29. Rosen CL, Storfer-Isser A, Taylor G, et al: Increased behavioral morbidity in school-aged children with sleep disordered breathing. Pediatrics 2004;114:1640-1648.
30. Gozal D, Daniel JM, Dohanich GP: Behavioral and anatomic correlates of chronic episodic hypoxia during sleep in the rat. J Neurosci 2001;21:2442-2450.
31. Bar A, Tarasiuk A, Segev Y, et al: The effect of adenotonsillectomy on serum insulin-like growth factor-I and growth in children with obstructive sleep apnea syndrome. J Pediatr 1999;135:76-80.
32. Williams EF, Woo P, Miller R: The effects of adenotonsillectomy on growth in young children. Otolaryngol Head Neck Surg 1991;104:509-516.
33. Marcus CL, Carroll JL, Koerner CB, et al: Determinants of growth in children with obstructive sleep apnea syndrome. J Pediatr 1994;125:556-562.
34. Yilmaz MD, Onrat E, Altuntas A, et al: The effects of tonsillectomy and adenoidectomy on pulmonary arterial pressure in children. Am J Otolaryngol Head Neck Med Surg 2005;26:18-21.
35. Brown OE, Manning SC, Ridenour B: Cor pulmonale secondary to tonsillar and adenoidal hypertrophy: Management considerations. Int J Pediatr Otorhinolaryngol 1988;16:131-139.
36. Sie KC, Perkins JA, Clarke WR: Acute right heart failure because of adenotonsillar hypertrophy. Int J Pediatr Otorhinolaryngol 1997;41:53-58.
37. Guilleminault C, Partinen M, Praud JP, et al: Morphometric facial changes and obstructive sleep apnea in adolescents. J Pediatr 1989;114:997-999.
38. Leighton BC: Cause of malocclusion of the teeth. Arch Dis Child 1991;66:1011-1012.
39. Gozal D, Wang M, Pope DW Jr: Objective sleepiness measures in pediatric obstructive sleep apnea. Pediatrics 2001; 108:693-697.
40. Owens J, Opipari L, Nobile C, et al: Sleep and daytime behavior in children with obstructive sleep apnea and behavioral sleep disorders. Pediatrics 1998;102:1178-1184.

41. Messner AH, Pelayo R: Pediatric sleep-related breathing disorders. Am J Otolaryngol 2000;21:98-107.

42. Mahboubi S, Marsh RR, Potsic WP, et al: The lateral neck radiograph in adenotonsillar hyperplasia. Int J Pediatr Otorhinolaryngol 1985;10:67-73.

43. Goldstein NA, Sculerati N, Walsleben JA, et al: Clinical diagnosis of pediatric obstructive sleep apnea validated by polysomnography. Otolaryngol Head Neck Surg 1994; 111:611-617.

44. Suen JS, Arnold JE, Brooks LJ: Adenotonsillectomy for treatment of obstructive sleep apnea in children. Arch Otolaryngol Head Neck Surg 1995;121:525-530.

45. Wang RC, Elkins TP, Keech D, et al: Accuracy of clinical evaluation in pediatric obstructive sleep apnea. Otolaryngol Head Neck Surg 1998;118:69-73.

46. Brietzke SE, Katz ES, Roberson DW: Can history and physical examination reliably diagnose pediatric obstructive sleep apnea/hypopnea syndrome? A systematic review of the literature. Otolaryngol Head Neck Surg 2004;131:827-832.

47. American Thoracic Society: Standards and indications for cardiopulmonary sleep studies in children. Am J Respir Crit Care Med 1996;153:866-878.

48. Sivan Y, Kornecki A, Schonfeld T: Screening obstructive sleep apnea syndrome by home videotape recording in children. Eur Respir J 1996;9:2127-2131.

49. Potsic WP: Comparison of polysomnography and sonography for assessing regularity of respiration during sleep in adenotonsillar hypertrophy. Laryngoscope 1987;97:1430-1437.

50. Brouillette RT, Morielli A, Leimanis A, et al: Nocturnal pulse oximetry as an abbreviated testing modality for pediatric obstructive sleep apnea. Pediatrics 2000;105:405-412.

51. de Serres LM, Derkay C, Astley S, et al: Measuring quality of life in children with obstructive sleep disorders. Arch Otolaryngol Head Neck Surg 2000;126:1423-1429.

52. Sohn H, Rosenfeld RM: Evaluation of sleep-disordered breathing in children. Otolaryngol Head Neck Surg 2003;128:344-352.

53. Ogden CL, Flegal KM, Carroll MD, et al: Prevalence and trends in overweight among US children and adolescents, 1999-2000. JAMA 2002;288:1728-1732.

54. Demain JG, Goetz DW: Pediatric adenoidal hypertrophy and nasal airway obstruction: Reduction with aqueous nasal beclomethasone. Pediatrics 1995;95:355-364.

55. Brouillette RT, Manoulkian JJ, Ducharme FM, et al: Efficacy of fluticasone nasal spray for pediatric obstructive sleep apnea. J Pediatr 2001;138:838-844.

56. Marcus CL, Carroll JL, Bamford O, et al: Supplemental oxygen during sleep in children with sleep-disordered breathing. Am J Respir Crit Care Med 1995;152:1297-1301.

57. Marcus CL, Ward SI, Mallory GB, et al: Use of nasal continuous positive airway pressure as treatment of childhood obstructive sleep apnea. J Pediatr 1995;127:88-94.

58. Downey R 3rd, Perkin RM, MacQuarrie J: Nasal continuous positive airway pressure use in children with obstructive sleep apnea younger than 2 years of age. Chest 2000; 117:1608-1612.

59. Massie CA, Hart RW, Peralez C, et al: Effects of humidification on nasal symptoms and compliance in sleep apnea patients using continuous positive airway pressure. Chest 1999; 116:403-408.

60. Li KK, Riley RW, Guilleminault C: An unreported risk in the use of home nasal continuous positive airway pressure and home nasal ventilation in children: Midface hypoplasia. Chest 2000;117:916-918.

61. Robertson NJ, McCarthy LS, Hamilton PA, et al: Nasal deformities resulting from flow driver continuous positive airway pressure. Arch Dis Child 1996;75:F209-F212.

62. Padman R, Hyde C, Foster P: The pediatric use of bilevel positive airway pressure therapy for obstructive sleep apnea syndrome: A retrospective review with analysis of respiratory parameters. Clin Pediatr 2002;41:163-169.

63. Suen J, Arnold J, Brooks L: Adenotonsillectomy for treatment of obstructive sleep apnea in children. Arch Otolaryngol Head Neck Surg 1995;121:525-530.

64. Mitchell R, Kelly R, Call E, et al: Quality of life after adenotonsillectomy for obstructive sleep apnea in children. Arch Otolaryngol Head Neck Surg 2004;130:190-194.

65. deSerres LM, Derkay C, Sie K, et al: Impact of adenotonsillectomy on quality of life in children with obstructive sleep disorders. Arch Otolaryngol Head Neck Surg 2002; 128:489-496.

66. Goldstein NA, Tatima M, Campbell TF, et al: Child behavior and quality of life before and after tonsillectomy and adenoidectomy. Arch Otolaryngol Head Neck Surg 2002; 128:770-775.

67. Weimert TA, Babyak JW, Richter HJ: Electrodissection tonsillectomy. Arch Otolaryngol Head Neck Surg 1990;116: 186-188.

68. Leinbach RF, Markwell SJ, Colliver JA, et al: Hot versus cold tonsillectomy: A systematic review of the literature. Otolaryngol Head Neck Surg 2003;129:360-364.

69. Koltai PJ, Solares CA, Koempel JA, et al: Intracapsular tonsillar reduction (partial tonsillectomy): Reviving a historical procedure for obstructive sleep-disordered breathing in children. Otolaryngol Head Neck Surg 2003;129:532-538.

70. Willging JP, Wiatrak BJ: Harmonic scalpel tonsillectomy in children: A randomized prospective study. Otolaryngol Head Neck Surg 2003;128:318-325.

71. Chang KW: Randomized controlled trial of coblation versus electrocautery tonsillectomy. Otolaryngol Head Neck Surg 2005;132:273-280.

72. Stoker KE, Don DM, Kang DR, et al: Pediatric total tonsillectomy using coblation compared to conventional electrosurgery: A prospective controlled single-blind study. Otolaryngol Head Neck Surg 2004;130:666-675.

73. Hultcrantz E, Erricson E: Pediatric tonsillotomy with the radiofrequency technique: Less morbidity and pain. Laryngoscope 2004;114:871-877.

74. Tom LWC, Dedio RM, Cohen DE, et al: Is outpatient tonsillectomy appropriate for young children? Laryngoscope 1992;102:277-280.

75. Reiner SA, Sawyer WP, Clark KF, et al: Safety of outpatient tonsillectomy and adenoidectomy. Otolaryngol Head Neck Surg 1990;102:161-168.

76. Guida RA, Mattucci KF: Tonsillectomy and adenoidectomy: An inpatient or outpatient procedure? Laryngoscope 1990: 100:491-493.

77. Ross AT, Kazahaya K, Tom LWC: Revisiting outpatient tonsillectomy in young children. Otolaryngol Head Neck Surg 2003;128:326-331.

78. Steward DL, Velge JA, Myer CM: Do steroids reduce morbidity of tonsillectomy? Meta-analysis of randomized trials. Laryngoscope 2001;111:1712-1718.

79. Moore MH: Upper airway obstruction in the syndromal craniosynostoses. Br J Plast Surg 1993;46:355-362.

80. Kosko JR, Derkay CS: Uvulopalatopharyngoplasty: Treatment of obstructive sleep apnea in neurologically impaired pediatric patients. Int J Pediatr Otorhinolaryngol 1995;32:241-246.

Approach to the Pediatric Neck Mass

RALPH F. WETMORE, MD

The presence of a malignancy is foremost in the minds of most parents when a mass is discovered in their child's neck. Fortunately, the incidence of a malignant neck mass in children is small (11% in one series) in contrast with that in the adult population.[1] In children, the vast majority of neck masses are congenital or inflammatory in origin. It is important to have a focused approach in the evaluation of a child with a neck mass. A detailed history and comprehensive examination of the entire head and neck and the body are essential first steps. Depending on the differential diagnosis, further evaluation may include laboratory and/or radiologic studies. At this point, if the diagnosis remains in doubt, surgical intervention in the form of biopsy or excision may be necessary. Following these steps in an orderly fashion will help the clinician reach a diagnosis sooner and allay some fears and concerns of the child's parents.

DIFFERENTIAL DIAGNOSIS

Congenital Masses

Thyroglossal Duct Cyst

During embryogenesis, the thyroid gland develops from primordial tissue at the foramen cecum. The thyroid diverticulum descends into the neck from this level, because the thyroglossal duct is in close approximation to the hyoid bone. A persistence of the thyroglossal duct at any point may develop into a thyroglossal duct cyst. The lining of the duct may be composed of squamous or respiratory epithelium, and it is not unusual for mucous glands or ectopic thyroid tissue to be found in the surgical specimen.

A thyroglossal duct cyst can appear at almost any age, but the average age is usually 5 years. Most thyroglossal duct cysts manifest as a painless mass in the neck (Fig. 15-1), although occasionally one may present as an acute infection in the neck at the level of the hyoid bone. Physical examination typically reveals a midline swelling near the level of the hyoid bone, although these cysts may appear as low as the level of the thyroid gland and, rarely, above the hyoid bone (Fig. 15-2). The mass usually elevates when the child is asked to swallow. Ultrasound examination of the neck not only identifies the presence of a cyst, as opposed to some other lesion such as a lymph node, but it also confirms the presence of a

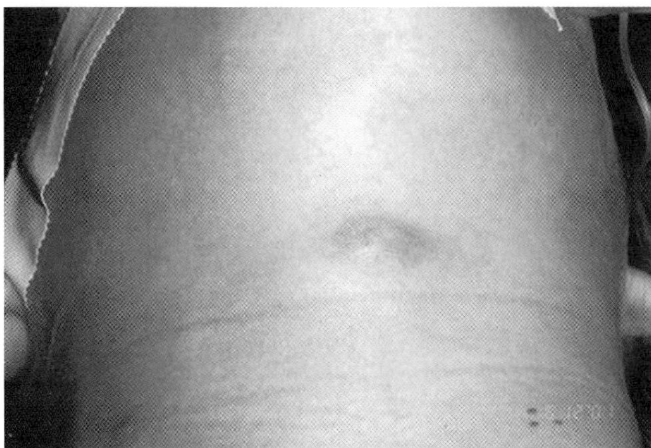

Figure 15-1. A thyroglossal duct cyst typically manifests as a painless midline neck mass between the levels of the hyoid bone and thyroid gland.

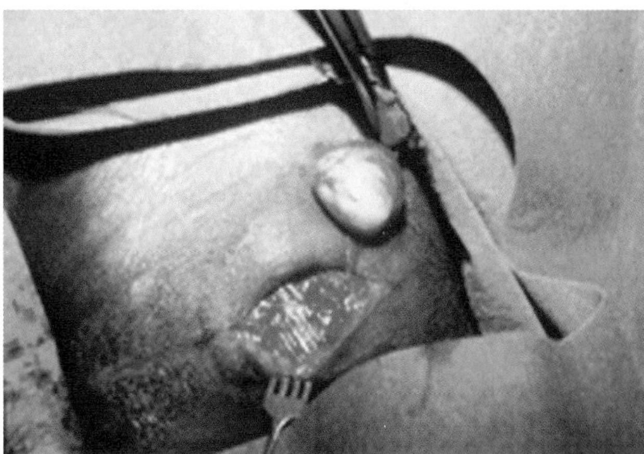

Figure 15-3. Excision of thyroglossal duct cyst, including cyst and tract (Sistrunk procedure).

normal thyroid gland, information that is helpful to know prior to surgical excision. A thyroid scan may also be used to confirm the presence of a normal thyroid gland.

The standard treatment of a thyroglossal duct cyst is surgical excision. Excision of the cyst alone usually results in recurrence, so the Sistrunk procedure, in which the cyst, any residual tract, and the central portion of the hyoid is excised, is the standard of care (Fig. 15-3).[2] Even with the performance of a Sistrunk procedure, there is a risk of recurrence of approximately 8%.[1] The development of papillary thyroid carcinoma within an nonexcised thyroglossal duct cyst has been reported.[3]

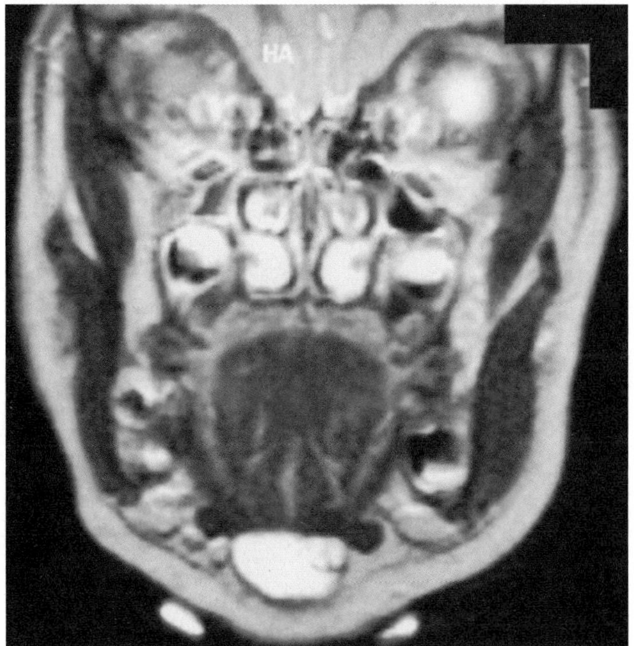

Figure 15-2. MRI scan demonstrates a thyroglossal duct cyst just below the level of the hyoid bone.

Dermoid Cyst

A dermoid cyst consists of tissue from all three germinal layers and may contain skin appendages, such as sweat glands and sebaceous glands. As with a thyroglossal duct cyst, a dermoid cyst typically manifests as a midline neck mass, although presentation with an acute infection is much less common than with a thyroglossal duct cyst. On physical examination of the neck, a dermoid cyst can be found in the midline at any level from the submental region to the suprasternal notch. Midline cysts above the hyoid bone and below the thyroid gland are more likely to be dermoid cysts. A dermoid cyst tends to be more superficial than a thyroglossal duct cyst and does not move with swallowing. Ultrasonography cannot distinguish between a dermoid and a thyroglossal duct cyst. Treatment of a dermoid cyst is by surgical excision.

Branchial Cleft Cyst

The branchial apparatus consists of arches, pouches, and grooves (clefts). The branchial or pharyngeal arches develop from mesodermal buds in the lateral walls of the fetal pharynx. Each arch contains a core cartilaginous skeleton, rudimentary muscle, a cranial nerve, and an artery. Development of each of these structures within the arch is variable. Ectoderm-lined clefts separate each arch externally, whereas endoderm-lined pouches separate each arch internally (Table 15-1). Maldevelopment of any of these structures may result in a neck mass.

First branchial anomalies comprise 1% to 8% of all branchial cleft anomalies.[4] First branchial anomalies can be divided into two types. A type I first branchial cleft cyst or sinus tract can be found as a swelling near the tragus or postauricular sulcus that runs parallel to the external auditory canal and usually ends in the canal or the middle ear. These tracts are lined with squamous epithelium and represent duplication anomalies of the

Table 15-1 Branchial Arch Derivatives

Branchial Arch	Cartilage	Muscle	Nerve	Artery	Pharyngeal Pouch
First	Meckel's cartilage—forms malleus and incus	Muscles of mastication—anterior belly of digastric, mylohyoid, tensor tympani, and veli palatini	Trigeminal	External maxillary	Eustachian tube, mesotympanum, mastoid antrum
Second	Reichert's cartilage—forms portions of hyoid bone, styloid process, and stapes superstructure	Muscles of facial expression—buccinator, platysma, posterior belly of digastric, stylohyoid	Facial	Stapedial	Mesotympanum, palatine tonsil
Third	Greater cornu and body of hyoid bone	Stylopharyngeus, superior and middle pharyngeal constrictors	Glossopharyngeal	Common carotid	Thymus, inferior parathyroid glands
Fourth	Thyroid cartilage, cuneiform cartilage of larynx	Cricothyroid, inferior constrictor	Superior laryngeal	Arch of aorta, proximal subclavian	Superior parathyroid glands
Fifth and sixth	Cricoid, arytenoid, and corniculate cartilages	Intrinsic laryngeal	Recurrent laryngeal	Ductus arteriosus, pulmonary artery	—

membranous canal. A type II first branchial cleft cyst or tract manifests below the angle of the mandible and is composed of both squamous epithelium and mesodermal elements, such as cartilage. Both types of first branchial lesions course near the facial nerve, but the type II lesions do so more often.

Second branchial anomalies are the most common form and result from a failure of obliteration of the cervical sinus of His.[5] This sinus forms as the second, third, and fourth branchial clefts become recessed by the growth of the second branchial arch superiorly and the epipericardial ridge inferiorly. Second branchial anomalies manifest as cysts, sinuses, or fistulas. Sinuses or fistulas occur in the lower third of the neck and may be bilateral in one third of cases (Fig. 15-4).[5] Second branchial cysts typically manifest along the anterior border of the sternocleidomastoid muscle during the second to fourth decades of life. Third branchial cleft anomalies are rare, and fourth branchial cleft anomalies may be theoretical.

Type I first branchial anomalies manifest as a sinus tract or area of swelling near the postauricular sulcus or anterior to the tragus. Type II lesions manifest as a superficial cyst or tract below the angle of the mandible but above the hyoid bone. Second branchial cysts manifest high in the neck, deep to the sternocleidomastoid

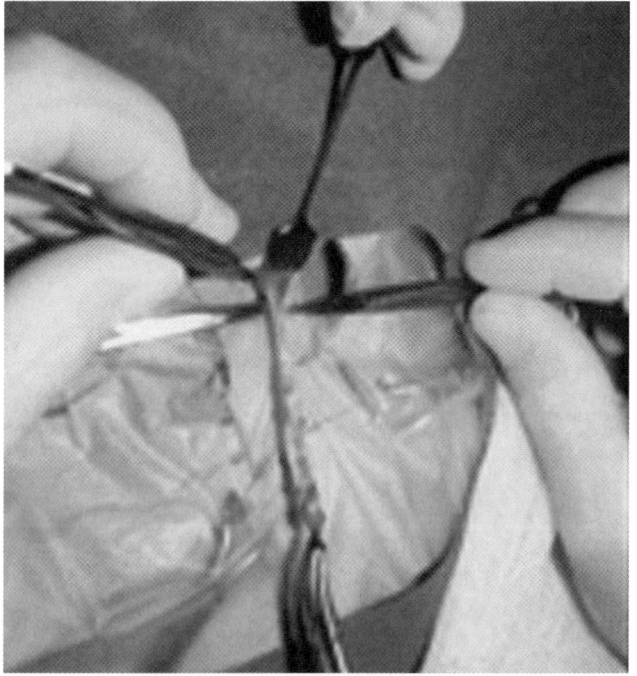

Figure 15-4. A second branchial sinus tract may extend from the lower neck to the pharynx, opening superiorly to the tonsil.

muscle and near the carotid bifurcation or in the parapharyngeal space. Second branchial sinuses or fistulas manifest lower in the neck. Third branchial cysts manifest as a mass low in the anterior neck, most often on the left side.

With the exception of small superficial branchial sinuses low in the neck, the evaluation of most branchial anomalies should include magnetic resonance imaging (MRI). This form of imaging is essential in the preoperative evaluation of first branchial sinuses and helpful in determining the extent of second and third branchial lesions. First branchial anomalies that involve the external auditory canal should also be evaluated by computed tomography (CT); squamous elements in the middle ear associated with these anomalies may be difficult to visualize by MRI alone. The definitive treatment of all branchial anomalies is surgical excision. First branchial anomalies may require a middle ear exploration to excise any squamous elements in the mesotympanum. Multiple stepped incisions in the neck may be necessary to excise second or third branchial fistulas.

Hemangioma

A hemangioma is a proliferative endothelial lesion that grows rapidly during the first 8 to 12 months of life and then slowly involutes over the next 5 to 8 years. They occur more commonly in females in a 3:1 sex ratio.[6] Use of the terms *capillary* for superficial and *cavernous* for deep hemangiomas is confusing and should be avoided, because both superficial and deep lesions show similar histopathology. Care must be taken not to confuse a venous or venolymphatic malformation with a deep hemangioma.

Hemangiomas are found most commonly in the head and neck.[7] Superficial lesions are usually obvious and present as well-circumscribed masses that may be vivid bright red if the skin is involved. Superficial hemangiomas are firm, rubbery, slightly raised lesions and are difficult to compress in contrast with vascular malformations. A superficial hemangioma may be confused with a capillary malformation, a congenital vascular lesion that grows at the same rate as the child. A hemangioma in deep tissues manifests as a mass that grows quickly during the first year of life. Cutaneous hemangiomas may be associated with similar lesions involving the larynx, trachea, orbit, liver, or brain.[8]

The diagnosis of a superficial hemangioma is usually obvious. Deeper masses may be evaluated by ultrasound, a study that is useful in distinguishing a slow-flow vascular malformation from a hemangioma. MRI is highly specific and sensitive and demonstrates the extent of involvement and flow characteristics. Because of spontaneous resolution, observation is the usual treatment option with most hemangiomas. Complete resolution occurs in 50% of cases by the age of 5, 70% by age 7, and continued improvement until 10 to 12 years of age.[9] Other treatment options, such as corticosteroid therapy (local injection or systemic), interferon alfa-2a or surgical excision should be considered if complications occur. Complications include visual disorders related to orbital involvement, airway obstruction secondary to subglottic involvement, ulceration and bleeding, congestive heart failure, and platelet-trapping coagulopathy (Kasabach-Merritt syndrome).

Vascular Malformations

Vascular malformations are structural lesions that are present at birth and grow with the child. Two major types are based on their flow characteristics, slow-flow and fast-flow lesions. Slow-flow lesions include capillary, venous, and lymphatic malformations. Capillary malformations (port wine stain) produce staining of the skin by abnormally dilated capillaries or venule-sized vessels that are present at birth and do not regress. In the Sturge-Weber syndrome, choroidal or intracranial extension may also be present. Superficial capillary malformations are usually treated with a pulsed dye laser.

Lymphatic malformations were previously known as lymphangiomas or cystic hygromas. These congenital lesions typically present by 2 years of age and may occur anywhere in the body, but more commonly in the head and neck. The histopathology of these lesions consists of multiple dilated lymphatic channels in two patterns—macrocystic lesions (formerly cystic hygroma), which appear in the anterior and posterior triangles of the neck (Fig. 15-5) and consist of large thick-walled cysts with little infiltration, and microcystic lesions, which extensively infiltrate the head and neck. A sudden increase in the size of these lesions may result from infection or intralesional bleeding. Depending on the extent of involvement, treatment may include observation, surgical excision, and sclerotherapy for macrocystic lesions.

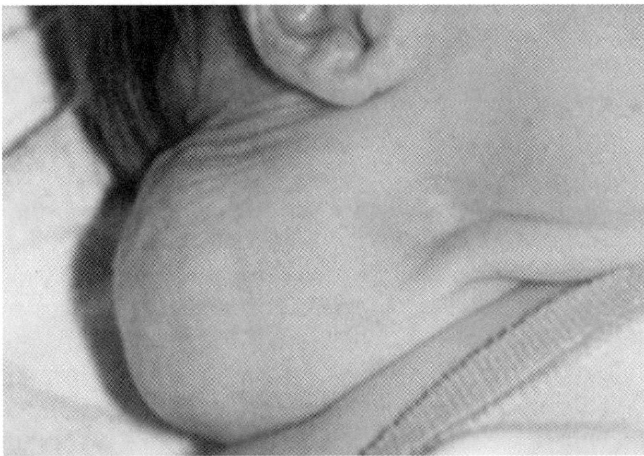

Figure 15-5. Macrocystic lymphatic malformation in the posterior triangle of the neck.

Venous malformations are a developmental anomaly of veins that include dilated or ectatic vascular channels. They are commonly found in the skin and subcutaneous tissues of the head and neck and manifest as soft, compressible, nonpulsatile masses. Some lesions may represent a combination of capillary and venous elements (capillary venous malformation) or lymphatic and venous elements (venolymphatic malformation). Treatment options include observation, sclerotherapy and, rarely, surgical excision.

Fast-flow lesions, arterial or arteriovenous malformations, are rare compared with slow-flow lesions and usually manifest in older childhood and adolescence with skin changes, including a warm, erythematous blush or port-wine stain. Affected children may complain of throbbing pain or exhibit a pulsatile thrill. Blood shunting may cause skin necrosis or ulceration; facial bone involvement may result in slow erosion. Asymptomatic lesions can be observed, but complicated malformations should be evaluated by MRI and treated with a combination of surgical excision following superselective angiographic embolization.

Congenital Torticollis

Congenital torticollis, also known as a sternocleidomastoid (SCM) tumor of infancy or fibromatosis coli, may be the result of one or a combination of several prenatal factors, including birth trauma and intrauterine malpositioning. This entity has been reported in siblings.[10] Other suggested causes include an ischemic injury or compartment syndrome of the SCM muscle and neurogenic or infectious insults to the muscle. Histopathologic examination of the affected muscle shows fibrosis and scarring. Neonates present with a mass in the SCM muscle during the first month of life that disappears after a few weeks. It may be associated with a slight head tilt or plagiocephaly and facial asymmetry. Most cases respond to physical therapy (active and passive stretching of the SCM muscle). Surgery is rarely necessary and only is undertaken if fibrosis and a persistent head tilt result.[11]

Thymic Cyst

Cysts of thymic origin can occur anywhere in the lower neck but predominantly on the left side, from the level of the pyriform sinus to the chest.[12] Thymic cysts are most often diagnosed during the first decade of life, with boys being affected twice as often as girls. These cysts appear as firm, compressible, rounded masses to palpation and may be confused with anomalies of the branchial apparatus. Depending on the size and location, additional symptoms include dysphagia, dyspnea, pain, and hoarseness. Extension into the anterior mediastinum may be demonstrated on chest radiograph or MRI. Treatment is surgical excision.

Infectious and Inflammatory Masses

Viral Adenitis

Common viral agents that result in lymphadenitis include rhinovirus, adenovirus, and enterovirus. The Epstein-Barr virus (EBV), the cause of infectious mononucleosis, is transmitted by mucous membrane contact; EBV infection manifests with the acute onset of lymphadenopathy in the neck, associated with splenomegaly. Cytomegalovirus (CMV) is another causative agent transmitted by mucous membrane contact, sexual contact, or transfusion of blood products. Another cause of lymphadenopathy, the human immunodeficiency virus (HIV), is transmitted by sexual contact, via blood products, or transplacentally. Other causative agents include measles, mumps, rubella, and varicella viruses.

Most cases of lymphadenitis follow a preceding viral upper respiratory infection. With infectious mononucleosis, the adenopathy may be extensive and associated with exudative, and almost necrotic, tonsillitis, fever, fatigue, malaise, and hepatosplenomegaly. With CMV infection, the symptoms and signs may be subclinical or may manifest as a mononucleosis-like illness, with fever and malaise along with the cervical adenitis. Acute HIV infection occurs as a flulike illness several weeks after inoculation with the virus. Associated signs and symptoms include fever, headache, diarrhea, malaise, and generalized adenopathy.

Most cases of viral adenitis are diagnosed by the clinical history and signs. Laboratory testing, including enzyme-linked immunosorbent assay (ELISA), latex agglutination, and viral cultures, provides confirmation of the causative agent. Increased atypical lymphocytes on peripheral smear, along with the presence of heterophile antibodies (positive mono spot), is highly suggestive of infectious mononucleosis. The diagnosis of infectious mononucleosis may be confirmed by obtaining titers of anti-EBV IgG and IgM antibodies.

The treatment of most cases of viral cervical adenitis is expectant. Enlarged cervical nodes may take weeks to months to return to normal size. In cases of infectious mononucleosis, massive lymphadenopathy may cause airway obstruction that can be overcome with the use of high-dose corticosteroids. Rarely, endotracheal intubation, emergent tonsillectomy, or tracheostomy may be necessary to relieve obstruction. Ampicillin or amoxicillin should be avoided in mononucleosis patients because of the association with a rash. In cases of HIV infection, early antiretroviral treatment may be important for long-term survival.[13]

Bacterial Adenitis

Bacterial infection of cervical lymph nodes usually stems from infection in the pharynx. Diffuse infection within a lymph node may resolve with or without treatment or may progress to a phlegmon (partially necrotic tissue) or to frank abscess formation. As the abscess forms, the nodal architecture becomes disrupted and, eventually, there is rupture of the nodal capsule, with spread of infection into the surrounding fascial spaces of the neck. Ultimately, this infection may result in systemic sepsis. In the preantibiotic era, spread of infection into the surrounding tissue and the resulting sepsis resulted in high morbidity and mortality.[14] The usual causative organisms include *Streptococcus*, *Staphylococcus*, and *Neisseria* species and anaerobes, including *Peptostreptococcus*, *Bacteroides*, and *Fusobacterium* species. Nodal areas that drain the pharynx are most commonly affected and include the submandibular and posterior cervical triangles.

Children with bacterial adenitis present with erythema and tenderness overlying the infected node in association with fever and other signs of systemic infection, including an elevated leukocyte count. There may be complaints suggesting pharyngitis. With parapharyngeal or retropharyngeal infection, the child may develop torticollis or complaints of neck pain and an inability to move the neck. The diagnosis is made on clinical history and findings, but use of contrast CT of the neck is helpful in distinguishing between nodes that have developed into a phlegmon and those that have formed an abscess. On a CT scan, a phlegmon appears as an area of hypolucency representing partial necrosis. Ring enhancement on contrast CT suggests formation of an abscess cavity.

Most cases of cervical adenitis require treatment with a systemic antibiotic, oral or parenteral, depending on the size and duration of infection and the presence of systemic symptoms. In cases of abscess formation, incision and drainage are often necessary, although intravenous antibiotics alone may be curative for a few cases of small abscesses. Needle aspiration, with or without CT guidance, has also shown to be effective in selected patients.[15]

Cat-Scratch Disease. Cat-scratch disease is cervical adenitis caused by *Bartonella henselae* infection transmitted by the scratch of a cat. Most patients provide a history of contact or scratch by a cat. In the typical patient, the infection manifests with unilateral adenopathy in the region of the cat scratch. There may be a papule at the site of the inoculum and associated low-grade fever and malaise. Before the offending bacterium was identified, the diagnosis of cat-scratch disease was difficult to confirm and often remained a diagnosis of exclusion. Fluorescent antibody and polymerase chain reaction (PCR) testing for *Bartonella* DNA have a high sensitivity and specificity for cat-scratch disease. In the past, treatment was expectant, with resolution in most cases, but treatment with antibiotics, including erythromycin, aminoglycosides, ciprofloxacin, rifampin, or trimethoprim-sulfamethoxazole, has been shown to be helpful in many cases.[16] In a small percentage of cases, adenitis progresses to frank abscess formation and requires surgical drainage.

Mycobacterial Infection. Most mycobacterial infections in the neck are caused by atypical (nontuberculous) mycobacteria (NTM) organisms that include *Mycobacterium avium-intracellulare*, *M. scrofulaceum*, *M. bovis*, and *M. kansasii*. Infection in the neck from *M. tuberculosis* is a more common cause of cervical adenitis in adults and is often associated with a known family contact.

Approximately 80% of NTM infections occur in children younger than 5 years, with girls more commonly infected than boys.[17] NTM organisms are ubiquitous in the environment and are found in soil and water. In contrast to tuberculosis, there is no evidence of human to human contact with NTM infection. Small mucosal breaks in the oral cavity, especially in teething children, serve as a portal of entry into the lymphatic system.[18]

Most children present with a slowly enlarging painless node in the submandibular or upper cervical regions. The preauricular, intraparotid, or posterior cervical nodal groups may also be involved. The skin overlying involved nodes often takes on a violaceous appearance. Chest radiographs are usually normal with NTM infection but may demonstrate positive findings in children with *M. tuberculosis*. Skin testing can be negative or weakly positive with NTM infection, whereas it is strongly positive with *M. tuberculosis* infection.

The diagnosis of NTM infection is suspected on clinical findings but confirmation may be difficult. Needle aspiration, surgical drainage, or excision yields material for culture or pathologic examination. Staining for acid-fast bacilli is not always positive, and NTM organisms can be difficult to culture, although the use of PCR testing may be helpful in identification.

M. tuberculosis is best treated with combination chemotherapy that includes isoniazid, ethambutol, and rifampin. NTM presents greater challenges for treatment. Untreated nodes frequently progress to suppuration, leaving a wound that may drain chronically for months. Cosmetic appearance may be improved by surgical treatment, which includes needle aspiration, incision and drainage, surgical curettage, and total excision. Chemotherapy is frequently ineffective, although use of some macrolides has had partial efficacy in some cases.[19]

Other Disorders

Lemierre's Syndrome. Involvement of the internal jugular vein with a septic thrombosis, Lemierre's syndrome, typically follows a pharyngeal infection or tonsillitis and is often caused by *Fusobacterium necrophorum*. Patients typically present with spiking "picket fence" fevers, along with tenderness or fullness in one side of the neck. The diagnosis can be confirmed by contrast CT or magnetic resonance venography. Treatment should include intravenous antibiotics, but the use of anticoagulants remains controversial. If repeated septic emboli occur, surgical ligation of the affected portion of the internal jugular vein may be necessary.

Bacillary Angiomatosis. Bacillary angiomatosis is an infection caused by *Bartonella henselae*, the same organism responsible for cat-scratch disease. Bacillary angiomatosis is found in severely immunocompromised patients and is associated with lesions in the skin, subcutaneous tissue, liver, and spleen. As with cat-scratch disease, treatment with one of the macrolide antibiotics is usually effective, although severe infection may require the use of an intravenous aminoglycoside.

Plague. Plague is an infection caused by *Yersinia pestis*. The reservoir of this organism is the rat, but other small mammals such as squirrels or prairie dogs may also carry the disease. Plague is transmitted to humans by the bite of an infected flea from an infected animal. Patients present with the sudden onset of fever, chills, weakness, and headache a few days following inoculation. The appearance of a bubo, an oval lesion from 1 to 10 cm in length that may be solitary or multiple, is frequently associated with very painful lymphadenopathy. Warm and edematous skin overlies the buboes that are found most often in the groin, axilla, or neck. The diagnosis is confirmed by staining the aspirated material from a bubo. Treatment regimens include chemotherapy with streptomycin, tetracycline (older children), or chloramphenicol.

Tularemia. Tularemia is caused by the gram-negative bacillus *Francisella tularensis* and can be transmitted in several ways—by insect bites (typically ticks), handling infected animals, or eating infected meat (usually rabbit). Tularemia may manifest in one of three ways: an ulceroglandular form, which includes a skin ulcer and adenopathy; oropharyngeal form, which includes an oral ulcer; or a glandular form, which manifests with adenopathy without an ulcer. In addition to the type of presentation, affected children may exhibit mild fever and headache. The diagnosis of tularemia is confirmed by agglutination titers. Treatment options include streptomycin, tetracycline (older children), aminoglycosides, and chloramphenicol.

Actinomycosis. Actinomycosis is caused by the gram-positive bacterium *Actinomyces israelii* and is most commonly found in young and middle-aged adults. Half of cases are cervicofacial, and the route of infection in most cases is through breaks in the oral mucosa. Typically, the patient presents with a slowly growing painless mass near the angle of the mandible that, if left untreated, progresses to chronic draining sinuses. The infection may also manifest as a warm, tender indurated mass associated with fever and chills. In 10% of cases, there may be brain or liver involvement. The diagnosis is confirmed by the presence of sulfur granules on histopathologic examination of surgical specimens. Treatment includes excision of infected tissue followed by a prolonged course of antibiotics, typically penicillin. Other antibiotic regimens include clindamycin, erythromycin, and tetracycline (older children).

Brucellosis. This infection is caused by *Brucella* species and is acquired by working with infected livestock or eating nonpasteurized dairy products. Manifests with fever, sweats, anorexia, fatigue, and lymphadenopathy. The diagnosis is confirmed by elevated *Brucella* titers or by culture. Treatment options include tetracycline (older children), streptomycin, gentamicin, and rifampin.

Toxoplasmosis. Toxoplasmosis is caused by *Toxoplasma gondii*, an obligate intracellular parasite. The organism reproduces in the gastrointestinal tract of cats, and infection is spread by the ingestion of oocytes following the handling of cat litter or by ingesting undercooked meat or dairy products that may be contaminated. Congenital toxoplasmosis causes multiple disorders in the developing embryo. Acute toxoplasmosis may manifest in an asymptomatic fashion or as a flulike illness. Approximately 80% to 90% of symptomatic patients have painless cervical adenopathy. The diagnosis is confirmed by serologic testing and histopathologic examination if a biopsy is performed. Treatment includes pyrimethamine plus sulfadiazine.

Kawasaki Syndrome. This disease of young childhood manifests as an acute multisystem vasculitis with no identifiable agent. Five of the following six criteria are necessary to make the diagnosis: (1) high fever (38° to 41°C); (2) conjunctival injection; (3) erythema of the lips, oral mucosa, and/or tongue; (4) polymorphous erythematous rash; (5) cervical adenopathy; and (6) edema, erythema, and desquamation of the skin of the hands and feet.[20] Cervical adenopathy has been shown to be present in as many as 83% of cases.[21] Neurologic, gastrointestinal, urologic, and cardiac involvement may also be seen. Untreated patients may go on to develop permanent cardiac damage in the form of coronary artery aneurysms. In addition to meeting the above criteria, the diagnosis is suggested by an elevated white blood cell count, increased sedimentation rate and C-reactive protein level, and abnormal liver function test results. The typical treatment regimen includes high-dose immunoglobulins and aspirin.

Sarcoidosis. Sarcoidosis is a chronic granulomatous disease of unknown cause that usually affects the lungs and lymph nodes, especially the intrathoracic lymph nodes. Patients present with fever, weight loss, dyspnea on exertion, cough, chest pain, eye involvement (retinitis and uveitis), neck masses, parotid masses, and facial nerve paralysis. Cervical nodes tend to be bilateral, nontender, and mobile. The diagnosis of sarcoidosis can be confirmed by biopsy, and treatment consists of corticosteroid therapy.

Sinus Histiocytosis. Sinus histiocytosis (Rosai-Dorfman Disease) is a benign idiopathic histiocytic proliferation that is seen most often in the first 2 decades of life. In addition to massive, nontender, cervical adenopathy, patients present with fever, leukocytosis, and an elevated sedimentation rate. Extranodal involvement includes the upper respiratory tract, orbits, and salivary glands. The diagnosis of sinus histiocytosis is confirmed by biopsy and treatment is expectant, because most patients undergo spontaneous regression.

Kikuchi-Fujimoto Disease. This idiopathic disorder is most common in young adults and women. In addition to fever, chills, night sweats, and nausea, tender lymphadenopathy is present in most causes. A biopsy is often necessary to exclude a malignancy. Treatment is expectant.

PFAPA Syndrome. PFAPA syndrome includes ***p***eriodic recurring ***f***ever, ***a***phthous stomatitis, ***p***haryngitis, and cervical ***a***denitis. The episodes last for several days and then recur periodically for years. Signs and symptoms include high fevers, chills, malaise, pharyngitis, aphthous stomatitis, and tender lymphadenopathy. The diagnosis is one of exclusion, and treatment is expectant.

Neoplastic Masses

Thyroid Malignancies

Approximately 10% of thyroid malignancies have been reported in patients younger than 21 years of age, with children of all ages being represented.[22,23] Females are more commonly involved than males by a 2:1 preponderance.[24] In the past, thyroid malignancies in children were associated with a history of low-dose radiation therapy for benign disease. Today, these malignancies are the result of exposure to radiation (industrial) or caused by treatment of other malignancies with radiation therapy.

Most thyroid cancers in children tend to be well-differentiated and of the papillary, follicular, or mixed type. Rarely, medullary thyroid carcinoma may be found. This latter tumor originates from parafollicular C cells that secrete calcitonin and may be associated with multiple endocrine neoplasia (MEN) types IIA and IIIB. Thyroid carcinoma may also be found incidentally in examination of thyroglossal duct cyst specimens.[3]

Most thyroid malignancies manifest as a painless mass in the lower neck. A thyroid nodule may or may not be palpable. Approximately 70% to 90% of children also present with cervical adenopathy.[24] Evaluation of a child with a thyroid malignancy should include the following laboratory studies: triiodothyronine (T_3), thyroxine (T_4), thyroid-stimulating hormone (TSH), calcitonin, antithyroid antibodies, and antimicrosomal antibodies. Radiopaque psammoma bodies may be demonstrated on chest and lateral neck radiographs in children with papillary carcinoma. Both technetium 99m and iodine 123 thyroid scanning can distinguish between hypofunctioning (cold) and hyperfunctioning (hot) nodules. From 17% to 36% of cold nodules are malignant, whereas most hot nodules are benign.[25] Ultrasound-directed fine needle aspiration of thyroid masses may identify cell types. If this is unsuccessful, a frozen section biopsy may be necessary.

The presence of a thyroid malignancy is an indication for total or near-total thyroidectomy and a modified neck dissection if palpable lymphadenopathy is present. Postoperative ^{131}I scanning is important to identify any residual thyroid tissue that may then be ablated with a therapeutic dose of ^{131}I. Thyroid hormone therapy is necessary to maintain an euthyroid state and suppress TSH. Medullary thyroid carcinoma is treated with total thyroidectomy and a modified neck dissection. Treatment of thyroglossal duct cyst carcinoma is controversial. Some experts have recommended observation and suppression following a Sistrunk procedure,[26] whereas others have suggested a total thyroidectomy if a palpable thyroid nodule is also present.[27]

Lymphoma

Lymphoma is the most common malignancy of the head and neck in children[28] and represents 11.5% of all childhood cancers.[29] Lymphomas can be divided into two major types, Hodgkin's disease (HD) and non-Hodgkin's lymphoma (NHL) (Table 15-2). HD is characterized by the classic histopathologic finding of Reed-Sternberg cells. Burkitt's lymphoma is a small-cell form of high-grade NHL that is related to Epstein-Barr viral exposure.

Children with lymphoma involving the head and neck present with a mass in one of the cervical lymph nodes groups. Nodes tend to be firm and rubbery, without fixation, and may be associated with systemic or B symptoms that include fever, night sweats, and weight loss, although children with disease localized to the head and neck tend not to have B symptoms.[28] Staging of HD and NHL is listed in Tables 15-3 and 15-4, respectively. Treatment of HD includes a combination of multidrug chemotherapy and concurrent localized radiation therapy.

Table 15-2 Classification of Lymphoma

Type of Lymphoma	Classification
Hodgkin's disease	Lymphocyte predominant
	Nodular sclerosing
	Mixed cellularity
	Lymphocyte depleted
Non-Hodgkin's lymphoma	
High-grade	Large cell
	Lymphoblastic
	Small noncleaved cell (Burkitt's)
Intermediate-grade	Follicular large cell
	Diffuse small cleaved cell
	Diffuse mixed cell
	Diffuse large cell
Low-grade	Small lymphocyte
	Follicular, small cleaved
	Follicular, mixed cell

Table 15-4 Staging of Non-Hodgkin's Lymphoma

Stage	Features
I	Single tumor or single anatomic area without abdominal or mediastinal involvement
II	Single tumor with regional lymphadenopathy
	Two or more nodal areas on the same side of the diaphragm
	Two single tumors with or without regional lymphadenopathy or on one side of the diaphragm
	Gastrointestinal tract tumor with or without mesenteric lymphadenopathy
III	Two single tumors on opposite sides of the diaphragm
	Two or more nodal areas above and below the diaphragm
	Primary intrathoracic involvement
	Extensive primary intra-abdominal involvement
	Paraspinal or epidural involvement
IV	As above, with initial involvement of the CNS or bone marrow

The treatment of NHL consists of multidrug chemotherapy that was initially developed for the treatment of acute lymphoblastic leukemia.[30]

Langerhans' Cell Histiocytosis

Langerhans' cell histiocytosis (LCH) encompasses a group of disorders that was previously called histiocytosis X and included eosinophilic granuloma, Hand-Schüller-Christian syndrome, and Letterer-Siwe disease. The histopathologic diagnosis of this disease is dependent on the identification of Langerhans cells, which evolve from T-cell immune-regulating dendritic cells.[31] Depending on the extent and location of the disease, children present with rashes, otorrhea, oral lesions, and hepatosplenomegaly. Cervical lymphadenopathy is present in 20% of cases.[32] The diagnosis of LCH is confirmed by biopsy, and additional studies include a complete blood count, liver function tests, and chest and skeletal radiography. Current treatment options are dependent on the extent of the disease and the clinical course; these may include surgical curettage, excision, intralesional or systemic corticosteroids, low-dose radiation therapy, and chemotherapy.

Table 15-3 Staging of Hodgkin's Disease

Stage	Features
I	Involvement of a single lymph node region (I) or single extralymphatic organ (IE)
II	Involvement of two or more lymph node regions on the side of the diaphragm (II) or one lymph node region and one extralymphatic organ on the same side of the diaphragm (IIE)
III	Diffuse involvement of one or more extralymphatic organs with or without lymph node involvement (IV)
A	No systemic symptoms
B	Weight loss, fever, or night sweats

Post-Transplant Lymphoproliferative Disorder

Post-transplant lymphoproliferative disorder (PTLD) is found in 2% of transplant recipients.[33] Suppression of T lymphocytes in transplant patients permits the proliferation of EBV-associated B lymphocytes, causing a disease that ranges from acute mononucleosis to lymphoma. The onset of PTLD is suggested by the sudden increase in the size of a tonsil, adenoid tissue, or cervical lymph nodes. Treatment is variable and may include decreasing immunosuppression or adding systemic corticosteroids or antiviral agents to the regimen.[34]

Neurofibromatosis

Neurofibromatosis (NF) may occur as an isolated process or as part of the neurofibromatosis genetic disorders. Neurofibromatosis type 1 (NF1), also known as von Recklinghausen's disease, is an autosomal dominant genetic disorder with variable penetrance that accounts for 85% of cases of NF, with an incidence of 1 in 4,000 live births.[35] Neurofibromatosis type 2 (NF2) occurs in 1 in 50,000 live births, and the other types (3 to 8) occur even less often. Malignant transformation of these tumors is seen in 3% to 15% of cases.[36] Children with NF1 present with skin discoloration, neck masses, airway compromise, or involvement of the larynx, parotid, or other structures of the head and neck. Patients with NF2 develop tumors of cranial nerve VIII along with meningiomas of the brain and schwannomas of the spinal cord. Neurofibromas exist as four types—cutaneous, subcutaneous, nodular plexiform, and diffuse plexiform. The plexiform lesions tend to infiltrate the surrounding tissue. Radiation and chemotherapy are not effective in the management of neurofibromatosis, leaving surgery as the mainstay of treatment. The goal of surgery is conservative resection with preservation of vital structures. If the neurofibroma is not affecting function, it is often prudent for treatment to consist of observation.

Neuroblastoma

Neuroblastoma is the second most common malignant tumor of childhood. Tumors originate in the neural crest cells of the adrenal medulla or in the sympathetic nervous system. Neuroblastoma may manifest in the neck as a solitary cervical mass or as metastatic cervical adenopathy. It may also manifest with Horner's syndrome or a metastatic mass in the orbit or nose. The diagnosis is confirmed by biopsy of the tumor mass or demonstration of tumor cells in bone marrow aspirates. Increased urine or serum catecholamine levels (e.g., homovanillic acid, vanillylmandelic acid, dopamine) are suggestive of the diagnosis of neuroblastoma. Depending on the clinical stage, treatment may include surgery, chemotherapy, and radiation therapy or myeloablative chemotherapy and radiation therapy followed by autologous bone marrow transplantation.

Rhabdomyosarcoma

Rhabdomyosarcoma is the second most common malignancy of the head and neck in children.[28] It typically manifests in the orbit, nasopharynx, or temporal bone, usually appearing in the neck as metastatic disease. Rarely, rhabdomyosarcoma may manifest as a primary in the neck. The signs and symptoms of rhabdomyosarcoma depend on the primary site of involvement, and treatment includes chemotherapy, radiation therapy, and surgery.

Salivary Gland Tumors

Salivary gland neoplasms are uncommon in children.[37] The parotid gland is seven times more likely than the submandibular gland to be involved with a neoplasm.[38] Benign salivary gland neoplasms include hemangiomas and pleomorphic adenomas. Hemangiomas are seen more commonly in females and in the left side of the neck.[38] MRI may help distinguish a hemangioma from a lymphatic malformation. Hemangiomas of the neck require treatment only if complications such as hemorrhage, ulceration, or platelet sequestration occur. Pleomorphic adenoma necessitates surgical excision with facial nerve preservation if the tumor is in the parotid gland and complete excision of the gland if the submandibular gland is involved.

Children exposed to radiation therapy early in childhood are more prone to develop salivary gland malignancies. Mucoepidermoid carcinoma occurs more commonly than acinic cell carcinoma, and both tumor types range in grade from low to high.[39] Ominous signs suggestive of malignancy include rapid growth, facial weakness, pain, and the sudden appearance of cervical adenopathy. Mucoepidermoid carcinoma affects older children, in contrast with sarcomas, which occur more often in young children. Most patients present with a neck mass in the parotid gland or submandibular triangle, sometimes associated with enlarged cervical nodes and facial nerve paresis or paralysis if the parotid gland is involved. Treatment includes surgical excision, with facial nerve preservation if possible. Surgical excision may be followed by radiation therapy if residual tumor is suspected, in cases with metastasis, or in cases with a high-grade lesion. Acinic cell carcinoma presents in a similar manner and requires the same level of treatment as mucoepidermoid carcinoma.

Metastatic Disease

Any malignancy in the body can metastasize to the neck. Squamous cell carcinoma, especially with the nasopharynx as a source, is aggressive in adolescents and often spreads to the neck. Management of cases of suspected metastasis to the neck should include a search for a primary site, although biopsy of the neck lesion may be necessary to establish the diagnosis.

EVALUATION

Symptoms and Signs

A detailed history from the parents or caregiver is the first essential step in focusing the differential diagnosis of a child with a neck mass. Determining the age of the child at the onset of the mass is an excellent place to start. The appearance of a mass in a neonate or infant may represent a congenital cyst or a vascular or lymphatic malformation. A source from a maternal infection, such as syphilis or HIV, must also be considered. During childhood, complications of an upper respiratory tract infection with the nose or pharynx as a source should be entertained as the cause of the neck mass. In adolescents, masses tend to be of inflammatory or malignant origin.

Temporal relationships are also helpful in narrowing the differential diagnosis. The appearance of the mass in close temporal relationship to an infection or an infectious agent may provide clues about the underlying cause. Eliciting a history of exposure to a cat, nondomestic animals, or insects such as ticks is an important part of the interview. The appearance of a neck mass soon after an episode of trauma to the neck suggests a vascular injury, whereas painful swelling of the face or upper neck with eating suggests a salivary gland origin.

Growth characteristics are also important. A slow-growing neck mass suggests a benign process, whereas rapid growth is usually seen in infectious or malignant processes. Fluctuating size may be seen in a mass that represents recurrent infection or, if associated with straining or crying, a hemangioma. Constitutional signs and symptoms of fever, weight loss, night sweats, and fatigue are often associated with a malignancy. A history of previous radiation therapy to the neck predisposes to thyroid or salivary gland malignancies.[40]

Physical Examination

The appearance of the mass may provide important clues about its origin. An attempt should be made to ascertain whether the mass is solid or cystic. Color may also be important; for example, a blue or purple color suggests a vascular lesion or hemangioma. Erythema, tenderness, or warmth of the overlying skin is strongly indicative of an infectious process. Masses that are fixed to underlying structures should suggest a malignancy. A draining fistula in association with a cystic mass suggests a branchial origin. A fluctuant mass is typical of an abscess or deeper cyst.

In addition to an examination of the neck mass, it is important to inspect the remainder of the head and neck carefully. A thorough examination of the remainder of the body may provide clues about a source. Particular attention should be paid to other lymph nodes groups in the axillae and groin and also to the spleen. Finding a skin lesion, such as a hemangioma or café au lait spot, may prove extremely valuable.

What makes a lymph node abnormal? Any node larger than 2 cm in diameter falls outside the range of normal and should be investigated. Infants often have shotty posterior cervical lymphadenopathy because this region is the site of drainage from the nose and nasopharynx, the locations of many upper respiratory infections in children younger than 2 years. Of infants younger than 1 year, 40% have clinically palpable nodes.[41] Because infections in older children tend to originate in the oropharynx, the anterior cervical nodes are more commonly involved than the posterior cervical group. Nodes in the supraclavicular and posterior cervical regions have a greater tendency to be associated with a malignant process.[1,42]

Other forms of examination such as flexible endoscopy may provide access to areas of the head and neck, such as the nasopharynx, that may provide clues about the origin of a mass. Purulent secretions in the nasopharynx may explain the appearance of lymph nodes in the posterior cervical chain, whereas a mass in the nasopharynx might suggest a malignancy with metastasis to the same region.[43]

Laboratory Studies

If the diagnosis of a neck mass is still in doubt at the completion of the history and physical examination, a decision may be made to proceed with laboratory testing. A complete blood count may provide an indication of systemic infection or malignancy. The presence of an increased number of atypical lymphocytes suggests acute infectious mononucleosis or a similar process. The sedimentation rate is a nonspecific indicator of a systemic process that may be infectious, inflammatory, or malignant.

Serologic testing is helpful in identifying various infectious agents and infections, including the Epstein-Barr virus, cytomegalovirus, toxoplasmosis, cat-scratch disease, syphilis, tularemia, brucellosis, and fungal infections. Abnormal chemistry results may provide clues about the cause of a neck mass. Children afflicted with sarcoidosis may have an elevated serum calcium level. Elevated urinary catecholamine levels, specifically vanillylmandelic acid (VMA), can be seen in patients with neuroblastoma. Depending on the pathology, certain thyroid masses may manifest with abnormal thyroid function test results. Although skin testing with purified protein derivative (PPD) is not as accurate as culturing of infected tissue, it may provide a clue about the cause of a neck mass, especially in cases of mycobacterial infection.

Radiologic Evaluation

Radiologic studies provide another diagnostic option. A lateral neck radiograph is helpful in demonstrating disease in the nasopharynx or oropharynx that may cause a mass in the neck. Specifically, a malignancy in the nasopharynx may be responsible for a metastatic mass in the posterior cervical region. Widening of the retropharyngeal space usually indicates an infectious process in that region and may suggest a source of the neck mass. Calcifications in involved lymph nodes may be diagnostic in patients with atypical mycobacterial infection. Similarly, a chest radiograph may provide important information about systemic processes, such as a malignancy, sarcoidosis, or tuberculosis.

CT with contrast is most helpful in the evaluation of infectious neck masses. The presence of ring enhancement surrounding an area of hypolucency on a contrast CT scan suggests abscess formation, whereas hypolucency alone is diagnostic of cellulitis.[44] CT is superior to MRI in the evaluation of processes that involve a soft tissue and bone interface. MRI provides better soft tissue resolution than CT. When combined with contrast, it may be diagnostic for vascular lesions. MRI is more expensive than CT, however, and the length of the study often requires the use of sedation in young children.

Other radiologic modalities helpful in the evaluation of a neck mass include ultrasonography and thyroid scanning. Ultrasound examination can be used to differentiate a cystic mass from a solid one. In an infant with a suspected sternocleidomastoid tumor, ultrasound may demonstrate a mass within the SCM muscle. Ultrasound is an easier to perform and more economical method of verifying the presence of a normal thyroid gland prior to excision of a thyroglossal duct cyst. Ultrasound-guided aspiration of pus from a neck abscess may provide material for culture and may be curative in selected cases. Ultrasound is also useful in the evaluation of thyroid masses. Thyroid scanning is essential in the management of any mass of the thyroid gland.

SURGICAL MANAGEMENT

In adults, fine-needle aspiration of suspected neck malignancies is performed often, especially if the diagnosis of squamous cell carcinoma is entertained. However, because many malignancies in children are not squamous, fine-needle aspiration of neck masses may not be as reliable. In addition, the pathology laboratory must be experienced in handling these types of specimens. Excisional or incisional biopsy allows careful inspection of the tissue, provides a layer of normal surrounding tissue for comparison, and provides a specimen for electron microscopy or tumor markers. If biopsy findings are negative for tumor, but all the clinical information is still suggestive of a malignancy, a repeat biopsy may be considered.

MAJOR POINTS

- Pediatric neck masses are rarely malignant.
- The differential diagnosis includes three major categories: congenital, infectious or inflammatory, and neoplastic.
- Many congenital masses arise from maldevelopment of the thyroid gland or branchial apparatus.
- Many infectious causes of a neck mass are viral or bacterial and resolve with observation or oral antibiotic therapy.
- Of thyroid malignancies, 10% occur in patients younger than 21 years.
- Lymphoma is the most common malignancy of the head and neck in children.
- Age at onset, temporal relationships, and growth characteristics are important factors to explore when eliciting a history.
- A thorough examination should include the entire head and neck and lymph node groups in the axilla and groin.
- Nodes in the supraclavicular and posterior cervical regions are more likely to be associated with a malignant process.
- Computed tomography is most useful for examining bone–soft tissue interfaces, whereas MRI is best for demonstrating soft tissue detail.
- If a biopsy result does not correlate with the clinical impression, a repeat biopsy should be considered.

SUMMARY

Although the incidence of malignancy in a child with a neck mass is low, this concern is usually what brings most parents and their affected child to a physician. By following an organized and thorough approach in evaluating a neck mass, the clinician can often narrow the differential diagnosis without resorting to a surgical biopsy. A comprehensive approach to a pediatric neck mass includes a detailed history, a complete physical examination, and radiologic and laboratory studies. If the diagnosis still remains in doubt at this point, a biopsy may be necessary to confirm the diagnosis.

REFERENCES

1. Torsiglieri AJ Jr, Tom LW, Ross AJ 3rd, et al: Pediatric neck masses: Guidelines for evaluation. Int J Pediatr Otorhinolaryngol 1988;16:199-210.
2. Sistrunk WE: The surgical treatment of cysts of the thyroglossal tract. Ann Surg 1920;71:121-122.
3. Chonkich GD, Wat BY: Papillary carcinoma arising in a thyroglossal duct cyst. Otolaryngol Head Neck Surg 1997;116:386-388.
4. Nofsinger YC, Tom LW, LaRossa D, et al: Periauricular cysts and sinuses. Laryngoscope 1997;107:883-887.
5. Chandler JR, Mitchell B: Branchial cleft cysts, sinuses and fistulas. Otolaryngol Clin North Am 1981;14:175-186.
6. Mulliken JB, Young AE: Vascular Birthmarks: Hemangiomas and Malformations. Philadelphia, WB Saunders, 1988.
7. Finn MC, Glowacki J, Mulliken JB: Congenital vascular lesions: Clinical application of a new classification. J Pediatr Surg 1983;18:894-899.
8. Healy GB, McGill T, Friedman EM: Carbon dioxide laser in subglottic hemangioma: An update. Ann Otol Rhinol Laryngol 1984;93:370-373.
9. Ezekowitz RAB, Mulliken JB, Folkman J: Interferon alpha-2a therapy for life-threatening hemangiomas of infancy. N Engl J Med 1992;326:1456-1463.
10. Tavill MA, Wetmore RF: A case of familial sternocleidomastoid tumor of infancy. Int J Pediatr Otorhinolaryngol 1996;38:163-168.
11. Tom LWC, Handler SD, Wetmore RF, et al: The sternocleidomastoid tumor of infancy. Int J Pediatr Otorhinolaryngol 1987;13:245-255.

12. Kelley DJ, Gerber ME, Willging JP: Cervicomediastinal thymic cysts. Int J Pediatr Otorhinolaryngol 1997;39: 139-146.

13. McKinney RE Jr: Antiretroviral therapy: Evaluating the new era in HIV treatment. Adv Pediatr Infect Dis 1996; 12:297-323.

14. Richards L: Retropharyngeal abscess. N Engl J Med 1936;215:1120-1130.

15. Brodsky L, Belles W, Brody A, et al: Needle aspiration of neck masses in children. Clin Pediatr 1992;31:71-76.

16. Maurin M, Birtles R, Raoult D: Current knowledge of *Bartonella* species. Eur J Clin Microbiol Infect Dis 1997;16:487-506.

17. Wolinsky E: Mycobacterial lymphadenitis in children: A prospective study of 105 nontuberculous cases with long-term follow-up. Clin Infect Dis 1995;20:954-963.

18. Suskind DL, Handler SD, Tom LWC, et al: Nontuberculous mycobacterial cervical adenitis. Clin Pediatr 1997; 36:403-409.

19. Rapp RP, McCraney SA, Goodman NL, et al: New macrolide antibiotics: Usefulness in infections caused by mycobacteria other than *Mycobacterium tuberculosis*. Ann Pharmacother 1994;28:1255-1263.

20. McLaughlin RB, Keller JL, Wetmore RF, et al: Kawasaki disease: A diagnostic dilemma. Am J Otolaryngol 1998;19:274-277.

21. Seicshnaydre MA, Frable MA: Kawasaki disease: Early presentation to the otolaryngologist. Otolaryngol Head Neck Surg 1993;108:344-347.

22. Buckwalter JA, Guril NJ, Thomras CG Jr: Cancer of the thyroid in youth. World J Surg 1981;5:15-25.

23. Winship T, Rosvoll RV: Childhood thyroid carcinoma. Cancer 1961;14:734-743.

24. Geiger JD, Thompson NW: Thyroid tumors in children. Otolaryngol Clin North Am 1996;4:711-719.

25. Hung W, Anderson KD, Chandra R: Solitary thyroid nodules in children and adolescents. J Pediatr Surg 1992;27:1407-1409.

26. Kristensen S, Juul A, Moesner J: Thyroglossal duct cyst carcinoma. J Laryngol Otol 1984;98:1277-1280.

27. Cote DN, Sturgis EM, Peterson T, et al: Thyroglossal duct cyst carcinoma: An unusual case of Hürthle cell carcinoma. Otolaryngol Head Neck Surg 1995;113:153-156.

28. Cunningham MJ, Myers EN, Bluestone CD: Malignant tumors of the head and neck in children: A twenty-year review. Int J Pediatr Otorhinolaryngol 1987;13:279-292.

29. Miller RW, Young JL, Novakovic B: Childhood cancer. Cancer 1995;75(Suppl 1):395-405.

30. Sandlund JT, Downing JR, Crist WM: Non-Hodgkin's lymphoma in childhood. N Engl J Med 1996;334:1238-1248.

31. Lieberman PH, Jones CR, Steinman RM, et al: Langerhans' cell (eosinophilic) granulomatosis. A clinicopathologic study encompassing 50 years. Am J Surg Path 1996; 20:519-552.

32. Irving RM, Broadbent V, Jones NS: Langerhans' cell histiocytosis in childhood: Management of head and neck manifestations. Laryngoscope 1994;104:64-70.

33. Ho M, Jaffe R, Miller G, et al: The frequency of Epstein-Barr virus infection and associated lymphoproliferative syndrome after transplantation and its manifestation in children. Transplantation 1988;45:719-727.

34. Sculerati N, Arriaga M: Otolaryngologic management of post-transplant lymphoproliferative disease in children. Ann Otol Rhinol Laryngol 1990;99:445-450.

35. Riccardi VM: Genotype, malleotype, phenotype, and randomness: Lessons from neurofibromatosis-1. Am J Hum Genet 1993;53:301-304.

36. Knight WA, Murphy WK, Gottlieb JA: Neurofibromatosis associated with malignant neurofibromas. Arch Dermatol 1973;107:747-775.

37. Krolls SO, Trodahl JN, Boyers RC: Salivary gland lesions in children: A survey of 430 cases. Cancer 1972;30:459-469.

38. Luna MA, Batsakis JG, El-Naggar AK: Pathology consultation: Salivary gland tumors in children. Ann Otol Rhinol Laryngol 1991;100:869-871.

39. Chong GC, Beahrs OH, Chen ML, et al: Management of parotid gland tumors in infants and children. Mayo Clin Proc 1975;50:279-283.

40. Favus MJ, Schneider AB, Stachura ME, et al: Thyroid cancer occurring as a late consequence of head and neck irradiation. N Engl J Med 1976;294:1019-1025.

41. Bamji M, Stone RK, Kaul A, et al: Palpable lymph nodes in healthy newborns and infants. Pediatrics 1986;78:573-575.

42. Moussatos GH, Baffes TG: Cervical masses in infants and children. Pediatrics 1963;32:251-256.

43. Jaffe B: Pediatric head and neck tumors: A study of 178 cases. Laryngoscope 1973;83:1644-1651.

44. Wetmore RF, Mahboubi S, Soyupak SK: Computed tomography in the evaluation of pediatric neck infections. Otolaryngol Head Neck Surg 1998;119:624-627.

CHAPTER 16

Pediatric Facial Trauma

KEN KAZAHAYA, MD, MBA

This chapter reviews of some of the more common pediatric head and neck traumas, including trauma to the ears, nose, facial bones, oral cavity, and neck. Foreign bodies of the upper airway are discussed in Chapter 12.

EAR TRAUMA

External Ear

The external ear includes the auricle and external auditory canal. The auricle is exposed on the side of the head, making it susceptible to physical and environmental trauma. Reflexive turning of the head to the side places the ear in direct line of injury. Blunt and sharp injuries to the auricle may require emergent management. Also, because of the exposed nature of the auricle, it is at risk for excessive sun and extreme cold exposures.

Injuries to the Auricle

Blunt Trauma

An impact on the side of the head may result in a blunt injury to the auricle. A superficial excoriation or contusion may occur, but requires only conservative management and wound care. However, more significant injuries may result. The injury can result in the formation of a hematoma in the auricle, which is an emergent situation and must be treated expediently. Hematomas should be suspected when there is a history of trauma and the formation of a soft, fluctuant swelling of the auricle with loss of the definition of cartilaginous contours, such as the helix or antihelix (Fig. 16-1). Pugilists and wrestlers frequently suffer this type of injury. Hematomas require urgent incision, drainage, bolster placement, and antibiotic coverage. Because the perichondrium is elevated away from the cartilage, the cartilage is devascularized during this injury, leading to its necrosis. Also, the hematoma itself may create scar tissue. An untreated auricular hematoma may result in a "cauliflower ear" because of stimulation of the perichondrium to create new cartilage.[1] Once the hematoma is evacuated, a drain and bolster dressing should be placed to prevent reaccumulation of blood. A broad-spectrum oral antibiotic that covers skin flora should be prescribed. Signs of increasing infection or perichondritis need to be addressed emergently.

A blow to the side of the head may also result in barotrauma to the tympanic membrane, causing a tympanic membrane perforation. Bloody otorrhea or a conductive hearing loss is not unusual. The external ear and tympanic membrane should be carefully evaluated in cases of trauma to the auricle.

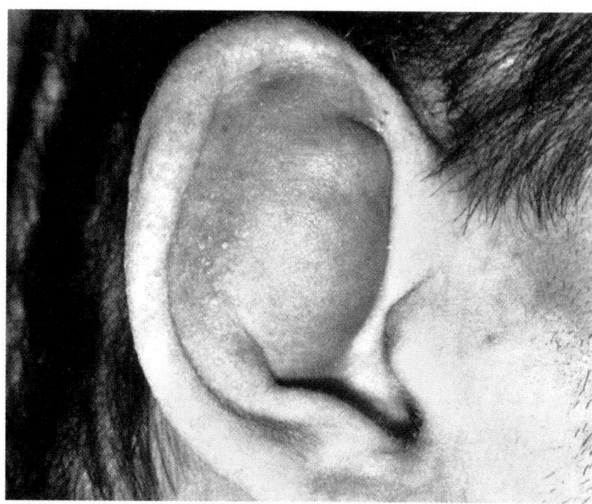

Figure 16-1. Auricular hematoma. (From Handler SD: Diagnosis and management of maxillo-facial injuries. In Torg J [ed]: Athletic Injuries to the Head, Neck and Face, 2nd ed. Philadelphia, Lea & Febiger, 1991, pp 611-634.

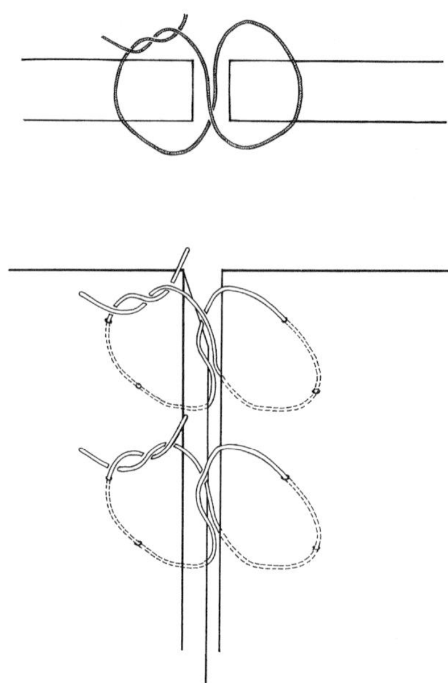

Figure 16-2. Figure-of-eight suturing of cartilage edges.

Sharp Trauma

Lacerations of the auricle can be divided into those involving the underlying auricular cartilage and those that do not. If the cartilage is not involved, the laceration may be closed primarily. In closing such a wound, care should be taken along the helix and lobule to approximate the edges closely, and a Z-plasty or broken line closure may be required to avoid notching of the edge of the auricle. If a defect is too wide to be closed without significant distortion, healing by secondary intention should be considered, with revision of the scar once the wound has healed.

If the cartilage is involved, the edges need to be reapproximated and the fragments accurately realigned as much as possible. A simple laceration of the cartilage can be reapproximated taking care to avoid overlapping the edges of the cartilage. It is sometimes helpful to consider using alternating figure-of-eight sutures to prevent the cartilage from overlapping (Fig. 16-2). This helps prevent the cut edges of the cartilage from overriding one another while still maintaining approximation of the edges. The wound should be irrigated copiously and conservatively débrided. A thin strip of cartilage may need to be resected to allow the skin to be closed over the cartilage. The overlying skin can then be approximated and closed with fine monofilament nonabsorbable sutures. A pressure dressing should be applied.

Loss of skin over cartilage with intact perichondrium may be treated with skin grafting, using postauricular skin, which has good color match. If perichondrium has been lost and vascularized tissue is required, a skin flap from adjacent skin or scalp may be used.

Auricular Avulsion Injury

In severe trauma to the ear, the pinna may be partially or completely avulsed. If it is only partially avulsed, the vascularity of the auricle needs to be assessed. If the arterial supply to the auricle has been transected, it should be evaluated to determine whether it may be reanastomosed using microvascular techniques. Often, the ear may be simply reattached, taking care not to strangulate the tenuous pedicle. Careful follow-up will be necessary to ensure that the tissue remains viable. Post-revascularization anticoagulation and antibiotic coverage are required. Medicinal leeches have been used in cases of venous congestion to assist with perfusion. Hyperbaric oxygen may also be considered in some cases. If the auricle is completely avulsed, the auricle may be deepithelialized, reattached, and then placed within a postauricular pocket. After 1 or 2 weeks, the buried portion is externalized and allowed to epithelialize.[2]

Thermal Injury

Because of its exposed position, the auricle is particularly at risk for thermal injuries, including frostbite in colder climates and burns. Signs and symptoms of exposure, such as pain, numbness, change in color, and loss of capillary refill, are of concern. Necrosis of the skin is an ominous sign. The treatment of auricular thermal injury should be treated in the same manner as for similar injuries to other parts of the body.

First-degree burns usually do not require any therapy. Pain relief with nonsteroidal anti-inflammatory drugs (NSAIDs), such as ibuprofen and acetaminophen, may be considered. Also, mild moisturizers may be used on the affected area. Second-degree burns should be treated with hydrotherapy, débridement, and topical antibacterials, such as silver sulfadiazine, bacitracin, or mafenide acetate. Treatment should continue for 10 days. At this point, the burns should be reevaluated to determine whether they are likely to complete healing or will require excision and grafting.[3] Third-degree or full-thickness burns will require excision and grafting. If ear cartilage is exposed, it may need to be placed in a postauricular pocket to provide coverage.

External Auditory Canal Foreign Bodies and Trauma

Foreign bodies in the external auditory canal (EAC) are common in children. They must be removed carefully as to avoid pain or injury to the EAC or tympanic membrane. Solid objects, such as beads, corn kernels, pebbles, and paper, are some of the more commonly encountered foreign bodies. Many foreign bodies may be gently rolled out of the ear canal with a cerumen curette or grasped with otologic forceps. Some objects may be gently irrigated out of the ear canal with body-temperature water. Irrigation should not be attempted if a tympanic membrane perforation is suspected. Insects in the ear canal may cause significant pain or discomfort if the insect is lodged medially against the tympanic membrane. Insects can be killed by filling the ear canal with alcohol or mineral oil, and then removed with forceps. If objects are against or adjacent to the tympanic membrane, irrigation of the ear canal may help avoid pain and/or injury to the tympanic membrane. If the foreign body cannot be easily removed, an otolaryngologist should be consulted and extraction may be attempted under binocular microscopy, with or without anesthesia. It is preferable to seek otolaryngologic consultation for an ear foreign body if the object cannot be removed easily, before the child becomes averse to allowing anyone near to examine their ear.

The medial portion of the external ear canal and the tympanic membrane are exquisitely sensitive and easily traumatized. Topical anesthetic emulsions can be attempted in cases with an intact tympanic membrane; however, the emulsions may not diffuse medially to the foreign body and may require significant time to anesthetize the canal skin adequately. If there is a tympanic perforation and the anesthetic gets into the middle ear, it may cause the child to have significant nausea and vomiting as a result of its effect on the vestibular system. After a foreign body has been removed from the ear, minor abrasions and trauma to the EAC should be treated with ototopical antibiotics to help prevent infection.

Tympanic Membrane

Perforation

Although the tympanic membrane lies nearly 1 inch inside the EAC, it is still susceptible to trauma from an internal cause, such as an acute otitis media, or an external cause, such as direct trauma (e.g., poking something into the EAC) (Fig. 16-3) or barotrauma (e.g., a slap to the side of the head, a fall into a swimming pool, exposure to rough waves, or scuba diving). Middle ear structures may be damaged by a penetrating object, resulting in fracture or dislocation of the ossicles or a perilymphatic fistula (PLF). Traumatic PLF typically manifests with the immediate onset of vertigo, nystagmus, and/or sensorineural hearing loss. There may be a mixed hearing loss if the ossicular chain has been disrupted. A penetrating object may also injure the facial nerve, resulting in facial palsy or paralysis. The injury can occur along the horizontal portion of the facial nerve, just above the oval window. Acute facial nerve paralysis following ear trauma requires urgent otolaryngologic consultation.

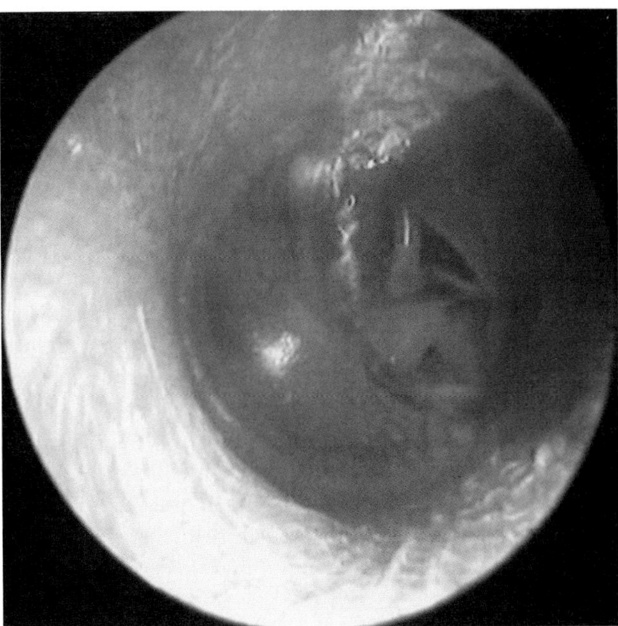

Figure 16-3. Traumatic perforation of the tympanic membrane.

Traumatic perforations of the tympanic membrane should be carefully examined, preferably with binocular microscopy. The perforation needs to be monitored to ensure that as it heals, the edges of the perforation do not curl medially into the middle ear space, risking the formation of a cholesteatoma. Most traumatic perforations of the tympanic membrane heal spontaneously within 2 to 3 weeks. If the injury was the result of water trauma, ototopical antibiotic drops should be used. Also, a child with a perforated tympanic membrane should be encouraged to keep the ear dry until closure of the perforation. If the ear is exposed to excessive water trauma, ototopical antibiotic drops should be used in the ear. Development of otorrhea may also be treated with ototopical antibiotics; however, if the otorrhea is temporally related to traumatic injury to the tympanic membrane or if the otorrhea is persistent, even with treatment, an otolaryngologic consultation should be sought.

Tympanic perforation with evidence of more serious injuries, such as a PLF, ossicular chain involvement, or facial nerve paralysis, may require urgent surgical exploration, and these children should be referred to an otolaryngologist.

Barotrauma

Barotrauma may result whenever there is a sudden change in environmental pressure, resulting in a significant pressure gradient across the tympanic membrane. This pressure gradient may arise from diving into a swimming pool or scuba diving, while flying in a plane, or from being slapped or struck on the side of the ear. Injuries are more likely to occur in the presence of eustachian tube dysfunction, because there is an inability to equalize the pressure in the middle ear to the ambient pressure (such as with a Valsalva maneuver). The eustachian tube is a natural conduit between the middle ear space and nasopharynx. When functioning properly, the eustachian tube promptly equalizes the pressure in the middle ear space to that of the atmosphere around the body. When it is not functioning well, changes in ambient pressure in the middle ear cannot be compensated for properly, and stress is applied to the tympanic membrane. If enough pressure is exerted, the tympanic membrane can rupture. Similarly, if the middle ear pressure is low and the ambient pressure rises suddenly, the pressure is transmitted within the vasculature and may result in rupture of the capillaries in the middle ear mucosa and acute hemorrhage into the middle ear space, resulting in a hemotympanum. Serous fluid may also accumulate in the middle ear in the presence of eustachian tube dysfunction.

In either case, the effusion in the middle ear should resolve spontaneously over several weeks. The use of oral antibiotics as prophylactic treatment against the development of infection is controversial. Lack of resolution of the middle ear effusion or hemorrhage requires otolaryngologic consultation. Barotrauma with acute onset of sensorineural hearing loss or severe vertigo may indicate a more severe injury and possible perilymphatic fistula, and should be evaluated by an otolaryngologist.

Inner Ear

Extreme sound levels and concussive impacts to the head may cause disruption of the delicate intracochlear structures, resulting in sensorineural hearing loss and/or vestibular symptoms. Most of these injuries leave permanent effects, but some losses can improve spontaneously. Constant exposure to loud noise or amplified sound may cause a progressive hearing loss, usually starting at the higher frequencies. There have been concerns raised recently with the increased prevalence of MP3 audio players and the potential for hearing loss that may result from exposure to high-intensity sound for extended periods. As a point of reference, a lawnmower creates approximately 85 dB of sound pressure, and studies have shown that hearing loss is likely to occur after 8 hours of exposure. Furthermore, for each 3-dB increase in sound pressure level, the time of exposure that may result in hearing loss is reduced by 50% (e.g., 8 dB may cause hearing loss after 4 hours).

Temporal Bone Trauma

Impact to the head may result in a temporal bone fracture. Of blunt head traumas, 30% to 75% result in a temporal bone fracture.[4,5] Once a trauma victim has been stabilized, a comprehensive neurologic evaluation should be completed, including assessment of facial nerve function. As part of the neuro-otologic examination, the child should be questioned with regard to hearing, dizziness, vertigo, and prior otologic history. Examination should include inspection of the ears, including the mastoid region. The ear should be evaluated for drainage and, if possible, the tympanic membrane should be examined. The ear should not be irrigated, because this may introduce contaminated material into the cranium. Acute neurological issues should be stabilized prior to imaging of the temporal bones for suspected fractures. Otolaryngologic consultation should be sought if a temporal bone fracture is suspected. Audiologic evaluation should be carried out once the child is stable and out of acute danger. Sudden onset of facial nerve paralysis may indicate transaction of the facial nerve and may require expedient intervention.

Temporal bone fractures are traditionally classified as longitudinal or transverse. Approximately 80% of temporal bone fractures are longitudinal, and usually are caused by an impact to the side of the head. Longitudinal temporal bone fractures typically avoid the otic capsule, parallel the internal auditory canal, and may disrupt the tympanic membrane and ossicles. Conductive hearing loss is common. A transverse fracture typically occurs as a result of a significant impact to the front or back of the head, and usually involves the otic capsule, with disruption of the internal auditory canal and facial and cochleovestibular nerves. Approximately 50% of transverse fractures have facial nerve involvement. Sensorineural hearing loss and facial nerve paralysis are more likely with transverse temporal bone fractures. Cerebrospinal fluid (CSF) leaks (rhinorrhea or otorrhea) are more common with transverse temporal bone fractures.

If a temporal bone fracture is suspected, a computed tomography (CT) scan of the temporal bones with 1-mm sections and with magnified axial and coronal views will

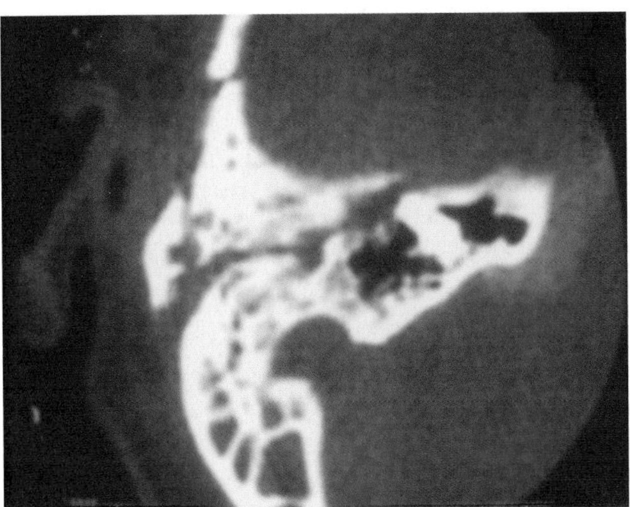

Figure 16-4. Axial CT scan of a temporal bone fracture.

allow for definitive diagnosis of the fracture (Fig. 16-4). Also, the scan may allow localization of sites of injury in the case of facial nerve paralysis or CSF leak. Audiologic evaluation should be obtained as soon as the child is medically stable to assess the child for possible hearing loss. Sensorineural hearing loss can be a result of a concussive injury to the cochlea or disruption of the cochlear nerve. Conductive hearing loss may be caused by disruption of the ossicular chain, a perforation in the tympanic membrane, or fluid (including blood and CSF) in the middle ear space.

Cerebrospinal Fluid Otorrhea

CSF otorrhea may be secondary to a temporal bone fracture in conjunction with a perforated TM. Although transverse fractures are more likely to result in a CSF leak, the TM is more likely to be ruptured in a longitudinal fracture. With an intact TM, a CSF leak may manifest as rhinorrhea if the CSF travels down the eustachian tube.

If otorrhea creates a bull's eye–like pattern on a piece of tissue or fabric or on the patient's sheets, CSF should be suspected. Fluid from the ear may be collected and tested for glucose and β_2-transferrin. Glucose may be found in many bodily fluids; however, β_2-transferrin is specific to CSF. Similarly, rhinorrhea fluid may be collected for similar testing.

Manipulation or instrumentation of the external auditory canal in the presence of CSF otorrhea is discouraged, because it could result in the introduction of bacteria and contribute to the development of meningitis. If a CSF leak from temporal bone trauma is suspected, bed rest with gentle head of bed elevation (approximately 30 degrees) and stool softeners are recommended. Neurosurgical consultation should also be considered. The use of prophylactic systemic and/or ototopical antimicrobials in the presence of a CSF leak is controversial.

Facial Nerve Paralysis

Temporal bone trauma may cause an injury to the facial nerve, resulting in facial nerve paralysis that may vary in severity and duration. Approximately 7% to 10% of temporal bone fractures are associated with facial nerve dysfunction.[6] In one study of 132 children with temporal bone trauma, 11 had unilateral facial nerve paralysis (8.3%).[7] Transverse fractures of the temporal bones can cause a disruption of the facial nerve within the intratemporal segment. Longitudinal fractures are less likely to cause facial nerve paralysis. When a temporal bone fracture is associated with a fracture, transverse fractures are much more likely to result in facial nerve transaction than longitudinal fractures.[6] Penetrating temporal bone trauma, especially as a result of gunshot wounds, typically causes more significant injuries. Whatever the cause of the temporal bone injury, the immediate evaluation of postinjury facial nerve function is imperative for appropriate management.

If there is normal facial nerve function immediately after injury, even though paresis later develops, there is excellent prognosis for a return to normal or near-normal function. Acute onset of partial facial nerve paralysis, without progression to complete paralysis, also has a good prognosis. In both of these cases, no surgical intervention or electrophysiologic testing is usually required.[6]

Sudden or immediate loss of facial motion may signify nerve disruption or transaction. Children who present with a complete facial nerve paralysis have a poorer prognosis. Once a child is stable, radiologic evaluation with CT and magnetic resonance imaging (MRI) may provide information regarding injury to the facial nerve. Electrical testing by electroneuronography may help identify denervation; more than 95% degeneration indicates significant injury to the facial nerve. If there is more than 95% degeneration within 6 days of injury, children typically have a poorer prognosis and surgical intervention may be warranted. If there is less than 95% degeneration at 14 days postinjury, there is a chance for good prognosis and surgical intervention is not indicated, even if there is degeneration of facial nerve function after the 14-day window.[6]

Surgical intervention may include decompression of the nerve and repair of complete nerve transections. There are no data on the efficacy of the use of steroids in children with facial nerve paralysis and temporal bone trauma; however, because of the anti-inflammatory activity of steroids and the assumption that neural edema is a primary factor in the progression of injury, a short course of steroids may be of benefit. Children with traumatic facial nerve paralysis should be referred to the otolaryngologist for evaluation, management, and possible exploration and nerve repair.[6]

FACIAL AND NASAL TRAUMA

Facial injury commonly occurs in the pediatric population as a result of play, contact sports, and motor vehicle accidents. Any child with significant facial trauma should be carefully assessed for other associated, and potentially more serious, injuries to certain regions of the body, such as the cervical spine, central nervous system, eyes, thorax, and abdomen. Facial trauma may be associated with ocular injury, such as a hyphema, retinal detachment, or fracture of the bony orbit. Contusions and lacerations may result in significant facial edema, which may have a rapid onset, and slow resolution.

Nasal Trauma

The nose, given its prominent position on the face, is subject to frequent trauma. In younger children, there is a more prominent cartilaginous portion compared with the adult nasal structure. Therefore, the cartilage can bend, allowing the force of the impact to dissipate across the midface, resulting in significant edema and ecchymosis. The swelling across the midface may make examination of underlying bony structures difficult. Significant facial injuries may result in orbital and nasoethmoid complex fractures and may require expedient evaluation and management.

Nasal Fracture

Impact to the nose may result in a fracture of the bony pyramid, and there may be a deviation or depression of the nasal bones (Fig. 16-5). The septal cartilage may also become fractured or deviated secondary to the trauma. The deviated or depressed bony fragments may be readily evident immediately after the trauma occurs; however, postinjury edema may prevent identification of these fragments. This may take several days, until the swelling subsides, before the injury may be accurately evaluated. Elevation of the head of the bed and application of ice or a cold pack to the site of injury may help reduce the posttraumatic edema. Once the edema has subsided, a step-off or bony irregularity may be detectable. Plain film radiographs are unreliable in the evaluation of nasal injuries and are not recommended in the management of simple fractures (Fig. 16-6). Epistaxis typically accompanies nasal bone fractures and is usually self-resolving. Persistent bleeding may require interventions such as direct pressure, topical vasoconstrictors, procoagulant topical medications (e.g., gelatin granules and topical thrombin [FloSeal]), or nasal packing. If there is no evidence of a septal hematoma (see later) or other associated traumatic injuries, the displaced nasal bone fragments may be reduced once the soft tissue edema has resolved enough to permit accurate evaluation of the deformity. Usually, a splint is placed over the dorsum to help stabilize the bony fragments and also to serve as a reminder. Broad-spectrum antimicrobials may be used following fracture reduction to prevent complications, given that the fracture is typically a compound fracture, with exposed bone intranasally. If more than 7 to 10 days elapse between when the nasal bones are fractured and an attempt is made for reduction,

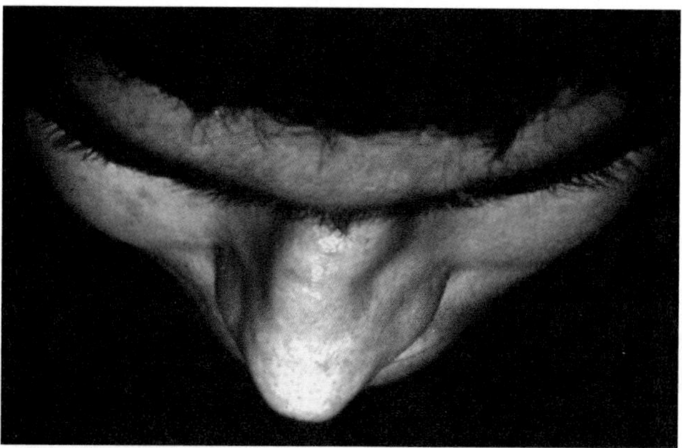

Figure 16-5. Nasal fracture with deviation of the nasal dorsum.

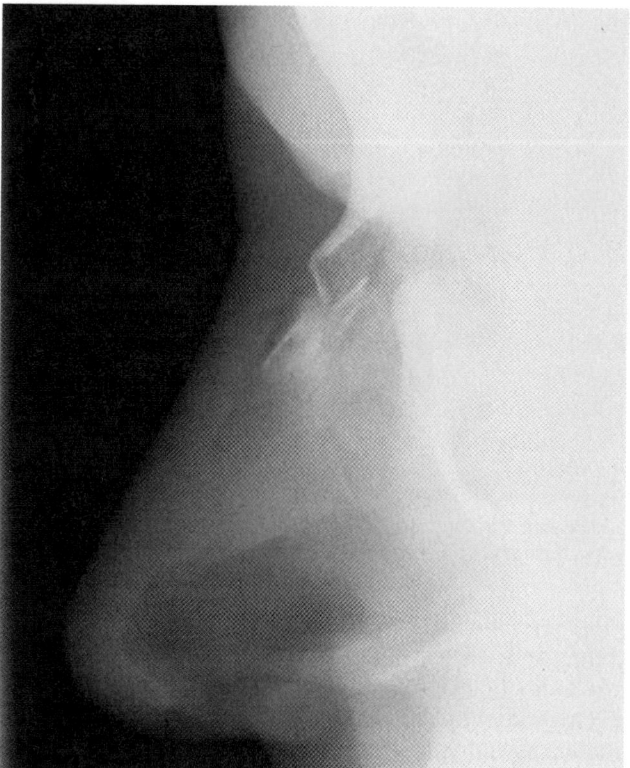

Figure 16-6. Nasal bone fracture radiograph.

the fragments may begin to form fibrous unions in the displaced positions, making reduction more difficult.

Septal Hematoma

Following trauma to the nose, the nasal septum should be evaluated for a septal hematoma. A septal hematoma can result if there is disruption of the septal perichondrium from the underlying septal cartilage when it is deformed by trauma; blood collects between the mucoperichondrium and the septal cartilage, depriving the cartilage of its blood supply. If the septum appears widened, boggy, or violaceous, it should be evaluated by an otolaryngologist to rule out a septal hematoma. A septal hematoma may be differentiated from the inferior turbinates, because the turbinates arise from the lateral nasal wall and septal hematomas are seen as bulging of the septum. Frequently, pain and fever will accompany a septal abscess (Fig. 16-7).

If there is a septal hematoma, it requires incision and drainage and placement of a drain, suturing, and packing within the nose to reapproximate the mucoperichondrium with the septal cartilage. A septal hematoma must be diagnosed and treated promptly to avoid a septal abscess, septal cartilage necrosis, or permanent deformity. A saddle nose deformity may result from an improperly managed septal hematoma.

Cerebrospinal Fluid Rhinorrhea

After nasal trauma, a clear, watery nasal discharge may represent a traumatic CSF leak. A CSF leak may result from a frontal bone or sinus or cribriform plate fracture. Less commonly, CSF rhinorrhea may be the result of CSF leaking from a temporal bone fracture and the fluid draining into the nasopharynx via the eustachian tube. As noted earlier in this chapter ("Cerebrospinal Fluid Otorrhea"), the diagnosis of a CSF leak may be confirmed by testing the fluid for β_2-transferrin. The use of prophylactic antimicrobials in the setting of CSF rhinorrhea is controversial. Thin-cut CT scans of the anterior skull base and sinuses with both axial and coronal views may help identify the site of leak; however, small defects may not be detected and may require multiple imaging attempts and perhaps different modalities, such as MRI or radioisotope scanning. When a CSF leak is suspected, otolaryngologic and neurosurgical consultations should be obtained. If a child does not have classic CSF rhinorrhea, but has had multiple episodes of meningitis, a CSF leak should be suspected.

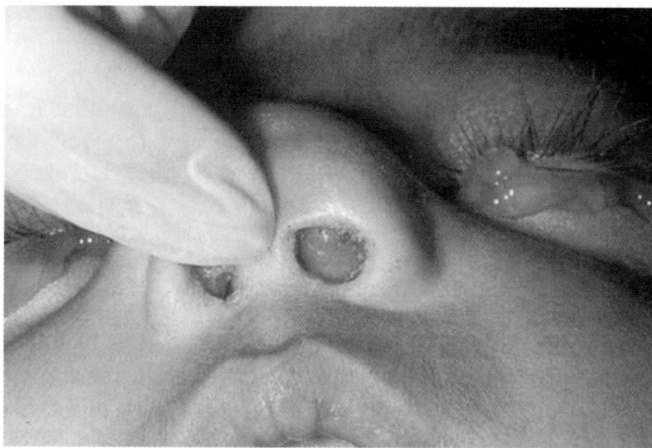

Figure 16-7. Nasal septal abscess.

Nasal Lacerations

The nose is a complex structure consisting of a thin layer of skin and soft tissue overlying a delicate skeleton of cartilages and bone, which is lined with mucosa within the nasal cavity. Lacerations and injury to the nose may require specialized attention because of its complexity and other factors that may complicate an injury to the nose. The nose not only is a prominent visual focal point, but also plays a significant functional role for smooth airflow during respiration and for the sense of smell. A consultation for otolaryngology or plastic surgery should be considered for open injuries to the nose.

If a laceration is over the dorsum of the nose and has not disrupted the underlying framework, it may be repaired primarily using facial plastic surgery techniques. Considerations of the esthetic unit of the nose need to be addressed, especially if there is a loss of skin and/or soft tissue from the dorsum. If necessary, various skin flaps are available for reconstructive purposes. Particular care is required at the nares because injuries in the area may create scar bands; these may be unsightly and result in obstruction of airflow because of narrowing of the nares.

Injury to the cartilaginous and/or bony framework of the nose requires urgent attention. Exposed bone and cartilage require expedient attention to reduce the risk of infection and prevent the loss of tissue. Additionally, débridement of the wound requires careful consideration of the framework so as not to remove or débride important structural elements. Soft tissue coverage may require local or regional vascularized flaps. Structural reconstruction may require bone and/or cartilage grafts. Depending on the extent of nasal trauma, staged procedures may be necessary to reconstruct the nose esthetically and functionally.

Facial Trauma

Facial Bone Fractures

Trauma to the face may result in fractures of the facial bones. Focal fractures may affect regions such as the nose, maxilla, orbit, mandible, or frontal bone, or may be more extensive and cover multiple regions, such as the maxillozygomatic region or nasoethmoid complex. Determination of the mechanism of injury and whether there was a loss of consciousness is helpful in assessing the severity of the impact. The initial physical examination is critical, especially with respect to the ocular examination and facial nerve function. Any unusual ocular finding, especially limited extraocular mobility, asymmetrical pupillary size, or reactivity or altered visual acuity or fields, may indicate an emergent intraocular and/or intracranial event. Ophthalmologic consultation should be considered. Typically, thin-cut CT scans of the skull, face, and brain can identify the fractures and intracranial processes and assist in developing a treatment plan. For mandibular fractures, a panoramic radiograph (Panorex) may also be helpful.

Force from an impact to the eye and orbit may result not only in ophthalmic injury but also in fractures to the surrounding bony structure of the orbit. The rim of bone around the orbit may be fractured and a step-off between the bone fragments may be palpable. If significantly displaced, the fracture may require reduction and plating. The impact to the orbit may result in the force being transmitted through the globe, resulting in a fracture of the orbital floor (maxillary sinus roof) or the medial orbital wall (lamina papyracea). These fractures are often referred to as orbital blowout fractures and may require intervention if there are signs of restriction of extraocular motion or diplopia.

Zygomatic arch fractures may cause trismus because of impingement on the temporalis muscle and its attachment to the mandible. A zygomatic fracture may manifest as a swelling or hematoma over the region or as a depression. A simple zygomatic fracture may be reduced via open reduction and plating. More significant fractures may require multidisciplinary cooperation among specialists, including but not limited to otolaryngology, ophthalmology, plastic surgery, oral maxillofacial surgery, and neurosurgery.

Fractures of the paranasal sinuses may occur as isolated injuries or in combination with other facial regions. In particular, the frontal, maxillary, and ethmoid sinuses are susceptible because of their anterior location. Trauma to the nose, cheek, or forehead region may result in ethmoid, maxillary, or frontal sinus fractures, respectively. Subcutaneous crepitation may be palpable. CT may demonstrate fracture lines with subcutaneous emphysema and/or air-fluid levels within the sinuses. As long as there are no ocular problems or significantly displaced fractures, conservative management with a broad-spectrum oral antimicrobial and observation may be considered. Isolated anterior maxillary sinus wall fractures rarely require intervention.

Frontal bone and sinus fractures may require special attention and otolaryngologic and neurosurgical consultation should be obtained. A nondisplaced or minimally displaced frontal bone fracture may be treated conservatively, whereas a more significantly displaced fracture may require open reduction and plating. Frontal sinus fractures are divided into two types, anterior table and posterior table fractures. The front or anterior wall of the frontal sinus, if fractured, may manifest as a depression or step-off. If the frontal recess and sinus are well pneumatized, an endoscopic intranasal reduction of the fracture may be considered. Otherwise, an open reduction of the fracture may be required. Posterior table fractures pose an additional complicating issue—a CSF leak. With disruption of the posterior table, the dura may be violated and CSF may leak through the defect, resulting in CSF rhinorrhea. Nondisplaced posterior table fractures may be followed conservatively. A displaced posterior table fracture may require an open procedure and potentially obliteration of the sinus. If there is evidence of frontal sinus outflow tract involvement, it is important to observe for obstruction of the frontal sinus. If medical management—empirical antibiotic therapy, topical nasal steroids, and systemic steroid taper—is unable to reopen the frontal sinus, endoscopic frontal sinus surgery may be required.[8]

Severe midface trauma may result in a nasoethmoid complex fracture and/or maxillary fractures. The airway needs to be stabilized in these children, because bleeding and swelling may cause airway problems. Nasoethmoid complex fractures should be suspected when there is significant midface swelling and increased intercanthal distance. Typically, with a nasoethmoid complex fracture, gentle traction on the eyelids laterally will cause widening of the intercanthal distance. CT is critical for accurate diagnosis of this type of fracture. Otolaryngology or plastic surgery consultation should be obtained for open reduction of the fracture.

Midface fractures that include the maxilla may affect the orbit and maxillary sinus. A complete malar fracture is sometimes referred to as a trimalar or tripod fracture when the fracture occurs along the orbital rim, zygomatic arch, and zygomaticofrontal suture line. Isolated malar region fractures can also occur at the zygomatic arch or lateral wall of the maxillary sinus. If there is no or minimal displacement, conservative management may be considered. The Le Fort fracture classification describes various degrees of fractures of the maxilla. Oral surgery, plastic surgery, or otorhinolaryngology should be considered for management of these fractures, which may require intermaxillary fixation and/or open reduction and internal fixation.

Sinus Barotrauma

Typically, there is a direct open connection between the paranasal sinus cavities and nasal cavity, which permits prompt equalization of ambient pressure changes. However, if the sinus ostia are obstructed, the changes in ambient pressure may not be able to equalize with the affected sinus cavity, and barotrauma can result. In an individual with congestion caused by a virus, descent while in an airplane or during an underwater dive, even in the deep end of a swimming pool, may result in a marked pressure change that cannot be relieved. Increased pressure is transmitted to the cardiovascular system and into the mucosal lining of the sinus. If the pressure within the sinus cavity does not match the pressure in the cardiovascular system and becomes high enough, the blood vessels in the mucosa of the cavity may rupture, fill the space with blood until the pressure developed within the cavity equilibrates with the cardiovascular pressure. Commonly, there are complaints of intense cheek or forehead pain when this occurs. Epistaxis may also occur. Conservative treatment with broad-spectrum prophylactic antibiotic coverage should be considered. Adjunctive therapy with topical nasal decongestant sprays (e.g., oxymetazoline) twice daily for 3 days, oral decongestants (if not contraindicated), topical nasal steroids (e.g., mometasone or fluticasone), and nasal saline sprays may also be considered in combination. Avoidance of further barotrauma until resolution of the injury is recommended. In the rare case of a lack of response to treatment or exacerbation or persistence of symptoms, the child should be referred to an otolaryngologist for further evaluation and management.

ORAL CAVITY AND PHARYNGEAL TRAUMA

Lip and oral cavity trauma can be the result of external forces or self-inflicted by biting. Lacerations and hematoma formation may result and may be painful. If the laceration is minor or superficial, treatment is rarely needed. Deeper lacerations may require suturing if there is excessive or persistent bleeding or if there is a significant flap of tissue requiring reapproximation. Lip lacerations can bleed profusely because of injury to the labial artery. Through-and-through lip lacerations should be irrigated copiously, and all three layers need to be reapproximated and closed completely and accurately. Lacerations involving the lip edge and vermilion border should be repaired carefully, taking extra care to reapproximate the vermilion border. Even a small misalignment of 1 mm may be evident.

Trauma to the mandible may cause injury to the tongue or buccal mucosa. Most tongue lacerations, puncture wounds, and buccal bites heal well without intervention. Even large wounds, up to 2 cm, often heal well by secondary intention. Larger wounds or those with gaping edges may require débridement and surgical management.

Oral cavity and oral commissure burns may occur when children bite electrical cords. After evaluation and stabilization of the cardiopulmonary system and for shock, injuries to the oral cavity can be assessed. Débridement and cleaning of the wound are recommended. Good oral hygiene is necessary; it should consist of use of toothpaste, with or without use of a toothbrush, and oral rinses with half-strength hydrogen peroxide or others available over the counter (e.g., a hydrogen peroxide rinse [Peroxyl]). Scarring of the oral commissure may cause microstomia. To help prevent this, oral appliances may be fashioned to separate the upper and lower portions of the oral commissure and provide lateral pressure to limit contracture.

Complaints of pain or malocclusion after a blow to the lower face may indicate a mandibular fracture. Trismus may result from splinting of the muscles of mastication. Fracture lines may be palpable, and gingival disruption may also be visible. Condylar displacement may cause anterior EAC lacerations, which might result in bloody otorrhea. A panoramic radiograph is best for evaluation of a mandibular fracture. Treatment of pediatric mandibular fractures is complicated by the presence of deciduous dentition and concern about the growth centers of the mandible; the mandible heals quickly, but rigid fixation may cause growth retardation. Typically, children older than 13 years may be treated as adults and intermaxillary fixation may be used. Other modalities are usually necessary for younger children. Consultation with a pediatric oral surgeon or dentist should be considered for younger children with mandibular fractures.

Deep lacerations to the cheek region may be associated with particular concerns—function of the facial nerve and integrity of the parotid duct. Facial nerve function distal to the injury must be assessed and documented expediently. Injuries to the facial nerve lateral to the lateral canthus should be repaired immediately. Injuries medial to the lateral canthus can generally be observed, because regeneration of the nerve typically provides adequate facial function. Lacerations and stab wounds to the cheek may also injure the parotid duct. The integrity of the duct must be determined if an injury is suspected. The duct may be cannulated with a small catheter or probe, and the wound explored. If the duct is transected, it can be repaired with small absorbable sutures and a small catheter may be left in place and sutured to the inside of the cheek for 2 weeks.

Children frequently suffer from oropharyngeal lacerations or puncture wounds as a result of running with an object in their mouths. If the trauma is restricted to the central portion of the palate, injury to vascular or neural structures is unlikely. If there is no significant flap of tissue as a result of the trauma, the child is usually safe to return home after it has been confirmed that there are

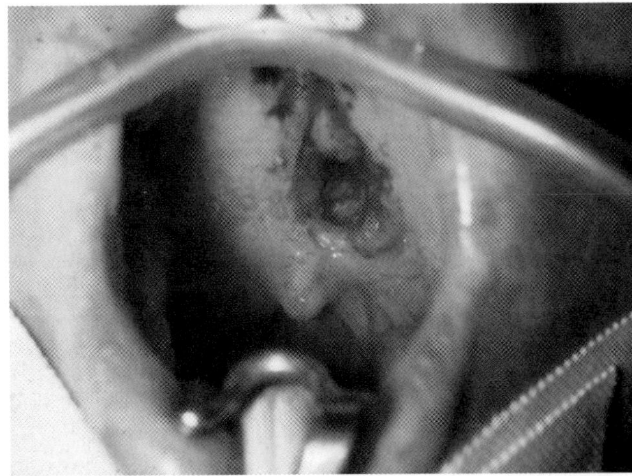

A

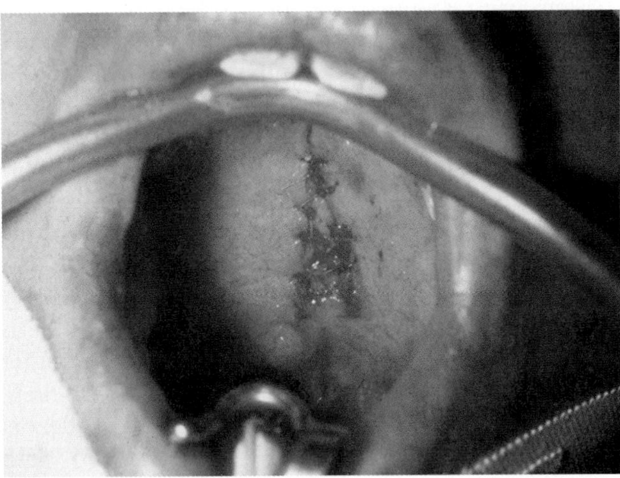

B

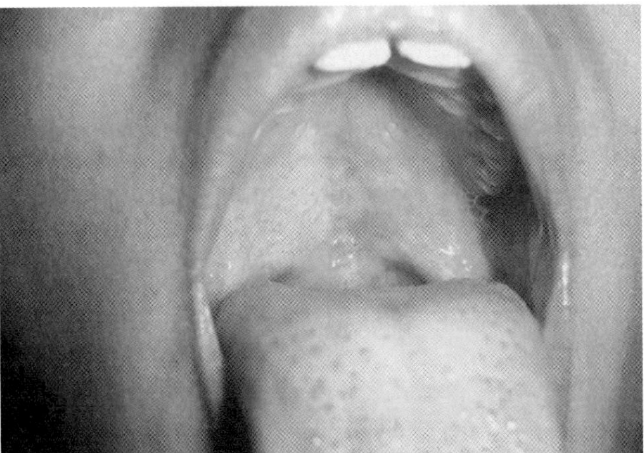

C

Figure 16-8. Palate laceration. **A**, Intraoperative—before closure of laceration. **B**, Intraoperative—after closure of laceration. **C**, Healed laceration at follow-up visit.

no retained foreign bodies and no other injuries. The junction between the soft and the hard palate is the most common location of injury, usually with a trap door-type wound. Most palatal injuries heal well without intervention other than good oral hygiene. A significant flap of tissue, deep puncture, or laceration of the palate, or a wound with significant debris, may require exploration, débridement, and repair (Fig. 16-8).

Trauma to the lateral aspects of the posterior palate or pharynx may be associated with vascular injuries to the carotid artery or jugular vein (Fig. 16-9). The lower cranial nerves are also at risk. An expanding hematoma of the neck or pharynx, continued intraoral bleeding, diminished pulse, and changing mental status are all potential signs of serious vascular injury. Affected children should have an urgent evaluation of the great vessels, either with conventional angiography or MRI (MR angiography [MRA]-MR venography [MRV]) and may require surgical exploration. A retained foreign body in these regions should be left in place until imaging can identify its location and the status of nearby vessels; CT or MRI may be helpful for localization of the foreign body (Figs. 16-10 and 16-11). Severe blunt injuries may also cause intimal damage to the carotid arteries. Neurologic impairment can occur immediately or can be delayed, manifesting 3 to 24 hours after trauma.[9] If a lateral pharyngeal or palatal puncture injury is present without evidence of vascular injury, the child should be observed closely in the hospital or at home for signs of neurologic deterioration. Conventional angiography should be considered in any child with highly suspicious injuries or with indication of injury on MRA.

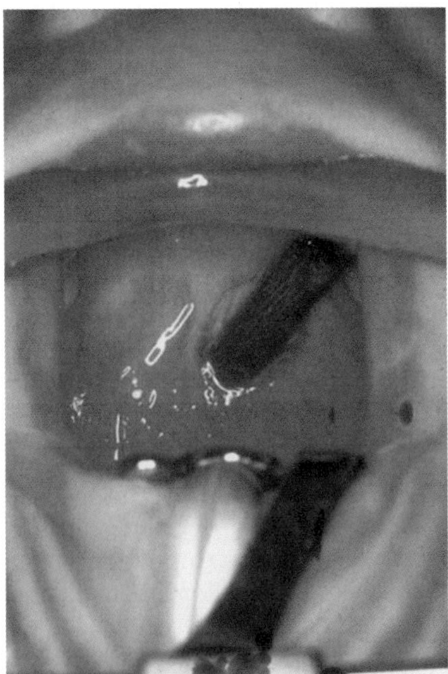

Figure 16-9. Stick penetrating palate.

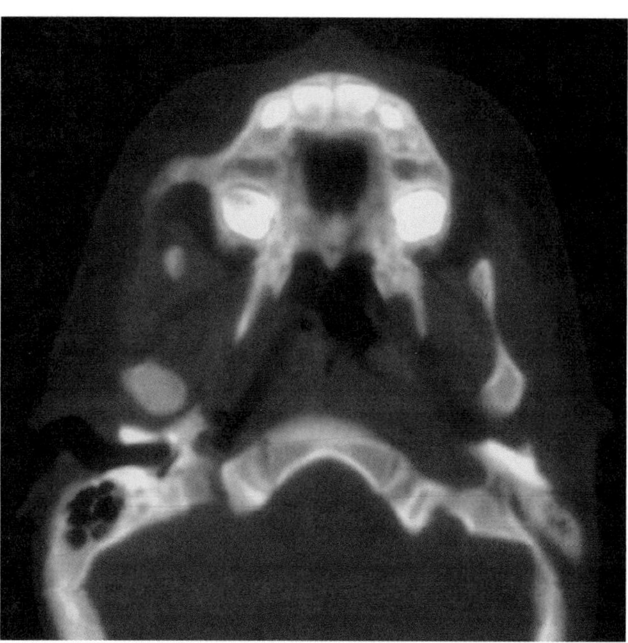

Figure 16-10. CT scan of child with penetrating stick shown in Figure 16-9. Note impingement on the right carotid artery.

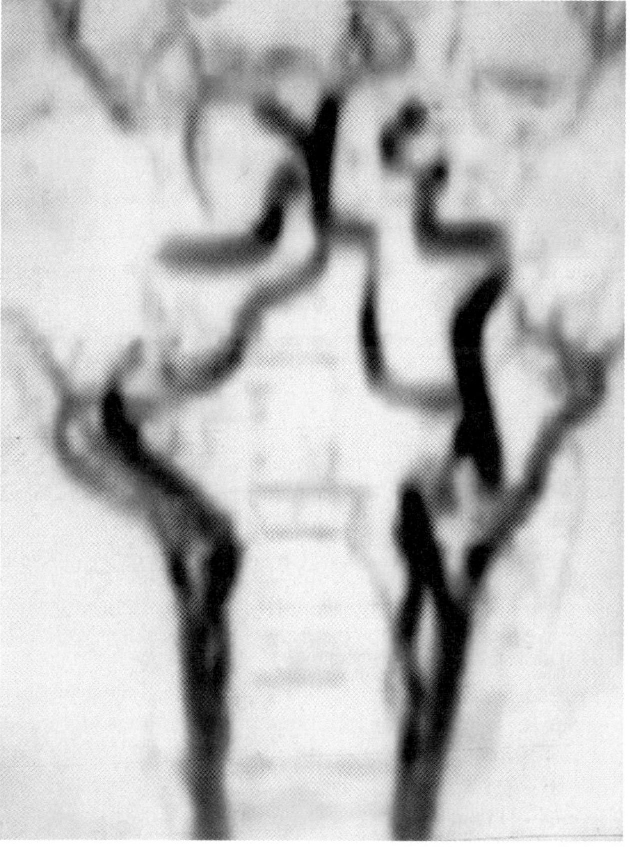

Figure 16-11. Angiography was performed in the same child as shown in Figures 16-9 and 16-10. Note the abnormal right carotid artery.

Neurologic consultation should be considered in cases of carotid involvement, especially in the presence of neurologic findings. Anticoagulation may be considered in cases of thrombosis; but this method of treatment remains controversial.

General management of intraoral injuries should include good oral hygiene. Warm saline and over-the-counter oral hygiene rinses (e.g., hydrogen peroxide rinse or chlorhexidine) may be used. Oral antibiotics should be considered for significant oral mucosal trauma.

NECK INJURIES

Neck injuries in the pediatric population are relatively infrequent. As with all traumas, the airway must be assessed and secured, and the cervical spine should be stabilized and cleared or immobilized. Injuries to the neck are at significant risk for compromising the airway. If there is a penetrating injury, the child should be placed in a slight Trendelenburg position to prevent the formation of an air embolism. Oxygen should be administered and the airway assessed. Evidence of hemoptysis or hematemesis suggests possible aerodigestive tract injury. Crepitation of the larynx, subcutaneous emphysema, and hoarseness may signify laryngotracheal injury. Intubation versus a surgical airway may need to be considered if the child is having respiratory difficulty. Fiberoptic evaluation of the upper aerodigestive tract may be performed and, if necessary, may assist in the establishment of a secure airway. Trauma, general, and otolaryngologic surgeons should be considered to assist with management of a traumatic airway.

Once the airway has been stabilized, ventilation needs to be assessed, because neck trauma may deflect into the chest and cause a pneumothorax. Bleeding from major vessel injury should also be addressed.

Once the child has been stabilized, a general physical examination, including assessment of cranial nerve function and neurologic status, can be performed. Neurologic status should be continually assessed to monitor for progression or change. Neurologic deficits may result from vascular compromise, intracranial processes, and/or systemic and metabolic factors. Neck wounds deep to the platysma should alert the clinician to more significant injury. Hematoma formation, crepitus, and loss of normal landmarks may indicate more significant injury.

The management of penetrating neck injuries depends on the child's symptomatology, findings on physical examination, and location of injury. The neck can be divided into three zones: Zone I is the area between the thoracic inlet and the cricoid cartilage, Zone II is the region between the cricoid cartilage and the angle of the mandible, and Zone III is the region between the angle of the mandible and the base of skull.

In adult studies, exploration has been recommended for Zone II injuries that penetrate the platysma. If an older child is hemodynamically stable, it is recommended that Zone I and III injuries be imaged by such methods as traditional angiography or MRA.

Children are not always cooperative with diagnostic studies, such as traditional angiography, CT and/or CT angiography, or MRI-MRA and may require sedation or general anesthesia. Sedation or anesthesia may not be possible or optimal, depending on whether the child is stable or if neurologic monitoring is required. In some studies, children with penetrating neck injuries were noted to be managed selectively in experienced trauma centers.[10] Criteria for mandatory exploration in these studies varied, but surgery was recommended for any child with a penetrating neck injury who had continued bleeding from the wound, hemodynamic instability, expanding or pulsatile hematoma, blood in the aerodigestive tract, subcutaneous emphysema, respiratory distress, neurologic deficits, and/or other injuries precluding observation or further study.[10]

MAJOR POINTS

As with any trauma, it is necessary to perform an appropriate primary survey, attend to the ABCs—airway, breathing, circulation—and stabilize the neck appropriately.

Once the patient has been stabilized, the examination may be completed, including an initial survey and documentation of cranial nerve function, especially optic nerves providing extraocular motion, and the facial nerve.

The presence of immediate facial nerve paralysis indicates probable injury to the nerve, which may require intervention, whereas delayed onset of facial nerve injury usually can be managed conservatively with oral steroids, such as prednisone 1 mg/kg/day, for about 1 week.

With nasal fractures, an intranasal examination should be performed to rule out a septal hematoma.

Oropharyngeal trauma should trigger a high index of suspicion for carotid artery injury, even with blunt trauma. Evidence of a reasonably forceful impact to the lateral aspects of the oropharynx may warrant further imaging to rule out carotid injury. Patients should be observed for neurologic sequelae if there is suspicion of carotid injury.

Surgical exploration should be considered in any child with a penetrating neck injury who has had continued bleeding from the wound, hemodynamic instability, expanding or pulsatile hematoma, blood in the aerodigestive tract, subcutaneous emphysema, respiratory distress, neurologic deficits, and/or an inability to be observed or studied because of other injuries.

REFERENCES

1. Ohlsen L, Skoog T, Sohn SA: The pathogenesis of cauliflower ear. Scand J Plast Reconstr Surg 1975;9:34-39.
2. Mladick RA, Carraway JH: Ear reattachment by the modified pocket principle. Plast Reconstr Surg 1973; 51:584-587.
3. Cole JK, Engrav LH, Heimbach DM, et al: Early excision and grafting of face and neck burns in patients over 20 years. Plastic Reconstr Surg 2002;109:1266-1273.
4. Hasso AN, Ledington JA: Traumatic injuries of the temporal bone. Otolaryngol Clin North Am 1998;21:295-316.
5. Wiet RJ, Valvassori GE, Kotsanis CA, Parahy C: Temporal bone fractures: State of the art review. Am J Otol 1985:6:207-215.
6. Chang CYJ, Cass SP: Management of facial nerve injury because of temporal bone trauma. Am J Otol 1999; 20:96-114.
7. Galangarner H, Meuli M, Hoff E, et al: Management of petrous bone fractures in children: Analysis of one-hundred twenty-seven cases. J Trauma 1994;36:198-201.
8. Smith TL, Han JK, Loehrl TA, Rhee JS: Endoscopic management of the frontal recess in frontal sinus fractures: A shift in the paradigm. Laryngoscope 2002; 112:784-790.
9. Hengerer AS, DeGroot TR, Rivers RJ, et al: Internal artery thrombosis following soft palatal injuries: A case report and review of 16 cases. Laryngoscope 1984;94:1571-1575.
10. Abujamra L, Joseph MM: Penetrating neck injuries in children: A retrospective review. Pediatr Emerg Care 2003;19:308-313.

SUGGESTED READING

Baker M: Foreign bodies of the ears and nose in childhood. Pediatr Emerg Care 1987;3:67-70.

Bressler K, Shelton C: Ear foreign-body removal: A review of 98 consecutive cases. Laryngoscope 1993;103(Pt 1): 367-370.

Burstein F, Cohen S, Hudgins R, Boydston W: Frontal basilar trauma: Classification and treatment. Plast Reconstr Surg 1997;99:1314-1321; discussion, 1322-1323.

Canty PA, Berkowitz RG: Hematoma and abscess of the nasal septum in children. Arch Otolaryngol Head Neck Surg 1996;122):1373-1376.

Cotton RT, Myer CM: Practical Pediatric Otolaryngology. Philadelphia, Lippincott-Raven, 1999.

Darrouzet V, Duclos JY, Liguoro D, et al: Management of facial paralysis resulting from temporal bone fractures: Our experience in 115 cases. Otolaryngol Head Neck Surg 2001;125:77-84.

East CA, O'Donaghue G: Acute nasal trauma in children: Causes, diagnosis and treatment. Ear Nose Throat J 1989;68:522-538.

Edmonds C, Lowry C, Pennefather J, Walker R: Diving and Subaquatic Medicine, 4th ed. New York, Arnold, 2002.

Handler SD: Maxillo-facial injuries. In Torg J (ed): Athletic Injuries to the Head, Neck and Face, 2nd ed. Philadelphia, Lea & Febiger, 1990, pp 611-634.

Handler SD, Wetmore RF: Otolaryngologic injuries. Clin Sports Med 1982;1:431-477.

Hester TO, Campbell JP: Diagnosis and management of nasal trauma for primary care physicians. J Kentucky Med Assoc 1997;95:386-392.

Kadish HA, Corneli HM: Removal of nasal foreign bodies in the pediatric population. Am J Emerg Med 1997;15:54-56.

Kadish HA, Schunk JE: Pediatric basilar skull fracture: Do children with normal neurologic findings and no intracranial injury require hospitalization? Ann Emerg Med 1995; 26:37-41.

Kim SH, Kazahaya K, Handler SD: Traumatic perilymphatic fistulas in children: Etiology, diagnosis, and management. Int J Pediatr Otorhinolaryngol 2001;60:147-153.

Liu-Shindo M, Hawkins DB: Basilar skull fractures in children. Int J Pediatr Otorhinolaryngol 1989;17:109-117.

Northern JL, Downs MS: Hearing in Children, 4th ed. Baltimore, Williams & Wilkins, 1991.

Potsic WP, Handler SD, Wetmore RF, Pasquariello P: Primary Care Pediatric Otolaryngology, 2nd ed. Andover, NJ, J Michael Ryan, 1995.

Rosenfeld RM, Sandhu S: Injury prevention counseling opportunities in pediatric otolaryngology. Arch Otolaryngol Head Neck Surg 1996;122:609-611.

Tong MC, Ying SY, van Hasselt CA: Nasal foreign bodies in children. Int J Pediatr Otorhinolaryngol 1996;35:207-211.

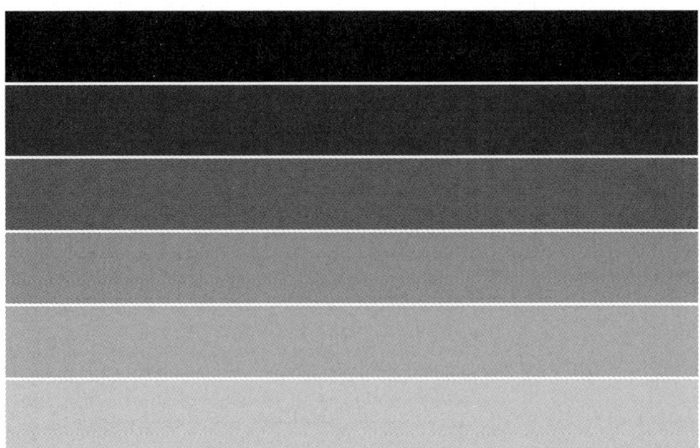

Index

Note: Page numbers followed by f or t refer to figures and tables, respectively.

D

E

F

G

H

I

J

K

L

M

N

O

P

Q

R

S

T

U

V

W

X

Y

Z